Health Visiting in Practice

Health Visiting in Practice

Carol Robertson BSc(Hons) RGN RM RHV CHNT RNT

Formerly Lecturer in Health Visiting at the Polytechnic of the South Bank, London

SECOND EDITION

CHURCHILL LIVINGSTONE
EDINBURGH LONDON MELBOURNE NEW YORK AND TOKYO 1991

CHURCHILL LIVINGSTONE
Medical Division of Longman Group UK Limited

Distributed in the United States of America by Churchill
Livingstone Inc., 1560 Broadway, New York, N.Y.
10036, and by associated companies, branches and
representatives throughout the world.

First edition 1988
Second edition 1991

ISBN 0-443-04137-7

A catalogue record of this book is available from the
British Library

Library of Congress Cataloging in Publication Data
Robertson, Carol, RNT.
    Health visiting in practice/Carol Robertson. — 2nd ed.
        p. cm.
    Includes bibliographical references and indexes.
    ISBN 0-443-04137-7
    1. Community health nursing.   I. Title.
    [DNLM: 1. Community Health Nursing.
    WY 106 R649h]
    RT98.R63   1991
    610.73'43—dc20
    DNLM/DLC   91-190
    for Library of Congress   CIP

Produced by Longman Singapore Publishers (Pte) Ltd.
Printed in Singapore.

Preface to the Second Edition

During the years that it took to write the first edition, health visiting's evolution continued apace. There were clear moves away from concentrating almost solely on individual families with occasional group work. Even as the original text went to the publishers, the need for a community perspective was obvious.

In this second edition, four new chapters, Chapters 12–15, present a community viewpoint and look at some of the recent innovations in our work. The three main frameworks continue as the underlying theme. They have been developed to accommodate the wider perspective. Most effort in this edition has been concentrated upon these new chapters. Some alterations to the content of the earlier chapters have been made, but mainly in the first and last chapters. Further reading lists have been added at the end of most of the original chapters.

All but one of the examples in the first edition were imaginary and drew mainly on the author's own experiences. The examples in the four new chapters describe the work of currently practising health visitors. These real-life examples fill about half of each new chapter in order to provide a strongly practical and easily understood basis from which to study the various themes.

The teamwork with other health visitors and the professional support I received whilst preparing this edition, were very much appreciated. They were particularly encouraging, educative and creative, just as they are in other aspects of health visiting practice.

Southampton, 1991   C.R.

Preface to the First Edition

A friend of mine remarked 'What a joy to be able to write whatever you like about health visiting!' and here lies the essential difference between her research and this book! This is, in essence, my opinion: the practice of health visiting as I have seen it and, to a fair extent, as I feel it ought to be. It is inevitable that it is a personal view, as there is very little research into the face-to-face, practical aspects of our work. However, that which is currently available has been incorporated.

Health visiting has remarkably wide potential and aims to accommodate and to provide for enormous variations in people's needs. Hoping to make this complex picture easier to understand, I have tried to muster the description into three main frameworks. They are founded on models which I have used both in practice and in teaching. The challenge of setting them out in print has caused me to refine them in a few small ways.

In essence, these frameworks show 'why', 'what' and 'how' in the work. A prevention model highlights the purpose of health visiting. Another model is one based on family health needs and highlights the various factors covered. The third, the health visitor cycle, outlines the mechanics involved and is derived from the nursing process.

Each model is particularly valuable in certain situations, that is, for considering the work over a period of time, for a particular visit, or for certain aspects of planning the care. After they have been introduced, each is given a chapter or two to show how they can help in thinking about and planning our work. Subsequent chapters continue the theme.

Besides looking at various philosophical aspects of health visiting, it seemed best to try to provide as much practical help as space would allow. Various aspects of the work have received only a cursory mention, others have been left out. It would take a book of encyclopaedic proportions to accommodate a full description. It has proved difficult to become properly informed across such a wide field — but that is a common problem in the practice of health visiting.

Southampton, 1987   C.R.

Acknowledgements for the Second Edition

I would like to thank:
- my husband John for his encouragement and financial support, without which this book would not have been possible
- my father Ken Moseley, and Bernadette, Sophie and Jack for dog-minding whilst I was away meeting health visitors at work
- all the people who spent so much time explaining about their role for the real-life examples of Chapters 12–15
- the tutors, managers and innumerable health visitors — well-experienced, newly-qualified and students — who helped by discussing topical issues and ideas
- members of the Health Visitors Association Special Interest Groups on Homelessness, Training, Older People and Community Development, for their support and encouragement
- the librarian and staff at the Royal Hampshire County Hospital in Winchester for their continued support and diligent searches
- Jane Paul, HVA Labour Relations Officer, for her ideas about workload and time management and Christa Wynn-Williams for her guidance on health visitor/client perceptions
- Sarah Cowley, Sheila Twinn, Liz Porter and Lindis Percy who bravely read through and made helpful suggestions for each of the new chapters, and Frances Appleby, Annette Furley and Jean Spray for their reassurance and advice over particular chapters
- all the people who helped with the first edition, especially Frances Appleby, Deborah Hennessy and Kate Robinson
- and my two computers for their flexibility and untiring willingness to keep revising the script!

Contents

This chapter gives a brief overview of health visiting and its origins and development. The main models used to describe the work in later chapters are introduced. They are demonstrated through an example of a visit to the home of a young mother.

1

Introduction

HEALTH VISITING IN OUTLINE

PREVENTIVE CARE

Health visiting is an aspect of nursing which concentrates upon preventive care. Pre-requisites for practice are registration as a general nurse and a year-long course, which provides an introduction to a wide range of studies. This includes topics such as psychology, social policy, sociology, as well as the theory and practice of health visiting.

The service, for which the health authorities are responsible, aims to improve community health by informing and encouraging people to remain healthy and by enabling them to make best use of the health and social services. The caseload is mainly defined by a GP's practice or a geographic area with the service theoretically available to everybody on the list or in the area. In practice, time limitations prevent this.

Health visitors try to select priorities which enable their preventive health care to have greatest effect and also provide most help where there is greatest need. Their community and caseload health profiles provide documented evidence about the most vulnerable groups, such as the homeless, the isolated elderly, low income families, ethnic minorities and single parents. Health problems associated with affluence are also highlighted. Many health visitors concentrate their effort on families with children under five years old. Increasingly, they are reaching out to other groups, especially to the elderly.

Education, surveillance and support

Health visitors are mainly concerned with three aspects of community health:

1. In their educational role, they attempt to promote positive health and to prevent the occurrence of disease by increasing people's understanding of healthy ways of living and their knowledge of health hazards. For example, they attempt to increase people's awareness of such diverse issues as coronary heart disease, childrearing practices or postnatal depression. The underlying idea is to enable people to have increased confidence in their own ability to improve their health circumstances. It is basically a facilitative and empowering role, rather than one which merely distributes information. This activity takes place in situations such as home visits and clinics and in various forms of group and outreach work.

   Another aspect of this educational role is to inform the relevant decision-makers about the health needs of the vulnerable groups with whom the health visitor is or should be in contact.

2. Health visitors undertake health surveillance, aiming to discover difficulties at an early stage and, through prompt attention, to prevent irreparable damage. This monitoring includes concern with families' environmental, physical, mental/emotional and social aspects of health. It also includes the surveillance of local community health needs and people's perceptions about them. This information plays an important part in the construction and keeping up to date of caseload health profiles. This work helps to guide ideas for the provision of relevant, acceptable and accessible services which enable early attention to incipient problems.

3. Where established conditions or situations already exist, health visitors can help to prevent further deterioration at an individual family level by giving supportive care. This is often by employing their listening skills to help their clients understand and take a positive approach to their problems. Health visitors can refer people to other health and social services and also encourage them to join or to establish self-help groups.

   At a broader level, it may be found that particular vulnerable groups, such as homeless families or the carers of elderly or handicapped relatives, face persistent and intractable difficulties. In this case, a more appropriate health visiting response may be to work behind the scenes with interested professionals and volunteers, helping *them* to provide improved supportive services.

Some health visitors have special assignments such as for homeless families, diabetics, families with a handicapped member or hospital liaison. Most continue to have a generalist remit with a caseload containing a variety of client groups.

Health visiting has changed in emphasis over the years, but its aim has always remained the same. This is to promote good health and to reduce the incidence of ill-health in the community through anticipatory and supportive care.

ORIGINS AND DEVELOPMENT

Preventive health guidance provided in people's homes can be traced back, through the infant welfare movement in the first half of this century, to voluntary work undertaken some fifty years earlier (Robinson, 1982; Connolly, 1980a; 1980b; Owen, 1977; Clark, 1973). Table 1.1 gives a thumbnail sketch of the development of health visiting and the influences that helped shape it.

Mid 19th century — the early days

By the middle of the nineteenth century, Victorian concern with the morality of the poor and the constant threat from epidemics of cholera and typhoid, gave rise to voluntary efforts to take education and relevant help into poor people's homes. In 1882, Manchester and Salford middle class volunteers supervised paid visitors who went from door to door on an organised basis. Similar schemes were set up in a few other towns, some workers being known as 'health missioners' and some as 'sanitary visitors'.

Table 1.1 Influences in the development of health visiting

Period	Attitudes	Pressures for action	Action	Administration by
Mid-19th century	Paternalistic welfare	Squalid town living Cholera and typhoid	Prevention of acute fatal diseases	Voluntary agencies
Turn of the century	Pragmatic: populate or perish	Infant mortality Boer War World War I	Teaching to prevent disease in the very young	
Post World War II	Egalitarianism: socialised medicine	Wartime experience: • separation • good nutrition Small family size	Social advice and health education for the whole family	
1960s–1970s	Cost consciousness Quality of life	Rising health service costs Increasing public expectations	As above and some: • specialisation • screening programmes	
Present day	Management efficiency Promote self-help and client participation	Unemployment Housing problems Increasing differentials in inequalities of health	As above and some more group work, community projects, health statistics used for analysis and action on priorities	State

The more pioneering medical officers of health encouraged the idea. With high levels of illiteracy and no mass media, individual tuition provided a useful tool for getting knowledge out to people. Gradually, visitors' training courses were set up. Some of the early visitors included doctors, nurses, people with various degrees and sanitary inspectors. Their work, which brought them into close proximity with social problems, led them to undertake supportive as well as health educational services.

Turn of the century — infant welfare movement

Robinson described how, with the turn of the century, attention focused on infant care. There was an increase in the already high death rates of the newborn. The poor health of the nation had been exposed, for example, when around half of the Boer War recruits were declared unfit for military service.

Concern about population trends led to the emergence of an influential infant welfare movement. Clinics were set up for the teaching and care of mothers with babies. Local Authorities became increasingly involved. The high death rate in World War I brought more concern. Compulsory notification of birth made it possible to visit all newborn babies. Preventive work was extended to include children under school age, and health visitors also took on work in Child Life Protection (Baly, 1980).

Post World War II

The voluntary element in health visiting disappeared once the welfare state was established after the Second World War. Local Health Authorities continued as the responsible bodies and remained so until 1974. In 1948, some of the health visitors' social service responsibilities, acquired in the previous period, were transferred to Children's Departments.

Ideas were changing. Jane Robinson outlined some of the factors which helped to shape post-war philosophies. Family unity was given high priority. The war had led many families to suffer complete separation through evacuation of children, as well as on account of military service. Small families had become commonplace. Child health was no longer such a problem, as it had been improved by good nutrition through rationing. It was therefore felt that health visitors should care for the family as a unit and not concentrate only on children. An inquiry in the mid-50s suggested health visitors should undertake 'social advice and health education for the whole family' (Ministry of Health, 1956).

1960s to 1970s

In the event, a very large proportion of the work still tended to be centred around preventive care for babies and young children, with some supportive care for their parents — especially the mother. But infant mortality figures did not dominate thinking to the same extent as before. Some specialisations emerged, such as in handicap, the elderly, diabetics and in hospital liaison. The service became taken over by District Health Authorities and was drawn even closer to other aspects of nursing, with inter-professional liaison playing an increasingly important role, through an Act of Parliament (DHSS, 1979).

The huge costs of the National Health Service caused increased interest in preventive health care. Screening was one area which received greater attention (DHSS, 1976). Pressure to visibly justify community health expenditure caused an emphasis on the more quantifiable activities in health visiting, such as screening and the number of times families were visited. Concentration on these issues overshadowed the less easily measured, but much more important educational and supportive aspects of our care. Researchers, in the meantime, were finding ways to investigate and to report on qualitative aspects of the work (Luker, 1982; Robinson, 1982; Orr, 1980). This kind of research is continuing (Luker & Chalmers, 1989; 1990).

Present day

Current important underlying influences include the preoccupation with making public services more efficient and more responsive to public wishes, together with encouraging greater public involvement. Recent reports such as the Griffiths Report (1983) and Cumberlege Report (1986) have been reflecting these ideas. A new style community nurse management has been developing. An increasing number of the newly appointed managers do not have a health visitor background. They need clear explanations about the aims and options for our service and about its achievements.

Another trend has been the significant increase in some areas, of people facing persistent difficulties with factors such as housing, single parentage, unemployment and/or a marginal income, all of which correlate with increased ill-health. On the other side of the coin are the health problems of affluence, such as coronary heart disease, for which the UK death rate is one of the highest in the world.

Happily, there has been a huge growth in the accessibility and computerisation of government survey statistics and health and illness data, enabling health visitors to draw up community and caseload health profiles. They can also undertake their own, and/or key into other, local health-based surveys. The resultant wealth of information can provide documented evidence of where special initiatives could and should be provided, and why. Increasingly managers are understanding the need for new initiatives, such as those using groupwork (Drennan, 1985; 1988), the community health development approach (see Chapter 12), the Child Development Project (1984) or strategies similar to those in Oxfordshire (Dauncey, 1987; 1988; 1989; 1990; Goodwin, 1988; Health Visitor Development Group, 1988; Deacon, 1989; Jackson, 1989; Nashe, 1990). 'Partnership' with clients and close work with other professional and voluntary agencies have been increasing.

Influence from acute medicine?

From its mid-century beginnings, right through to the current period, few of the major pressures for the preventive work of a health visitor seem to have come directly from the sphere of acute medicine. However, the current need to contain the costs of acute care and the clear pictures coming from ill-health statistics, seem to be providing a modern stimulus to achieve positive preventive goals. For example, the recent changes to the GP contract are increasing the preventive role of GPs (Cameron, 1990; Turner, 1990). These changes bring an increased possibility of creative cooperation in our preventive care, provided that health visitor 'screening' activities are kept in perspective (Barker, 1988). For example, it would be a derogatory step if over-concentration on the case-finding aspects of surveillance left us little or no time for the allied educational and supportive work, and for outreach and group activities. Using a more specific example, it is more logical to spend time encouraging the development of children's speech, perhaps through some form of group work with mothers, than to chase round merely trying to pick up delayed speech.

Health visiting has come a long way, but has had a clearly recognisable structure throughout its development. Health promotion, the timely discovery of problems and concern for emotional well-being and social support, have been the basis of the work. The profession has been strongly involved in the health and welfare of families with young children, but has also responded to several other groups' needs for preventive health care.

FRAMEWORKS FOR DESCRIBING THE WORK

A detailed account of health visiting includes an enormously wide and diverse range of factors in family health and social welfare. In this book, certain categorisations or models have been used to bring some order to the description and to help the reader think about the work. The main three are the 'prevention', the 'family health needs' and the 'health visitor cycle' models.

Models simplify and clarify

When trying to describe something complex, it is helpful to find some means of untangling its intricacies to present the information more clearly. Various forms of categorisation and listing may help. There are, of course, limitations on these models or frameworks as they necessarily present a simplistic version. However, even though they can only tell part of the story, they are generally easier to remember and to contemplate than the diffuseness and complexity of reality. The reader can benefit by thinking about health visiting through the perspective of several different models. This way it becomes possible to highlight a variety of features. Depending on the context, a particular model may be chosen for its ability to emphasise certain basic and important characteristics. Also, as will be seen later in the book, the models are very easily adapted. They are not a once-and-for-all immutable idea. Anyone can create any modification they find useful.

THE PREVENTION MODEL

One of the underlying models used in this book has already been met earlier in this chapter (see

Table 1.2 A basic version of the prevention model showing the health visitor's role in some of the person-to-person aspects of the work

Aspect of prevention	Mainly through	Examples of activities
Prevent occurrence of condition	Teaching	Discussing: • rights and benefits • safety • nutrition • immunisation • child behaviour • adult health
Prevent development of condition	Surveillance	Of children's: • neurological development • possible CDH • hearing and vision • environment Of adults': • health and social circumstances
Prevent deterioration of established condition	Support	Sympathetic listening: clients clarify and decide Giving information about services Catalyst: encouraging self-help groups

p. 2). The three aspects of community health described in the introductory definition are based on Caplan's (1961) model of primary, secondary and tertiary prevention. An example of the basic framework is presented in Table 1.2. This version concentrates mainly on person-to-person aspects of health visiting and is used later, in the central part of this book.

Box 1.1 Visit to Mrs Smith: a basis for demonstrating the models

Prevention model	Needs model*	The visit	Prevention model	Needs model*	The visit
	1	The house is situated in a suburban estate built in the 1930s. It is a mile from the nearest shops and services. The health visitor arrived on the afternoon arranged by appointment. She was welcomed in and the conversation turned quickly to child care.	Education — to **prevent occurrence** of problems	4	The health visitor gave Mrs Smith a Health Education Council pamphlet on safety, emphasising Charles' needs over the next few months.
			Test — to **prevent development** of problems	5	The appointment for the hearing test in two weeks' time had arrived and Mrs Smith promised to attend.
Observation, aimed at early diagnosis — to **prevent** (potential) **development** of problems	2	It seems that Mrs Smith had enjoyed using the developmental assessment format, previously suggested by the health visitor. She was delighted to show how Charles was progressing. She said he was now capable of sitting alone for around 15 minutes and holding a cup for drinking.	Listening skills —knowledge of local facilities **preventing deterioration**	6	Just as the health visitor was starting to go, Mrs Smith mentioned a personal problem — extreme loneliness and 'missing work'. She looked rather tired as she described her worries and fears. The health visitor quietly listened and occasionally asked a question which seemed to help Mrs Smith come nearer the core of her concern.
		The health visitor heard him say 'dada' and he held two small cubes, one in each hand, in a palmar grasp. He required reassurance before really accepting the visitor but played the game with the cubes quite sociably.	As above	7	A newly set up local mother and toddler group was suggested. A promise was made to introduce Mrs Smith, at the hearing clinic, to another mother who was already attending.
Health education—to **prevent occurrence**	3	The conversation led on to expectations in the future: the emergence of conscience and the effect of mobility in toddlerhood. They talked of the sort of discipline and play appropriate to that period. Mrs Smith's expectations seemed balanced. She had found one of the recommended child care books especially easy to read and helpful. She remarked on how much her husband enjoyed playing with Charles.	As above	8	Local schemes for minding children of working mothers were discusssed. However, Mrs Smith rejected this idea, saying that now she had put it all into words, it did not seem so bad.
			As above	9	Her husband, she said, had a good job. She preferred, for the present, to be at home with her baby and would take steps to get adjusted.
				10	The visit ended amicably and with a wave from Charles.

* See Box 1.3

1. Health promotion

Primary prevention is *preventing the occurrence* of ill-health and promoting good health. Health visitors achieve this mainly through some enabling form of teaching or informing. This may be during individual contacts in homes or clinics and, for example, through participative groupwork or through outreach work such as at a health stall at a fair or in a market place.

A very wide range of health promotional issues is discussed. For example, adequate income and accommodation are basic requirements for healthy living. For this reason health visitors seek to find ways of helping people who may need it, to know all about their rights and entitlements. General health education tends to be in some form of anticipatory guidance on issues such as safety, nutrition or general child care, both physical and behavioural, and immunisation. Any aspect of positive health relevant to the adult members of the family being contacted, such as diet, stress management and exercise, might be included. Health visitors' educational style aims to be facilitative and certainly not that of an all-knowing expert.

2. Early discovery

Preventing the development of problems is generally achieved through some aspect of surveillance within routine visiting or other contacts with families. This surveillance pertains to 'social' as well as to 'medical' factors, once again because social factors have such an influence in levels of health. Sometimes surveillance and/or screening is undertaken in a specifically planned clinic. The aim of this secondary aspect of prevention is to discover difficulties early, enabling them to be dealt with before any irreversible or debilitating damage can be done.

Some models of prevention used in medicine (Williamson, 1981) classify secondary prevention in a different way. They see it as the search only for the precursors of disease in symptom-free people, and not the search for early stages of difficulty. An example of this would be cytology screening, in which the precancerous condition is sought.

With the exception of congenital dislocation of the hip (CDH), health visitors rarely take part in screening at pre-symptomatic stages. Most are involved in seeking, for example, children's neurological, visual or hearing defects and in keeping an eye open to behavioural, social and environmental difficulties. Here, the aim is to bring to light conditions which would benefit from early attention.

Health visitors are in a good position to keep an educated and informal eye on both the physical and mental health of the adults they visit, in particular the emotional well-being of the young mother.

3. Supportive care

Tertiary prevention is *preventing the deterioration* of an established condition. The aim is not only to contain the problem but also to achieve rehabilitation, where this is possible.

Listening skills are perhaps health visitors' most useful tool, and particularly in this aspect of care. Using them in non-directive counselling, health visitors can encourage people to talk through their problems, helping them to gain a better understanding of the difficulties involved and to come to terms with the situation. This sort of approach can also help people clarify their ideas and decide on the sort of solution they would like to seek.

A good knowledge is needed of people's entitlements and of local voluntary and statutory services to enable people to be informed about agencies that would be able to offer appropriate help. Timely and up-to-date information can help people facing difficulties, such as unemployment or caring for a gravely handicapped member of the family. This knowledge can help people start to take positive steps towards coping with and containing their problem.

Health visitors sometimes take a background and/or a catalytic role in the creation of self-help groups. People with major problems, such as those who are bereaved or who have a handicapped baby, often find these groups an excellent source of sympathetic understanding and of basic, practical suggestions for everyday problems. The professional contribution is mainly through bringing people together, helping them to find information about similar ventures and by offering encouragement and occasional help.

Using the model

It may help to have an example of the use of the model. A description of a visit to a young mother and her baby will be found in the right hand half of Box 1.1. The column on the far left has each of the three aspects of the prevention model set against certain activities — health education, surveillance or screening, and supportive care. The numbers in the central column pertain to the family health needs framework which is explained below.

The model highlights important points, but there can be minor complexities. Things do not always unambiguously fall into the pigeon-holes chosen. For example, some might argue that the mother in the case described did not have a problem. Therefore, helping her find a group of like-minded mothers would be more likely to prevent its occurrence and so would be regarded as primary, not tertiary, prevention. Others might suggest that the health visitor would be on the look out for early signs of emotional difficulties and that her response deserves to be classified as secondary prevention!

Borderline delineations, however, are not of great importance. A model is devised only to draw attention to noteworthy features and is successful if it can be used as a tool to clarify thinking and aid learning.

Also, overlaps are inevitable. Teaching, surveillance and supportive work are inseparable in health visiting. For example, health education is necessarily inter-linked with screening and surveillance activities. When discussing current child developmental progress with parents, health visitors help the parents to know about factors such as the child's future expected behaviour and achievements and what signs of poor vision or hearing to look out for. Parents themselves are then better able to monitor their children's future

progress. In addition, discussion of future needs, such as for safety, feeding or social contact at the next stage of development, is an integral part of the surveillance procedure. Equally, supportive work frequently runs concurrently with discussion of the difficulties associated with a child's current attainments and behaviour. The separation of education, surveillance and support in the models is merely a conceptual exercise.

The model is developed

In the last quarter of the book, this model is developed to accommodate the community perspective in our work.

1. Health education is extended to include health visitor communications *informing* decision-makers about relevant health and welfare factors. Knowledge of local data, for example on homelessness or coronary heart disease, can help these people come to well-informed conclusions about the use of relevant resources and services, thereby helping to prevent the occurrence of these difficulties.
2. Surveillance is extended to include the gathering of local health and welfare statistics and *discovering* local opinion about health and preventive health services. This surveillance of community health levels and local perspectives aims to identify problematic factors as early as possible and to know how to provide prompt access to care through services sensitive to and tailor made for local need.
3. Supportive work includes activities such as inter-professional *teamwork* on specific issues seen to be harmfully and significantly affecting the health of particular groups of people. For example, if there were difficulties due to a failure in the normal provisions, such as in services for homeless families, the team's aim would be to change and to improve the situation through influence and coordinated action.

The prevention model is particularly useful in broad explanations of the role and in helping to describe ways health visitors can organise their work. We return to it in Chapters 5, 6, 7, 9 and 11. The 'developed' model will be met in the subsequent chapters, particularly in Chapter 13.

THE FAMILY HEALTH NEEDS MODEL

Of more practical value to student health visitors preparing their early fieldwork practice visits, is an approach which centres round the health needs of a family. Features pertaining to family preventive health care are brought together under headings of general environment, social, mental/emotional and physical factors. Health is emphasised and facets of daily life and general social needs are included. Box 1.2 gives an outline of this approach. Specific examples will be found in the chapters on visiting antenatally and on the first visit after the birth.

Four areas of health need

1. The section for *general environment* can give an outline of the local area, its facilities and services, the basic social situation of the family, their accommodation and their standard of living.
2. Aspects of the family's *physical health* and daily life, such as nutrition, home safety, hygiene, developmental attainments (in children), medication and other facets of general health, are in one section.
3. Factors such as parental knowledge and attitudes and family members' *mental and emotional health* needs are included in another.
4. The last grouping is for family *social aspects of health*, such as hobbies, child care facilities and support from family, friends or community organisations.

As in the prevention framework, deciding exactly what fits best under any particular category is a matter of personal preference. The way that the visit to the Smith household (Box 1.1) would be viewed from the standpoint of this model is demonstrated in Box 1.3.

In the last few chapters of this book, this model is used to demonstrate the community perspective in health visiting. In several of the examples there, the family health needs models are presented in matched pairs, the first model showing what health needs the health visitor found and the second the activities that were initiated in response to these findings.

THE HEALTH VISITOR CYCLE

A third way of analysing the work of a health visitor is by looking at the behind-the-scenes planning processes. These are not easily detected in an example such as the visit to the Smiths, as this

Box 1.2   Some aspects of family health need

General environment	Physical health	Mental/emotional health	Social aspects of health
Community/area	*Parents and children*	*Parents*	*Mother*
Social mix of locality	General health	Knowledge	Support from:
Urban, suburban, rural	Nutrition	Attitudes	• family
Special features	Safety	• expectations	• friends
	Hygiene	Psychological illness	• community
Home	Developmental progress	• postnatal depression	Group activities
Proximity to:	Special screening	Emotional stability	
• transport	• vision		*Family unit*
• shops	• hearing	*Child*	Emotional support
• health services	• chiropody	Play needs	Housing
Availability of:	Medication	• equipment	
• garden/play area		Normal discipline	*Child*
• lift/stairs for flats		Affection	Play — with other children
Standard of living			Stimulation

Box 1.3 Visit to Mrs Smith's home: 'family health needs' analysis

General environment	Physical health	Mental/emotional health	Social aspects of health
Community 1 1930s estate housing, a preponderance of elderly people Relatively remote	*Mother* 6 Seems tired *Child* 2 Developmental assessment: reported and observed characteristics	*Mother* 3 Well-read, attitude to discipline relaxed *Father* Involved	*Mother* 7 ? Mother and toddler club 8 Information: local child-minding facilities
Family 9 Adequate income	4 Safety discussed 5 Hearing test arranged	*Baby* Sociable *Mother*	
Father In employment	10 Developmental attainment observed	6 Loneliness discussed	

Numbering of the factors corresponds to that in the centre column in the example on p. 7, Box 1.1

Features of the *general environment* are important because they make Mrs Smith more vulnerable to loneliness. *Physical* aspects of health covered on this visit were biased towards the baby: observed and reported developmental attainments, safety and Charles' hearing. The *mental/emotional* factors — the mother's knowledge and attitudes, the father's involvement and the baby's social reactions — were all normal and augured well for the future. Mrs Smith's emotional problem of loneliness may be helped by *social* activities with a group of local mothers. Although she misses work, she is not keen to use the child-minding facilities and return to employment at the moment. The family seems to have an adequate income and the father satisfying employment.

model, outlined in Figure 1.1, is concerned with the way the health visitor works out how best to help the family.

Planning processes

The basic problem is to:

(i) assess the family's health needs
(ii) then plan action to be taken (set objectives)
(iii) set about implementing the plan and
(iv) then evaluate the effect of the action.

The information needed to make the assessment and choose priorities for action, comes from several sources:

a. background reading during and after training and knowledge of the locality
b. prior to the visit, from records and inter-professional communication
c. the client's viewpoint and observations during the visit and
d. the synthesis and outcome of work with the family on previous visits guiding plans for future contact.

The example

The description of the visit to Mrs Smith (p. 6, Box 1.1) does not state how the health visitor was actually thinking. It does seem, however, that (i) the assessment led to (ii) and (iii) high priority being given to child health matters and the mother's emotional welfare. It also seems that (iv) previous contact with Mrs Smith resulted in her positive involvement in her child's developmental assessment.

Sources of information which help the planning processes, both before and after the visit, are not specified. There is (a) no indication of the health visitor's general background knowledge of relevant research results acquired either during or since her training, or of her understanding of local health policies based on local community health profiles. However, there is evident awareness of local agencies. It seems likely that (b) the record system triggered the appointment for the hearing test and provided a reminder for the assessment of developmental attainments and safety literature. The description does clearly show, however, that (c) the health visitor's objectives and subsequent ac-

Fig. 1.1 The health visitor cycle

tions were modified during the visit, on hearing the mother speak of her loneliness. There is (d) no explanation in the case history of how previous visits influenced this one or what is planned beyond the appointment at the hearing assessment clinic.

The health visitor cycle is explained in detail in the next chapter. This model looks at the underlying processes of planning and action: an entirely different perspective from (i), the broad overview which can be provided by the prevention model,

and (ii) the more specific and individual approach of the family health needs model. Each scheme makes a useful contribution towards highlighting important aspects of a health visitor's work.

This chapter has been concerned with a brief description of health visiting, a historical perspective and an introduction to the three basic frameworks used in later chapters to help think about and describe the work.

REFERENCES

Baly M B 1980 Nursing and social change, 2nd edn. Heinemann, London, p. 137

Barker W 1988 The myth of prevention. Nursing Times Community Outlook 84, 41: 4–10 — Strongly recommended.

Cameron J 1990 Unpopular practices. Nursing Times 86, 15: 18

Caplan G 1961 An approach to community mental health. Tavistock Publications, London

Child Development Project 1984 Child development programme. Early Childhood Development Unit, Senate House, University of Bristol, Bristol BS8 1TH

Clark J 1973 A family visitor. Royal College of Nursing, London, ch. 2

Connolly M P 1980a Health visiting 1850–1900: a review. Midwife, Health Visitor and Community Nurse 16: 282–285

Connolly M P 1980b Health visiting 1900–1910: a review. Midwife, Health Visitor and Community Nurse 16: 375–378

Cumberlege Report 1986 Neighbourhood nursing — a focus for health care. Report of the Community Nursing Review. HMSO, London

Dauncey J 1987 (letter) Health visiting in Oxfordshire. Health Visitor 60, 6: 181

Dauncey J 1988 A positive response. Nursing times 84, 42: 75–77

Dauncey J 1989 (letter) Oxfordshire's health visiting strategy. Health Visitor 62, 12: 388

Dauncey J 1990 (letter) A plea for the future of health visiting. Health Visitor 63, 3: 104

Deacon G 1989 (letter) Metamorphosis of a health visitor. Health Visitor 62, 5: 165

DHSS 1976 Report of the Committee on Child Health Services. Fit for the future. Cmnd 6684 HMSO, London (Court Report)

DHSS 1979 Nurses, Midwives and Health Visitors Act, 1979. HMSO, London

Drennan V 1985 Working in a different way. A research project examining community work methods and health visiting. Community Nursing Service Paddington and North Kensington Health Authority, London

Drennan V (ed) 1988 Health visitors and groups — Politics and practice. Heinemann Nursing, Oxford

Goodwin S 1988 Whither health visiting? Keynote speech: Health Visitors' Association Annual Study Conference. Health Visitors' Association, London — Clear and concise coverage of many issues regarding change in health visiting.

Griffiths Report 1983 NHS Management Inquiry. Letter to Secretary of State, Department of Health and Social Security, London

Health Visitor Development Group 1989 A change for the better. Oxfordshire's strategy for health visiting, 2nd edn. Oxfordshire Health Authority, Oxford. c/o Jane Dauncey, East Oxford Health Centre, Cowley Road, Oxford OX4 1XD

Jackson C 1989 Wherefore to Oxfordshire? Health Visitor 62, 5: 159–160

Luker K A 1982 Evaluating health visiting practice. Royal College of Nursing, London

Luker K A, Chalmers K I 1989 The referral process in health visiting. International Journal of Nursing Studies 26, 2: 173–185 — Strongly recommended.

Luker K A, Chalmers K I 1990 Gaining access to clients: the case of health visiting. Journal of Advanced Nursing 15, 1: 74–82

Ministry of Health 1956 An inquiry into health visiting. HMSO, London (Jameson Report)

Nashe S 1990 (letter) Oxford responds. Health Visitor 63, 3: 104

Orr J 1980 Health visiting in focus. Royal College of Nursing, London

Owen G M (ed) 1977 Health visiting. Bailliere Tindall, London, ch. 1

Robinson J 1982 An evaluation of health visiting. Council for the Education and Training of Health Visitors, London, ch. 1

Turner T 1990 The new GP contract. A case for concern? Nursing Times 86, 20: 27–29

Williamson J 1981 Screening, surveillance and casefinding. In: Arie T (ed) Health care of the elderly. Croom Helm, London

This chapter expands on the health visitor cycle, outlined at the end of the introductory chapter. Making contact with a family is discussed using this framework because it draws attention to important underlying processes that take place. The model highlights health visitors' need to plan their work by gleaning information from various sources and situations, in order to choose whom to visit, to assess their needs and to provide health care.

2

Making contact

THE FRAMEWORK

A particular advantage of the framework is that it concentrates on a range of information sources available at various times to the health visitor. It highlights the everchanging pattern of information on which health visiting decisions are made. It is able, specifically, to draw attention to the family's viewpoint and perspective. This should be a major factor in health visitor planning and care. Success in the work depends upon:

- building up a good relationship
- making it easy for the family to understand how the health visitor is aiming to help
- ensuring that the family feels the appropriateness of that help.

The diagram in Figure 2.1 shows the four sources of information required in the provision of a good health visiting service. The first three sources are:

1. *Background information acquired over time* Knowledge of health visiting priorities, and including practical knowledge of how families can be helped

2. *Information acquired before the visit* Written/verbal communications about each individual family to be visited

3. *Information available when meeting the family* Information from the family itself, for example any particular wishes, viewpoint, cultural background or situation.

Fig. 2.1 The health visitor cycle.

These three together form the basis for assessing health needs and for planning and implementing health care at the first visit.

A fourth source, the last in the diagram in Figure 2.1, is:

4. *Information emerging as a result of the visit*
   Closer understanding of the particular family's circumstances and requirements and, as far as possible, assessment of the effect of the health care given.

This sort of evaluation provides part of the basis on which to plan for care in later encounters, helping to form the health visitor's tentative longer-term and short-term objectives for further work with the family. These objectives are borne in mind and, together with additional information available between visits and at the time of the next visit, they help towards further assessment and provision of care. This is then, in essence, a continuous cycle of drawing together information, planning, action and assessment. The framework is derived from the nursing process.

Use of the health visitor cycle is demonstrated in two examples of a health visitor making contact at a first visit. The matter is then discussed in the rest of the chapter, with this framework providing the format.

EXAMPLES OF FIRST VISITS

The first example is about making contact with a recently bereaved lady in her late 50s. The other is a visit to a young family who have just moved into the area. In each case, the planning processes for the visit and the four sources of information are plotted on health visitor cycle diagrams, Figures 2.2 and 2.3.

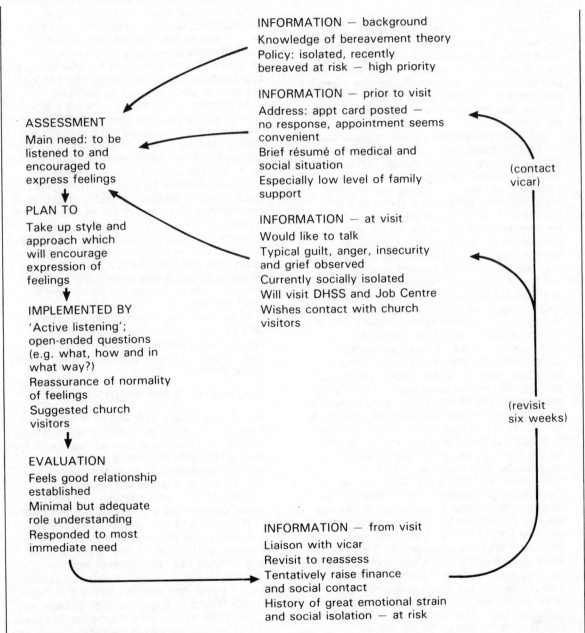

INFORMATION — background
Knowledge of bereavement theory
Policy: isolated, recently
bereaved at risk — high priority

INFORMATION — prior to visit
Address: appt card posted —
no response, appointment seems
convenient
Brief résumé of medical and
social situation
Especially low level of family
support

INFORMATION — at visit
Would like to talk
Typical guilt, anger, insecurity
and grief observed
Currently socially isolated
Will visit DHSS and Job Centre
Wishes contact with church
visitors

INFORMATION — from visit
Liaison with vicar
Revisit to reassess
Tentatively raise finance
and social contact
History of great emotional strain
and social isolation — at risk

ASSESSMENT
Main need: to be
listened to and
encouraged to
express feelings

PLAN TO
Take up style and
approach which
will encourage
expression of
feelings

IMPLEMENTED BY
'Active listening';
open-ended questions
(e.g. what, how and in
what way?)
Reassurance of normality
of feelings
Suggested church
visitors

EVALUATION
Feels good relationship
established
Minimal but adequate
role understanding
Responded to most
immediate need

(contact
vicar)

(revisit
six weeks)

Fig. 2.2 Example one: Miss Denby.

EXAMPLE ONE: MISS DENBY

An 'attached' health visitor, Harry Vosper (HV), had experience in bereavement counselling and knew local health policy on visiting recently bereaved people — particularly those with minimal family and social support. The initial visit was usually about two weeks after the death, when family and friends would probably be becoming less involved.

Dr Golding, a GP, referred Miss Denby, aged 58, whose mother had died. The health visitor learned that Miss Denby had given up work four years previously to care for her mother. They had had little contact with the surgery until four weeks before the death. The home was a small Victorian terrace house near the shops. Dr Golding said few people were expected to attend the funeral.

The visit was made on the day suggested on the card the health visitor had posted to Miss Denby. A slim, grey-haired woman with upright posture answered the door. She was very welcoming and offered a cup of tea. This HV accepted, as he wanted Miss Denby to feel there was plenty of time to talk if she wished to. He listened attentively as she spoke, and he concentrated on helping her to express her feelings. He was successful in this and felt the grief and insecurity she showed were normal and typical features of the grieving process.

When Miss Denby hesitated over speaking angrily against her mother and about her guilt feelings, HV responded by saying she need not tell him anything she did not wish to. He went on to explain that such feelings are perfectly normal and that many people find it helpful to talk about them. He reassured her, too, of the confidentiality of their conversation. Miss Denby thanked him and added, a little despairingly, that there was no one else she could tell about such things. In order to help her recontinue, he tried to summarise briefly what she was feeling and saying. Little by little, she explained about her situation, her wishes and how she felt.

Her story was that having taken over care of her increasingly immobile mother, Miss Denby had been left to cope. It seems Mrs Denby had refused all treatment for her Parkinsonism. Her daughter's social life had almost ceased on account of the 24 hour obligations. They did not know about the attendance allowance or what services there might have been available to help. Finally, the old lady had required a very great deal of nursing care. Under great emotional strain, Miss Denby over-rode her mother's wishes and called the doctor.

Admission to hospital had been a traumatic experience for them both and the old lady deteriorated fast.

The neighbours had called on hearing of the death. Miss Denby was no longer a church attender, but when HV told her about the local church bereavement visiting service, she said she would like them to call. As he got up to go, HV promised to contact the vicar. He suggested he should come again in six weeks, when, as she had said, she would have had a chance to seek advice on her financial position and entitlements and, perhaps, her chances of finding employment. He drew her attention to the telephone number on his visiting card and told her at what times he could be contacted.

As he reflected on the visit, HV felt a friendly working relationship had been established and she seemed to understand the purpose of his work — at least to the limited extent of his work with her! She had said how much better she felt for having talked about the bereavement. Six weeks would allow the church bereavement visitors time to befriend her and, perhaps, draw her into their circle. He felt the experiences and life-style of the past few years might impede her recovery. She had no close family and had been very isolated. He therefore intended to keep in touch for a while in order to make further assessment until it was obvious she had adequate support or was well on the way to a good recovery.

In the event, the church group proved to be very helpful, and after the second visit which included a full health assessment, the health visitor made no further calls until the anniversary of the death.

EXAMPLE TWO: THE TRENT FAMILY

Miss Hazel Vickery (HV) worked in a Health District in which, as is common practice, young families who have newly moved in are visited as soon as possible after notice of their new address is received. The general practice to which she was attached was running an experiment on developmental assessment of young children, using Professor Barber's (Barber et al, 1976) Woodside visual display charts.

A note in the practice manager's 'transfer in' file informed HV that a young family, parents and children, had just registered with the surgery. Within days, this family's health visitor record cards were received from the previous Health District, noting the change of address.

According to the notes, the mother had been a very regular attender at the clinic with her first

ASSESSMENT

Current need:
- to continue decorating
- social contacts
- knowledge of local services
- information on tests

Safety measures good

PLAN TO

Estimate whether visit
ill-timed

Inform re services

Arrange for test

IMPLEMENTED BY

Short visit

Describe local services,
lists given, promise
further inquiry

Health education re
child development

Congratulations on
safety

EVALUATION

Seemed very welcoming

Already understand role

Barber forms as spring-board
for involvement
and health education
- successful

INFORMATION — background

Policy: young family new
to area, high priority

Practice: experimenting
with 'involvement'
assessment

Information on local
services

INFORMATION — prior to visit

Address, age of children

Résumé of previous health
visitor contact

Attendance at clinic
mother and toddler group

Immunisations

Developmental assessments

INFORMATION — at visit

Evidently busy, but keen
for visit

Safety good

Father's role: involved

Assessment forms stimulate
questions

Seeks educational group

INFORMATION — from visit
- return for two year test
- ring library service
- tentatively — issue of
  playgroup for 3 year old

(ring
'Help for
Health')

(revisit
two weeks)

Fig. 2.3 Example two: the Trent family.

baby, now just over three years, and rather less
so with her second, now nearly two. The most
recent entry pertained to the three year
examination by the clinic doctor. Immunisations
for both children were up to date and the mother
seemed to have been a staunch supporter of her
previous health visitor's mother and toddler
group.

Having a 'birth visit' in that area, HV decided
to make a brief visit to the Trent household in
order to make contact. They were at home. She

introduced herself and found the couple in the
middle of decorating. She said she would call
back at a more convenient time, but they
insisted she come in.

The couple had made the room which
overlooked where they were working into a huge
safe area by using wide, temporarily fitted gates.
Here the children were playing and HV was
invited to step over the gates to meet them. She
congratulated the Trents on their safety
precautions. Mr Trent, who was taking a holiday

prior to starting his new job, was evidently proud of his children — and his safety measures. It seems the idea had evolved from a discussion at the clinic mother and toddler group.

Not wanting to outstay her welcome, HV asked when she might return to undertake the two year developmental assessment test. In response to a query from the couple, she showed them a copy of the stepladder centile charts used for recording attainments. These led to more questions and discussion on child development.

A date was arranged for HV to return. She gave Mrs Trent a list of child health centres and another of mother and baby groups. Mrs Trent asked about groups with an educational bias. Thinking that the information service, 'Help for Health', might know of some, HV undertook to make enquiries. On parting, the couple were reminded that they could contact HV through the surgery.

As the Trents returned to their wallpaper stripping, HV walked away hoping they had shown their true feelings about her unexpected visit. She felt that it was likely that she would develop a good working relationship with this family. They had made her very welcome and had found their previous health visiting service very useful. The Barber assessment scheme had, as usual, encouraged parental involvement and understanding. Interaction with their children was calm and caring and the children were lively and creative.

Miss Vickery planned, at the next visit, to discuss two year attainments using the Woodside charts (see pp. 91–92) as visual aids, and to see what views Mrs Trent had about playgroups as preparation for schooling. She made a note in her diary to ring the library 'Help for Health' service the following morning about mothers' health educational groups.

WHO ..... AND HOW?

Making contact with families is necessarily preceded by decisions on *who* is to be visited. Reading and discussion can generate useful ideas on *how* these families might be helped and keep up to date the wide range of knowledge needed in the practice of health visiting. They both form an important part of background understanding in health visiting.

BACKGROUND INFORMATION — FOR PRIORITIES

With a remit as broad as a health visitor's, the first question is 'to whom do I give priority, how do I apportion my time?' As in most professions, accustomed patterns of practice play an important role in such decisions, but local health policies and local environmental and health factors also influence the priorities chosen.

Customary patterns of practice

These patterns are learned during training. Students gain experience alongside their fieldwork teachers. They become conversant with current

common practice and will probably see some experimental projects. Research suggests that some 70% of health visitors' time is spent on work with children, proportionately more of it in activities associated with the young infant. Time is spent on advice, counselling, reassurance and education. That in child health or well baby clinics, for example, was found to be 26% on diet and infant feeding, 21% on parentcraft and children and 12% with people's personal problems. Developmental assessment accounts for 11% of the time, hearing and vision 5% and immunisation 4%. On average, care for the elderly takes up 6% of the time available (Dunnell & Dobbs, 1982).

The aim is to provide a service at various 'critical periods' (Council for the Education and Training of Health Visitors, 1977), such as ante- and postnatal phases, old age and bereavement. Ann Stanton (1982) has drawn up an outline suggesting one way a new health visitor might arrange her activities, and included some hours set aside for planning, thinking and reading. Ideas are constantly being modified in the light of new research findings, and it is important for health visitors to organise for both keeping up to date and forward planning in their work.

Jean Orr (1982) has described the influences of recent reports and governmental advisory documents. A lack of money and manpower has stifled many of the developments suggested. Inspired local initiatives, however, have led to improvements in aspects of the work such as antenatal care, child abuse, the elderly, inner city work, 'positive discrimination', out of hours service, 'outreach programmes' and group work. Many are described in the later chapters of this book. The implementation of newer trends and ideas varies from area to area.

Local health policy

Many factors influence the number of health visitors employed per head of population and an important one is the willingness of the health authority to allocate resources for training and staffing. Metcalfe (1983) points out that, currently, the number of health visitors is regrettably low. It varies quite markedly between some regions (Orr, 1982). Health visitors may find themselves in quite stressful situations, trying to choose how best to spend their time (Schofield, 1982, 1983). Some are obliged to cover two or more caseloads for quite lengthy periods (Thompson, 1983). As Alison Norman (1982) points out, there is a need for more discussion and investigation of the way caseload size and environmental factors affect health visiting practice.

In most Health Districts, health visitors can decide their own priorities (Fitton, 1983, 1984a, 1984b). Rather than directing the work, many nurse managers use their monitoring role more as that of a consultant advisor and act, to some extent, as a sounding board. In this way, they enable their health visitors 'to come to their own professional decision' (Dingwall et al, 1983). When this works well, it can help them develop new and useful approaches.

There has been some apprehension within the profession because, in some Districts, structured visiting programmes have been drawn up and the health visitors directed to complete them (Health Visitor, 1983). It is feared that some such schemes will result in 'doorstep-hopping, superficial health visiting' (Goodwin, 1982). An obligation to call on a prescribed number of homes each day may increase the number of visits recorded and counted in management terms, but it is unlikely to increase the fruitfulness of the work. The fear is that doorstep visiting will prevent the chance to establish meaningful relationships, the key to useful health visiting, and in the pressure to complete a particular visiting target each day, vital cues to problems may be lost (Health Visitor, 1983).

Gradually the concept of 'contact' on a basis agreed with clients, is gaining ground (Goodwin, 1988; Dauncey, 1989). This leaves time for group work or other forms of contact, which have been found to be more effective and preferred by clients. It also makes it possible to rearrange priorities in favour of particular groups needing special effort and attention. In essence, common sense prevails, rather than some prescribed and imposed visiting pattern.

Local statistics

In order to choose the most important preventive health priorities, it is necessary to know the particular problems prevalent in the locality. Students gain experience of enquiring into environmental and health statistics by undertaking a neighbourhood study. Many now complete a caseload profile (Hunt, 1982a; 1982b; see Ch. 15).

Baroness MacFarlane (1982) suggested that the health visitor should become the primary health care team epidemiologist. Many do become very aware of the environmental, social and health problems of their area and try to tailor their work accordingly. Sheila Jack (1983) has outlined the range of statistics available to the health visitor. Small-scale, local epidemiological information, though, is not a reliable guide (Robinson J, 1983).

Computers can now be used to process the social and environmental data from the 1981 census enumeration district statistics, defining characteristics of small areas with a population size of only a few hundred. From these, quite detailed Health District social profiles can be mapped out. Jarman (1983; 1984; 1989) and Irving (1983) give examples of how this has been done.

The correlation between levels of health and social circumstances is now well known. Where local health statistics are post-coded, they could also be mapped and used to overlap the District profile. Such maps, when they are drawn up, are able to provide District Health Authorities with documentary evidence of what health visitors tend already to know: the areas needing special initiatives and, perhaps, proportionately greater investment in primary care services.

There is some debate over the extent to which health visiting should be provided equally to all, or slanted towards those with potentially greater health problems. The Cumberlege Report (1986) has helped to stimulate greater acceptance of new and better ways of assessing priorities and of the need to implement new initiatives. We will look at some examples of these ideas in the later chapters.

BACKGROUND INFORMATION — FOR PRACTICAL WORK

Students quickly realise that the health visitors course, although tightly packed with information about, for example, nutrition, psychology and social medicine, and thought-provoking ideas on how to help people, can only be an introduction. Reading, practical experience, advice from colleagues and the search for services and ideas, are all important sources of background information (see Fig. 2.1).

Journal articles

The breadth of the work means health visitors will need to continue to read widely, in order to keep up to date and also to enquire into particular aspects of the work as they are encountered. Professional journals like the *Health Visitor*, the *Nursing Times' Community Outlook*, *Midwife*, *Health Visitor and Community Nurse* and — as will be seen from the lists of references in this book — many others, provide background sources of information.

It is not always easy to maintain a high level of reading alongside the obligations associated with a full caseload. With this in mind, some nurse managers build up and make available a file of useful literature.

Research and library facilities

One of the services some medical libraries provide is access to the Health Visitor Association's *Current Awareness Bulletin* — a very good source for updating work practice. It is important constantly to be seeking the latest and most reliable research results which pertain to practical aspects of the work, in order to provide people with the best possible information.

Hours can be spent by individual health visitors and social workers trying to search out information on, for example, meeting times and places of special interest groups appropriate to individuals they are trying to help. If a small team can be specially employed to build up a library of such information and have it available as a telephone, postal or call-in service, it can help provide a much more efficient service.

Robert Gann (1983) has described how the Regional Health Authority set up such a service called 'Help for Health'. It provides patients and all health and welfare workers with accurate and up-to-date information on voluntary organisations (Gann, 1988). It is especially helpful to health visitors. There is also a wealth of educational material available to both professionals and patients.

Some health visitors accumulate their own small library of favourite reference books which they can lend, for brief periods, to the families they visit (see Ch. 4, Table 4.1 and Ch. 5, Box 5.1).

Discussion and support groups

There are other ways health visitors can share their discovery of useful literature. For example, some meet on a regular basis, perhaps with allied professionals, in order to tell each other of research findings and new ideas that have come to their notice. Working with colleagues on exploratory studies or new projects can also stimulate further thought on how to respond to people's needs. Where they exist, research liaison officers could be invited to help think through ideas for setting up local research into aspects of health visiting.

Clulow (1982, pp. 80–99), Appleby (1987a; 1987b), Rowe (1988), Pittaway and others (1988) and Vizard (1983) have described how health visitors meeting together as a support group has helped them cope with, and gain a better insight into, their day-to-day work. Sharing some of their difficult experiences with sympathetic colleagues can lead to new depths of understanding on how to help families. A National Association for Staff Support has now been set up (Swaffield, 1990). Stress management is mentioned towards the end of Chapter 15. Refresher courses and classes, such as those aimed at improving counselling skills, are also ways of gaining knowledge in order to improve practice.

This section has looked at sources of information for decision-making on priorities and for the knowledge needed for day-to-day work. Both of them are basic to the practice of health visiting and are categorised and shown as 'background information' at the top of Figure 2.1.

PREPARING FOR THE VISIT

INFORMATION — PRIOR TO THE VISIT

Before health visitors can call on any particular family, they need to know where to call and to have, if at all possible, at least an outline of the family size and age structure. Prior warning of any particular needs there might be, means that some forethought can be given to the sort of assistance that might be offered. This information, acquired before the visit and seen in the second grouping in Figure 2.1, shows records, referrals and liaison as important sources of information.

Health visitor records

Record cards give incoming health visitors a picture of the families currently being visited. The cards tend to be filed by one of the following:

- street and neighbourhood
- family surname, in alphabetical order
- age of the youngest child in each family.

Whichever system or combination of systems is chosen, the aim is to facilitate plans to make more frequent visits to families with younger babies and to save time by visiting people living fairly close to each other. Sometimes small sections of the file are set aside for families who for some reason

might benefit from more frequent visiting, such as one with a handicapped member.

Annual 'birth books' are used by many health visitors to list, month by month, the births that have occurred within the caseload. These lists make an excellent quick guide to the babies due for hearing tests and other assessments falling at a particular age.

Administrative schemes and referrals

Some Districts use computers for making appointments for developmental assessment and/or for their immunisation programmes. These schemes make it easy to inform health visitors of the families who, for example, have missed three appointments. Follow-up visits can then be arranged.

Notification of the birth enables the District Health Authority to send a health visitor record card for each baby on the GP list of 'attached' health visitors and each one born in the 'geographic patch' of those who are not. There are not such clear-cut arrangements for those who were born outside the area and have 'transferred in'. 'Attached' health visitors may have a special arrangement with the practice manager to have, for example, families newly added to the GP's practice listed in a notebook. In many cases the newly moved in families may be unknown to the health visitor until the old notes are sent on from the previous area. Getting to know about elderly people and other client groups is different again and is discussed elsewhere (Robertson, 1984).

Liaison

Where a family is known to the

- midwife
- social worker
- district nurse
- liaison health visitor
- general practitioner
- community psychiatric nurse
- voluntary worker or
- some other agency,

it might be helpful to meet or phone so that, within the rules of confidentiality (see Ch. 8), the situation may be discussed. Contact with other people working with the family lessens the chance of conflicting advice and gives the benefit of the other worker's perspective of the family's needs. However, care needs to be taken that when professionals work in concert like this, they do not become so united in their plan of action that they then take no account of their clients' perspectives and wishes.

In this small section we have had an introduction to the main sources of information acquired before the visit, that is, through records, referral and liaison. These will be touched on again in subsequent chapters.

THE VISIT

A major part of the activity in the health visitor cycle takes place during the visit itself and many interacting factors are at work. For this reason, this section is the longest. Three important elements of success are identified and each is discussed in depth. The two main information sources are, as shown in Figure 2.1, the client's opinion and viewpoint, and the health visitor's own observations.

INFORMATION — WHILST VISITING

The health visitor arrives at a first visit to, for example, a family with young children, a handicapped member or an old person, having given a grading of priority, as explained above, to their potential need for preventive health care. Depending on the depth of information on the family that is available, some ideas will have been formed on the sort of help that might be offered. These are tentative objectives for the visit, but they may be altered radically during the meeting, once the family's own perspective is taken into account and an 'on site' assessment has been possible.

These factors — the client viewpoint and the health visitor's observations — equate, in the health visitor cycle, to the 'subjective' and 'observed' or so called 'objective' elements of the SOAP model of the nursing process (see Ch. 8, p. 147).

The client viewpoint

A great deal is being written now on the importance of client opinion and involvement (Warnock Report, 1978; Department of Health and Social Security and Child Poverty Action Group, 1978; National Children's Bureau, 1981; Dowling, 1983). Health care is no longer seen as something which is 'done to people'. Client or parental views and feelings provide what is, basically, the most important information for the health visitor. It is the main springboard from which to begin to plan possible ways of offering help. The Children's Committee (1980) proposed, for example, that parents and professionals should have a partnership in which there is:

- regard for the parents' key position in the life of the child
- sensitivity to the family's social and cultural situation
- parental understanding of the services and
- encouragement for parents helping parents.

In writing about teaching and learning, Elizabeth Perkins (1980) drew attention to the two way processes involved, the need for professional sensitivity to the particular needs of each individual and the central contribution of the parent in preparatory education for childbirth and parenthood.

Health visitor observations

People's beliefs and attitudes are not communicated by the spoken word alone. Betty Raymond (1983) describes how non-verbal signs convey information to the health visitor. The way a door is opened, clothing and general appearance, posture, gesture and mannerisms, facial expression, eye contact and tone of voice, all give an impression of how people are feeling and their approach to life.

It might please some to think of the health visitor as an objective observer of these matters. The fact is, as Betty Raymond points out, there may be several possible interpretations of any given gesture or action. Social science research has shown the inevitability of personal bias. Health visitors as observers are not exempt. The way they view what happens at a visit will be heavily influenced by their background, their training and their various preconceptions. Equally, the behaviour and style of the health visitor also creates an impression, and itself influences the way people feel and act.

Some of the visible information available to health visitors, such as babies' weight and appearance, presents more clear-cut evidence. This type of evidence is likely to be perceived in the same terms by all the parties involved and is not so open to misinterpretation.

There are, of course, enormous limits on the extent to which health visitors may observe the physical surroundings in which they find themselves. They are guests in people's homes and their demeanour needs to be appropriate to the situation. They may not, for example, feel free to allow their gaze to wander around the room, in case this is interpreted as an inspection — and even, perhaps, an intrusion upon privacy. Raymond mentions the need for clients to feel accepted. A non-patronising, non-judgemental relationship in which the people being visited really feel they are, and are being treated as, equals, is the key to this.

There is sometimes talk of 'seeing people as they really are' as a consequence of the health visitor's calling unexpectedly. However, the Rcn Health Visitors Advisory Group (1983) felt that 'checking up' on people or 'catching them unawares' and other aspects of what might be seen as 'social policing', are no part of the health visitor's role. Appointments systems can help avoid this problem and save time and money (Reynolds & Hay, 1986).

There will be an attempt to show, in the rest of this section, that successful communication be-

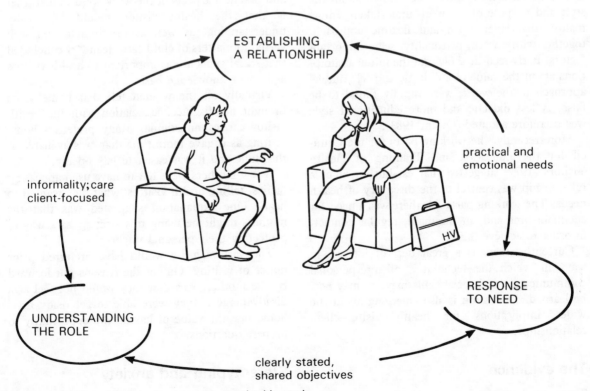

Fig. 2.4 Elements of success in communicating health needs.

tween the health visitor and the family about health needs and problems, depends mainly on the three interdependent and interlinked factors depicted in Figure 2.4. These are the quality of the relationship, the extent to which the role is understood and the sort of help that is given. Each is considered in depth.

It could be said that they are, all three, an essential part of all health visiting. However, I feel that it is in making contact, particularly at a first visit, that (i) establishing a relationship, (ii) trying to portray the role and (iii) responding, where possible, to the immediate needs of the family, come very much to the fore — both for health visitors and those they visit.

1. ESTABLISHING A RELATIONSHIP

The key to effective health visiting has always been seen as the development of a good relationship, one in which the worker's attitudes are acceptable and in which there is mutual agreement about the style and purpose of the work undertaken. Informality, that is an open and flexible approach, together with a warm personality, seem important factors. Early records show that the initial assumptions about the value of a didactic and 'charitable' approach to the work, were rapidly found to be false. A less didactic and more educational style was therefore adopted (Owen, 1983).

More recently, the working party for the Council for the Education and Training of Health Visitors (1977) suggested that establishment of a relationship was central to the discovery of health needs. The working party felt there was a need for adequate time and, in the main, regular contact, in order to achieve this.

Currently, there is a great deal of interest in ways in which the techniques of interpersonal communication and social skills may, or may not, be learned. Discussion is also emerging about the wider implications for health visitor–client relationships.

The evidence

There are two main ways in which to investigate the relationship between health visitors and the members of the families they visit. One way is to observe and/or tape-record what actually happens. The other is to ask participants to describe it.

There is very little published evidence, yet, on what is actually said and takes place during the conversations between health visitors and their clientele. With the advent of small-sized tape recorders, quite detailed studies have become possible (Dingwall, 1977; Clark, 1984). Several are under way. However, there are some descriptive studies.

Research undertaken by Jean Orr (1980) used an interview method in seeking clients' opinions. It was an exploratory study in which 68 wives of semi-skilled workers were interviewed in depth. The study highlighted important factors about the relationship. For example, over 80% of the mothers felt the health visitor understood and was interested in their particular problems. A large proportion, some 66%, felt they would not like to do without their health visitor. Both supportive and practical aspects of the work were valued, that is that the health visitor should be 'really understanding' as well as up to date and well versed in matters of child care. Jean Orr concluded that social skills are as important to health visitors as is their knowledge base.

Virtually all the women felt that home visits brought no disgrace: association with the health visitor carries no stigma. Many preferred home visiting as it gave more time than was available at the clinic and it was easier to talk openly.

A few mothers were felt to have used appeasing tactics, telling health visitors 'what they wanted to hear'. One explanation suggested was that the mothers might be using this strategy as a way of protecting their personal integrity.

The vast majority would have preferred prior notice of visiting. One of the reasons put forward by the mothers was that they would not feel at a disadvantage if they were able to get ready first. Some saw the value of having the opportunity to prepare questions.

Stereotyping and anxiety

Eighteen mothers in Orr's study felt that an 'ideal

health visitor' would be married and have children. Marjory Adams' (1982) personal experience of the helpfulness of a childless, unmarried health visitor, led her to propose that this stereotyped opinion is misplaced. She said that merely having children does not make a person more feeling and thoughtful towards others, and suggested too, that indiscriminate complaining about health visitors often reflects the speaker's own anxieties and inadequacies regarding parenthood. Whatever the basic cause, health visitors should always try to discover their own part in any customer dissatisfaction. The suggestion does remind us, however, as does the example in Clulow's study discussed later in this chapter (p. 29), that the health visitor–client relationship is not always a simple one.

Early motherhood

Field et al (1982) interviewed 78 women. A third were early in their first pregnancy and a third were newly delivered of their first baby. The rest had a first baby of 12–15 months. These researchers also found the same stereotyping about childless health visitors. Most of the mothers were happy with their health visitor.

Valued attributes were:

- readiness to answer questions
- speedy response to requests for help
- preparedness to listen to problems
- boosting confidence in mothering abilities
- friendliness and
- approachability.

Health visitors who were not liked tended to be seen as:

- interfering
- out of touch
- unsympathetic and
- authoritative.

Again, social skills and relationship play an important part.

Interviewing women from the chosen three stages of early motherhood enabled the researchers to see the value of getting to know the health visitor in the antenatal period, a matter taken up at the beginning of the next chapter.

Observations of style

An American researcher (Mayers, 1973) observed the conversations between public health nurses and some of their patients. It was found that whatever the nurses' style of intervention, whether it was information giving, directive or non-directive (or any mixture of the three), each nurse maintained the same individual interactional style for everyone visited. Whichever the approach, a positive and involved response from the patient was found to relate to the extent to which the nurse paid attention to the patient's point of view.
'Patient-focused nurses'

- demonstrated a sense of concern
- showed personal interest
- engendered a feeling of mutuality in the relationship
- gave the opportunity for their patients to be involved in decisions about solutions to their problems.

'Nurse-focused nurses', on the other hand, reacted to patient initiatives by interpreting them according to their own point of view or frame of reference. These nurses relied on their own perspective too, for decisions on solutions to patients' problems.

The sort of relationships that work well have been discussed and listed (see Fig. 2.5), but how do they come about? How can they be achieved?

Some theories

The way people feel and behave towards each other involves deep labyrinths of intricate variation, far too complex for a single, simple explanation. There are, however, a number of useful theories which provide a degree of partial understanding, by piecing together certain observed patterns of behaviour. Many of them are of interest to health visitors. For example, there are the theories on learning and group behaviour and explanations of child abuse.

Eric Berne (1968) likens social transactions between people to games, pastimes, rituals and procedures. This theory provides very interesting and useful perspectives on social custom and prac-

Fig. 2.5   A good relationship.

tice. Both Berne and Harris (1973) believe that tendencies towards what they classify as the 'Parent', 'Adult' and 'Child' in people, are present in all our behaviour. Harris suggests that by understanding these processes, people can improve their quality of social interaction and attain an 'I'm OK — you're OK' approach to life.

Learning communication skills

Another theory suggests that social skills can be learned through practice, very much as can the motor skills of riding a bicycle or driving a car (Argyle, 1978). This notion has an important role in health visitor social skills training. Enid Lythgoe

(1983) has described how communication skills are taught in the Leeds course, using role play and video equipment. With these, the students get feedback on their achievements as well as all the other benefits of experiential learning.

These communication skills are sometimes referred to as counselling skills. Courses aim, not at training professional counsellors, but at helping students develop particular aspects of interpersonal skills. It is hoped that these can be used to help facilitate people's understanding of their own view of their situation and enable them to explore and decide on possible solutions to their problems and needs. Also, all health education and supportive care has to be founded on and tailored to each individual's preconceptions and understanding. The need, therefore, to help people express these thoughts, permeates the whole of a health visitor's work.

Students are given hints on the sort of remarks that can detract from people's ability to give their view or explore their problem. It is generally suggested that untimely advice and opinion giving, and other strategies which draw attention away from the speaker, are best avoided in the early, exploratory stages when the problem or notion is being thought through. A warm, caring and un-judging manner is a basic necessity. Students discuss the sort of non-verbal stance and mannerisms that portray these attitudes.

Learning about these skills and the effect and implications of using them, can be achieved properly only through guided practice and through broadly-based discussion. As a back-up, there are several useful books on counselling and interpersonal skills which give, for example, good introductions for nurses (Tschudin, 1982; Scottish Health Education Group, 1989), suggest simple exercises to increase self-awareness and to develop particular skills (Munro et al, 1983; Burnard, 1985), and provide a problem management model (Egan, 1981) and a discussion of research into the field alongside a description of the range of social skills needed (Hargie et al, 1981). Listening and questioning are key elements in counselling techniques. Examples of the advice that health visitor students might be given on how to help people to

---

Box 2.1 Listening — some points to remember

Environment
If possible, *choose* a situation reasonably
- free from distractions
- comfortable for both
- close to each other

Non-verbal responses
It may help to *show interest* by
- nodding your head in agreement and understanding
- using good eye contact
- indicating with 'A-ah' and 'M-mm' sounds that the client should continue to talk

Verbal responses
You may be able to *encourage* the client to continue by
- echoing back last word/words e.g. 'I wish I'd called for mother' 'Mother?'
- reflecting back feelings e.g. use of analogy (as the encounter continues)
- paraphrasing talk so far, perhaps summarising
- appropriate use of questioning
- making sensitive use of silence — to allow client thought to develop uninterrupted

You should be aware that you will *detract* from the client's view or problem by
- stating your opinion
- giving advice — 'if I were you . . .'
- over-sympathising — 'me too . . .'

These draw attention away from your client and towards you and your own perceptions and ideas

---

Box 2.2 Questioning — some points to remember

You may find it helpful to ask:
Open questions
which encourage your client to take the lead in the dialogue, for example
- How . . . .
- What . . . .
- In what way . . . .
- When . . . .
- How do you feel about . . . .

Your approach should neither be, nor sound, inquisitorial

Care should be taken that your questions are geared only for the benefit of the client and not, for example, to satisfy your curiosity or any other matter centred on yourself

You should be aware of the effect of:
Leading questions
indicating particular conclusions, e.g.
- Don't you think that . . . .

Closed questions
able to be answered by 'Yes' or 'No', e.g.
- Would you like to . . . .
- Do you get . . . .

These questions can tend to shut off conversation and limit client talk express themselves can be found on p. 27, Boxes 2.1 & 2.2.

It will be interesting to see to what extent these listening and questioning techniques are used in practice — and with what effect. Research is needed in the field because these techniques are so widely advocated. Some recently published, in which tape-recorded health visitor clinic conversation was studied (Warner, 1984), did not report on this specific issue. One of the health visitors in the project was found to be particularly skilled at getting the mothers to ask the 'right' question. However, the researcher was not able to see how she achieved this, despite the availability of the tape recording for analysis. Interpersonal skills do not seem to hinge on any simple and trite formula.

Kate Robinson (1983) is concerned that communication has now become a task to be performed on people. She suggests that treating talk with clients as a professional skill and seeing it as a 'problem', may detract from the basic issue of whether or not the conversation and the visit has relevance and value to the participants.

Relationship and clarity about role are linked

The relationship between health visitors and the people they visit necessarily affects the way their role is understood by those families. Both client-focused care and informality are shown in Figure 2.4 as linking factors. Obviously, people who have an involved and participating interaction with their health visitor, will gain direct insight. Working together 'in partnership' means aims and intentions are explained on both sides. As the subsequent health visiting is based on the clients' wishes and perspectives, it is naturally more meaningful, of more value to them and better understood.

Similarly, the feeling of informality and approachability in a good, supportive relationship leads to a closeness in which wider purposes of the visit and the function of a health visitor can be more readily discussed. A brief introduction to the role is, of course, all that can be hoped for on a first visit.

2. UNDERSTANDING THE ROLE

'Role' in this context means 'one's function, what (a) person is appointed or expected to do' (Oxford Dictionary). The role in health visiting is a particularly broad one. The Mayston Committee (1969) listed some 60 separate and varied aspects of the work. Just a glance at this formidable description shows it is no easy task to give clients a succinct résumé. More commonly used, shorter descriptions, for example those by the Council for the Education and Training of Health Visitors (1967, 1977), have tended to be broad and non-specific. Alison Norman (1982) says that in her explanations to clients she concentrates on the more practical aspects of the work. These are likely to be much easier for people to understand (see Mayers (1973), later in this chapter on p. 30).

The Health Visitor Association has produced a colourful and practically based pamphlet which can be used on visits to give clients an idea of the health visitor's role. Ann Stanton (1982) suggested that a tailor-made hand-out could be made up by health visitors where no suitable one is available. Not everyone feels such pamphlets are necessary (Schofield, 1982) and many health visitors rely on demonstrating their role through their work.

Research findings

Research on the way health visiting is perceived has looked at three aspects: client opinion, psychological explanations about role, and the way a changing role may be emerging with recent policy and structural changes.

Mothers' opinions

About 80% of the mothers Jean Orr (1980) interviewed knew their health visitor by name. The locally used visiting card may have helped this. The card also stated nursing and midwifery qualifications, but this does not seem to have prevented the health visitors from being perceived as social workers or 'a lady from the welfare', almost as often as a nurse.

All of the mothers in this sample had one pre-school child. The health visitors' work was seen, therefore, in terms of care for children. Over a third seemed unaware of any function pertaining to other members of the family. However, a very wide variety of health and welfare aspects of care were mentioned as having been discussed with the health visitors.

Jean Orr drew attention to the health visitors' use of tact and discretion in advice giving. This and their style of helping people to come to their own conclusions, naturally means that their contribution is not always fully evident to their clients. Health visitors face the dilemma of wanting to make their role understood but, at the same time, finding it necessary to provide a self-effacing and background style which itself makes too many assertive statements about the work impracticable.

Ascribed role

In a study of the effects on marriage of the first baby and preparation for parenthood, Clulow (1982) set up workshops where health visitors could discuss issues arising out of their work with such couples. Clulow said that often families who wanted help had mixed feelings about whether they really did want it. Others who clearly wanted it, were unsure of what help they needed and therefore what role their health visitor should perform. The ambivalence, it seems, could be conveyed in a variety of ways, through both overt and covert communications. Clulow showed how parents might ascribe a role for the health visitor, of which neither she nor the couple were aware.

In an example (pp. 83–5) a health visitor had been chided by a new parent she was visiting over her own abilities as a mother, and was made to feel an inadequate parent. Clulow said these parents had needed the health visitor, not as an expert in child care, but as 'the parent who was found wanting'. He went on to say that they had been comparing themselves against a model of ideal parenthood. He suggested that the 'ascribed health visitor role', by comparison, helped to reduce their anxiety and contributed to building up their confidence.

Many inherent complexities in the role were discussed by Clulow. He felt ideas about the role should not be too rigidly interpreted, in order to give scope for health visitors to be involved with and have better understanding of the people they visit.

Administrative effects on function

The role of the health visitor is to provide a service offering advice and help which families are free to accept or reject as they wish. Dingwall (1982) suggests that the success and continuance of health visiting depend on this non-authoritarian approach to people. Having studied health visiting in depth (Dingwall, 1977; Dingwall et al, 1981), he observed that close supervision and detailed accountability, which tend to be associated with a bureaucratic hierarchy, can undermine this relationship and muzzle professional freedom to react towards clients in the traditional intuitive way. There have been administrative changes in recent years towards a more hierarchical structure for health visiting.

Jane Robinson (1982a) feels that the voluntary relationship that exists between health visitors and those they visit, one in which advice from the so called 'expert' may be accepted or rejected, may be under threat. She is apprehensive about the implications of some recent reports from governmental committees. They urge child health workers to take various initiatives to 'persuade' people to attend clinics and to take other steps towards activities that might be regarded as coercion and as 'social policing'. Structured visiting programmes and 'checking up' on people have both been mentioned earlier in this chapter.

Role and response to need are linked

Clearly stated and shared objectives are shown at the bottom of Figure 2.4 as linking factors. People being visited can understand the role better if the aims and intentions of the health visitor can be made quite clear. Understanding these enables clients to be consulted on and involved in any proposed course of action. Actions mutually decided upon are both more acceptable and meaningful and, themselves, lead to a greater appreciation and understanding of the part played by health visitors.

3. RESPONDING TO NEED

Ways that health visitors may be able to help people are discussed in greater detail in most of the later chapters. This section looks at the processes involved in carrying out the work, particularly at the setting of objectives, and draws on some research findings.

The studies

The ways in which health visitors respond to people's health requirements need, of course, to be as effective as possible and to be felt by the people involved to be useful and worth trying. Several research projects have studied health visitors' attempts to respond to people's needs. These have involved short-term, regular visiting, problem and relationship-based responses, and the need for clear explanations about, and agreement on, short-term goals.

Short-term regular visits

In research into the evaluation of health visiting, Karen Luker (1982) looked at the way goals for the work might be measured against results. The study looked at the effect of four consecutive monthly visits on samples of elderly ladies (see Luker, 1982, Ch. 7, pp. 117, 119–120). A significant improvement in their problems was found to have occurred. Much of this was maintained at least six months after visiting ceased. Dr Luker has now turned to researching in detail the behind-the-scenes processes in referral (Luker & Chalmers, 1989) and in gaining access to clients (Luker & Chalmers, 1990).

Two approaches

Looking at young mothers' perceptions of health visiting (see earlier this chapter, p. 25), Jean Orr (1980) identified two basic health visiting responses to their needs. These were, firstly, practical aspects such as advice giving and developmental checks and, secondly, relationship-based responses such as willingness to listen to problems and giving support. These

were partially mirrored in Jane Robinson's (1982b) study of non-attendance at developmental assessment sessions, as she felt that the health visitors caring for the people in her small sample tended to polarise towards either one or the other of the above approaches to health visiting. To what extent this polarisation is common in the practice of health visiting is not known.

Robinson found failure to attend at clinics tended to be related to the parents' seeing the service as an agency of social control. The case of one mother, 'Mrs Graham', serves very well as an example. She very much resented her first health visitor 'prying' into her private life. Enquiries were made about her husband's income and employment and their food supplies. This discourteous health visitor was asked not to return. Their next health visitor was very friendly — she maintained a low profile and was consulted by 'Mrs Graham' (p. 79). Jane Robinson suggested the first of the health visitors had a 'problem-oriented' approach, whilst the second had a 'relationship-centred' one.

The health visitors in Orr's sample tended to give the mothers satisfaction and seemed to have been functioning from an adequate knowledge base, which gave them the ability to respond to the mothers' requirements. Robinson's 'problem-oriented' health visitor may well have worked from a predetermined list of items, based rather more on bureaucratic notions than on what the family saw as problems. The second was much more sensitive to family feelings and priorities — and was much more effective in being able to provide a preventive health service.

Conversations studied

In her study of health visitor conversations in clinics, Una Warner (1984) showed agreement on goals was associated with success in the work. She found these goals were explained and negotiated in the normal course of conversation.

Marlene Mayers (1973) in her research into public health nurse–patient conversations found that patients who had a better understanding of how the nurse was aiming to help, were those who were cared for by the nurses who thought theoretically mostly in terms of specific, short-range goals — 'keep six weeks appointment' or 'get needed medical care'. Where nurses explained objectives to the researcher in more abstract ideas of personal-social goals — 'adjustment to new culture' or 'achieve stable home life' — there was a lower level of understanding by the patients.

Objectives

Aims, goals, plans, intentions and objectives are words commonly used in health visiting to describe what is proposed and what it is hoped to achieve. A time-scale dimension is sometimes used. An example suggesting long- and short-term and immediate objectives is set out in Table 2.1. Intermediate plans for the medium term, many months or a year ahead, become relatively short-term when visiting is infrequent. For this reason, they have not been assigned a special category.

Table 2.1 Time-scale for health visiting objectives

Objectives	Concerned with	Examples
Immediate	Current meeting	Answering queries that arise during the visit Informing family of appropriate services available
Short-term	Present and near future	That the infant receives the full course of immunisations That the mother understands the basic principles of weaning
Long-term	Philosophical aims	That the family attain their full potential for social, mental and physical health Early discovery of family health needs

Long-term objectives in this model include the broad-based, largely unattainable ideals for which to aim. These describe the purpose of health visiting and provide the philosophical framework within which the more tangible and practical objectives are set. It is debatable as to whether these philosophical ideals are better classified as 'aims' or as 'objectives'.

If short-term objectives are made clear and immediate objectives are tailored to what the family feels is important, then client understanding of the aims of health visiting and the extent to which the health visitor can help the family are all likely to be enhanced. This is especially important when making initial contact with the family, such as at a first visit.

The health visitor cycle

Deciding on objectives for a family's care is a complex matter. Three of the sources of information that can help make these decisions — background knowledge and those sources available prior to and during the visit — have already been discussed. The sequences of thought in the health visitor cycle (Fig. 2.1) are, of course, the same as for the nursing process and any other form of management by objectives. These are that an assessment has to be made, based on the information available, so that plans or objectives can be drawn up and put into action. Evaluation and further planning follows. In intuitive, creative activities and in all everyday decision-making, the same processes are gone through but in an unplanned, informal sort of way.

Families are highly individual and present a diversity of environmental and social situations. Also, seemingly routine conversations constantly introduce new notions and perspectives. This brings a need for wide variation in and continually changing objectives. The advantage of the health visitor cycle, as a framework, is that it concentrates on the *sources* of changing ideas — the origins of the subsequent processes of planning and implementation. It has the benefit, too, of being able to highlight the clients' opinions.

Inevitably, objectives have to be founded on inadequate knowledge, but that is a problem common to most spheres of management and decision-making. It is a question of making the best possible use of what is available, and being prepared to vary objectives as new information comes to light.

A checklist

A working party in Northumberland (McClymont, 1983) set out to draw up a standard for measuring health visiting practice (see Ch. 8). They aimed to list criteria for the first visit to a family with a new baby (pp. 9–12). It was hoped these items would provide a framework within which help could be given.

They listed statements (p. 7) about the purpose of health visiting and its objectives in general, philosophical terms similar to those Marlene Mayers had found were not satisfactorily explained to, nor understood by, the people visited.

Lists of specific items were drawn up. These included:

- factors that should be known prior to the visit
- observations and examinations deemed necessary during the visit and
- matters needing to be clarified.

Some of these 'criteria' would convert quite well into easily understood short-term or immediate objectives for the time-scale model shown in Table 2.1, for example, 'clarification' of the method and routine of feeding and the infant's behaviour, or the suggestions for a physical examination of the baby. The lists had good and poor points and are returned to in Chapter 4.

Health visitor style

Care has to be taken that a predetermined checklist of objectives does not dominate health visitor thought and become counter-productive. A good relationship and sensitivity to the wishes of the family could well prove to be the most important of all objectives.

Figure 2.6 shows a continuum of possible health visitor intention and style. At one end, lack of well thought-out objectives would be likely to result in a confused client, wondering about the purposes of the service.

At the other extreme, where pre-set objectives are rigidly and unthinkingly adhered to, the response would more likely be one of irritation and a strong suspicion of 'social policing' — the experience of 'Mrs Graham'!

In the central range, health visiting is able to respond to clients' wishes, as far as this is possible. Being prepared to vary objectives gives the opportunity for both practical and supportive care, according to what seems to be needed.

Limits on response

Whatever objectives may be drawn up and planned, there are limits on time, and choices have to be made. Jane Schofield (1982) points out that it is *quality* and not quantity that is central to the work. Particularly in places with large numbers of problems, such as inner city areas, some aspects of the work will have to be foregone, in order to provide an adequate depth of service for those with outstanding need.

Karen Luker's study of old people's problems showed focused health visiting, regular and concentrated over a few months, to be productive. Fears about shallow, 'doorstep-hopping health visiting' were mentioned earlier in this chapter (p. 19).

Response to need and relationship are linked

This section has looked at research on approaches to responding to people's health needs. Once again client opinion needs to be central, this time with regard to planning objectives. If health visitors are able to respond to requirements of a practical nature and to the emotional needs of the people they visit (the linking factors shown to the right in Fig-

Fig. 2.6 A continuum of possible approaches. A range of health visitor method is shown above the line, whilst below is health visitor style.

ure 2.4), then this is likely to be appreciated and to further improve the health visitor–client relationship.

In summary, it is the proceedings during the visit itself which should most influence decisions on how best to help the family. The main information source is the people themselves. Encouragement and explanation by the health visitor can play an important part. There needs to be great sensitivity to non-verbal and other signs which express needs and wishes.

Relationship, role and response are all basic and, in many ways, inseparable parts of health visiting. Running through them all is the need for involvement for the client, and for the health visitor, approachability, responsiveness, well thought-out objectives and a flexible and adaptable style. All these are, of course, necessary throughout all aspects of health visiting, but it is obvious that they are urgently required when making contact at a first visit.

PLANS FOR SUBSEQUENT VISITS

Many of the objectives for further visits result from an evaluation of the meeting and discussion with the client. Short-term objectives form an important part in the planning process of the health visitor cycle. Longer-term objectives, more concerned with the underlying philosophical aims of health visiting (see Table 2.1), may rarely be achieved. They can, however, provide useful guidelines and pointers for planning the more day-to-day aspects of the work.

During the visit, several immediate objectives will probably have been achieved. For example, in a first visit it is likely that there would have been explanations about health visiting and how the health visitor can be contacted. There may have been provision of information about local health and welfare services and/or a response to requests for advice and discussion of various issues of importance to the people being visited.

SHORT-TERM OBJECTIVES

As these immediate objectives are identified and, hopefully, satisfied, other objectives come to light in the course of the conversation. Short-term objectives, those concerning matters which will need attention either between this visit and the next, or at some subsequent visit, can be agreed between the parties. For example, the health visitor may promise to return with information on some special topic or problem. There might be plans for a list of queries to be jotted down by the client as they are thought of, so they can be discussed at the next visit.

Another future goal might be assessment of a baby's developmental progress or of an old person's functional ability. These matters might be noted on the record card and/or in the health visitor's diary.

Client perspective

An assessment of the visit will be being made by *all* the participants involved. Both during and after the visit, the health visitors and people they visit will give some thought to how to approach the next encounter in the light of how this one is perceived. These and other assessments of health visiting are very important. However, evaluation is a very complex matter. It is returned to in Chapter 8. The significant point in this discussion about planning objectives for future visits, is that the clients' evaluation and perspectives are clearly important. These need to be understood for the health visitor's work — be it discussions, explanations, assessment or referral — to be either relevant or useful.

It is not easy to assess people's true feelings, but the better the relationship, as already described above, the greater the likelihood of success.

LONG-TERM OBJECTIVES
Aims or objectives

All planning in health visiting is based on the philosophical aims of the work. These have been expressed in different ways. In the time-scale model for health visiting objectives in Table 2.1, these are classified as long-term objectives. This could include, for example, McClymont's (1983, p. 7) list of aims of health visiting

- promoting overall health and preventing disease
- concern with developing and continuing professional help
- assessment of health and ability to cope
- provision of health education

or the Council for the Education and Training of Health Visitors' (1977) four basic principles:

- search for health needs
- stimulation of the awareness of health needs
- influence of policies affecting health
- facilitation of health-enhancing activities.

The prevention model

The health visitor role model in Table 1.2 may provide a particularly useful basis for thinking about overall and long-term objectives. Its three basic aims are described in Chapter 1:

1. *Preventing occurrence* of conditions or problems
2. *Preventing development* of conditions or problems
3. *Preventing deterioration* of established conditions.

This framework can be used to cover the main practical and everyday aspects of the work and can readily convert into more specific longer-term objectives. For example:

1. *Preventing occurrence* of conditions or problems:
   - improvement of the local environment, e.g. smoke-free zones in public places
   - to provide health education, e.g. on safety, nutrition, immunisation and welfare rights
2. *Preventing development* of conditions or problems:
   - to seek conditions which will benefit from early attention, e.g. hearing and visual defects, functional disability in old people, developmental delay in babies, and family emotional problems

3. *Preventing deterioration* of established conditions:
   - to enable clients to express and talk through their problems
   - to help clients know which agency can offer appropriate help
   - to encourage and facilitate emerging self-help groups.

This model also seems capable of providing a guiding framework for some short-term and immediate objectives specific to a particular family. Under '2. *Preventing development* of conditions or problems', for example, can be derived:

- to explain six month developmental assessment to parents
- to involve parents in noting down developmental attainments
- to answer queries raised by these discussions
- to undertake developmental testing, by appointment.

It can be seen that the concepts in this model are pragmatically based. They can tie in with those in the family health needs model, the format used in the following two and some later chapters. They provide a useful basis for planning future encounters in practical terms which could be easily understood by the families involved, as the example in the paragraph above demonstrates.

To conclude, contact has been made and plans are under way for future meetings. By the next visit there may be more information available from the several sources described in this chapter. For example, at the level of background information new pamphlets and other literature may be acquired and, later, used to help a family understand a difficult problem. Liaison with other workers between the visits may give rise to useful guidance.

It is quite likely that by the next visit the clients' circumstances will have changed in some way and some new objectives will need to be drawn up. Mostly, however, the basic and fundamental theme of the objectives tends to remain fairly constant, especially with regard to the underlying long-term philosophical aims and objectives which run throughout this book.

A repeated theme in this chapter has been the

need for client involvement and understanding. The importance of a good working relationship, comprehension of role and appropriate response to need, have been demonstrated. The health visitor cycle was proposed as a way of thinking about planning processes. It draws attention to and concentrates on the various sources of information on which health visiting decisions are made — including those when first making contact.

USEFUL ADDRESS

Help for Health
Grant Building,
Southampton General Hospital
Southampton SO9 4XY
Tel 0703 779091

REFERENCES

Adams M 1982 Health visitors — a tribute from a mother. Health Visitor 55: 661

Appleby F M 1987a Stress in the first year of health visiting. Health Visitor 60, 2: 39–40

Appleby F M 1987b Professional support and the role of support groups. Health Visitor 60, 3: 77–78

Argyle M 1978 The psychology of interpersonal behaviour, 3rd ed. Penguin Books, London, p. 63

Barber J H, Boothman R, Stanfield J P 1976 A new visual chart for preschool developmental screening. Health Bulletin 34: 80–91

Berne E 1968 Games people play. Penguin Books, London

Burnard P 1985 Learning human skills. A guide for nurses. Heinmann Nursing, London

The Children's Committee 1980 The needs of under fives in the family. The Children's Committee, London

Clark J 1984 Recording health visitor–client interaction in home visits. Health Visitor 57: 5–8

Clulow C F 1982 To have and to hold. Marriage and the first baby and preparing couples for parenthood. Aberdeen University Press, Aberdeen

Council for the Education and Training of Health Visitors 1967 The function of the health visitor. CETHV, London

Council for the Education and Training of Health Visitors 1977 An investigation into the principles of health visiting. CETHV, London, p. 31

Cumberlege Report 1986 Neighbourhood nursing — a focus for care. Report of the Community Nursing Review. Department of Health and Social Security, HMSO, London

Dauncey J 1989 (letter) Oxfordshire's health visiting strategy. Health Visitor 62, 12: 388

Department of Health and Social Security and Child Poverty Action Group 1978 Reaching the consumer in the antenatal and child health services. Report of the conference, April 1978. DHSS CPAG, London

Dingwall R 1977 The social organisation of health visitor training. Croom Helm, London, p. 109

Dingwall R 1982 Community nursing and civil liberty. Journal of Advanced Nursing 7: 337–346

Dingwall R, Eekelaar J, Murray T 1981 Care or control. Decision-making in the care of children thought to have been abused or neglected. A summary of the final report.

Social Science Council Centre for Socio-Legal Studies, Wolfson College, Oxford

Dingwall R, Eekelaar J, Murray T 1983 The protection of children: state intervention and family life. Basil Blackwell, Oxford

Dowling S 1983 Health for a change. The provision of preventive health care in pregnancy and early childhood. Child Poverty Action Group in association with National Extension College

Dunnell K, Dobbs J 1982 Nurses working in the community. HMSO, London

Egan G 1982 The skilled helper, 2nd ed. Brooks/Cole Publishing Company, Monterey, California

Field S, Draper J, Kerr M, Hare M J 1982 A consumer view of the health visiting service. Health Visitor 55: 299–301

Fitton J M 1983 Policy constraints on HV practice (letter). Health Visitor 56: 229

Fitton J M 1984a Health visiting the elderly: nurse managers' views. One. Nursing Times Occasional Paper No 10 80, 16: 59–61

Fitton J M 1984b Health visiting the elderly: nurse managers' views. Two. Nursing Times Occasional Paper No 11 80, 17: 67–69

Gann R 1983 It's your line to the health computer. Health and Social Services Journal XCIII: 782–783

Gann R 1988 Self help is at hand. Nursing Times 84, 10: 61–62

Goodwin S 1982 A partnership to promote self help. Nursing Mirror 155, 24: 63–65

Goodwin S 1988 Whither health visiting? Health Visitor 61, 12: 379–383

Hargie O, Saunders C, Dickson D 1981 Social skills in interpersonal communication. Croom Helm, London

Harris T A 1973 I'm OK — you're OK, Pan Books, London

Health Visitor 1983 Quality visits, not quantity (editorial). Health Visitor 56: 225

Hunt M 1982a New approaches in health visiting 2. Caseload profiles — an alternative to the neighbourhood study. Health Visitor 55, 11: 606–607

Hunt M 1982b New approaches in health visiting 3: Caseload profiles: their implications for evaluating health visiting practice. Health Visitor 55: 662–665

Irving D 1983 How statistics can plot areas of need. Health and Social Services Journal XCIII: 1262–1263

Jack S 1983 Research and vital statistics for the health visitor. In: Owen G (ed) Health visiting, 2nd ed. Bailliere Tindall, London

Jarman B 1983 Identification of under-privileged areas. British Medical Journal 286: 1705–1709

Jarman B 1984 Underprivileged areas: validation and distribution of scores. British Medical Journal 289: 1587–1592

Jarman B 1989 General practice. In: While A (ed) Health in the inner city. Heinemann Medical, Oxford

Luker K A 1982 Evaluating health visiting practice. Royal College of Nursing, London

Luker K A, Chalmers K I 1989 The referral process in health visiting. International Journal of Nursing Studies 26, 2: 173–185 — Strongly recommended reading.

Luker K A, Chalmers K I 1990 Gaining access to clients: the case of health visiting. Journal of Advanced Nursing 15, 1: 74–82 — Strongly recommended.

Lythgoe E J 1983 Teaching health visitor students to communicate. Health Visitor 56: 368–369

McClymont A 1983 Setting standards in health visiting practice. National Board for Nursing, Midwifery and Health Visiting for Scotland, Edinburgh

MacFarlane of Llandaff 1982 Responsibility for the future development of health visiting. Health Visitor 55: 273–277

Mayers M 1973 Home visit — ritual or therapy? Nursing Outlook 21. 5: 328–331

Mayston Committee 1969 Report of the Working Party on Management Structure in the Local Authority Nursing Services Department of Health and Social Security, London (Chairman E L Mayston)

Metcalfe D 1983 Trends in the utilisation of the National Health Service. Journal of the Royal College of General Practitioners 33: 615–617

Munro E A, Manthei R J, Small J J 1983 Counselling. A skills approach. Methuen, Auckland, New Zealand

National Children's Bureau 1981 Parents as partners. Intervention schemes and group work with parents of handicapped children. National Children's Bureau, London

Norman A 1982 When sticky plaster is not enough (letter). Nursing Mirror 154, 22: 22–24

Orr J 1980 Health visiting in focus. Royal College of Nursing, London. p 60–64

Orr J 1982 Health visiting in the U.K. In: Hockey L (ed) Primary care nursing. Churchill Livingstone, Edinburgh

Owen G 1983 The development of health visiting as a profession. In: Owen G (ed) Health visiting, 2nd ed. Bailliere Tindall, London, p 5

Perkins E 1980 Education for childbirth and parenthood. Croom Helm, London

Pittaway C, Sinker C, Wood A 1988 Health visitor workshops: a method of support. In: Drennan V (ed) Health visitors and groups: politics and practice. Heinemann Nursing, Oxford

Raymond E 1983 The skills of health visiting. In: Owen G (ed) Health visiting, 2nd ed. Bailliere Tindall, London

Reynolds M W, Hay H S W 1986 Health visiting by appointment. Health Visitor 59, 8: 252–254

Robertson C A 1984 Old people in the community. One: Health visitors and preventive care. Nursing Times 80, 34: 29–31

Robinson J 1982a The health visitor — an authority on child rearing or an agent of social control? Health Visitor 55: 113–116

Robinson J 1982b An evaluation of health visiting. Council for the Education and Training of Health Visitors, London

Robinson J 1983 The role dilemma of health visiting. Health Visitor 56: 22–24

Robinson K 1983 Talking with clients. In: Clark J, Henderson J (eds) Community health. Churchill Livingstone, Edinburgh

Rowe J 1988 Health visitors talking. In: Drennan V (ed) Health visitors and groups: politics and practice. Heinemann Nursing, Oxford

Rcn Health Visitors Advisory Group 1983 Thinking about health visiting. Royal College of Nursing, London, p 46

Schofield J 1982 Health visiting — quality not quantity (letter). Nursing Mirror 155, 25: 37

Schofield J 1983 Visiting can be stressful too. Nursing Mirror 157, 13: 20–21

Scottish Health Education Group 1989 Sharing counselling skills. A guide to running courses for nurses, midwives and health visitors. Scottish Health Education Group, Edinburgh

Stanton A 1982 The listening, liaising, counselling health visitor. Nursing Mirror 155, 22: 57–59

Swaffield L 1990 Built in support. Nursing Times 86, 29: 19 — Strongly recommended

Thompson J 1983 Health visiting: the quality does count (letter) Nursing Mirror 156, 7: 18

Tschudin V 1982 Counselling skills for nurses. Bailliere Tindall, London

Vizard E 1983 Twenty months of Fridays — a support group for health visitors. Health Visitor 56: 255–256

Warner U 1984 Asking the right questions. Nursing Times Community Outlook 80, 24: 214–216

Warnock Report 1978 Report of the Committee of Enquiry into Education of Handicapped Children and Young People. Cmnd 7212, HMSO, London

FURTHER READING

Guldager E 1988 Do health visitors improve children's health? Nursing Times 84, 18: 58

Chapter 3 describes the value of antenatal health visiting and the importance of liaison. It looks at some of the environmental and physical health factors and mental/emotional and social aspects of family health which might receive attention during an antenatal visit.

3

Antenatal visiting

POLICIES AND PRIORITIES

Increasingly health visitors are encouraged to make contact during the antenatal period. These visits have been shown to be a very sound investment, particularly for the post-natal phase (Field et al, 1984), as they provide the opportunity to establish a good working relationship and as part of this, to explain about health visiting and, of course, to offer health education.

The relationship

In a small, in-depth study, an association was found between the extent of the contact with the health visitor in the antenatal period and the degree of support the women felt they had once the baby was born (Field et al, 1982a, 1982b). The researchers pointed out that a brief encounter or two is not enough to establish a good relationship. They found many of the mothers they interviewed had not met their health visitor before the birth of the baby. Two weeks into motherhood, a very vulnerable and emotional time in the adjustment to this new role, these mothers had to face setting up a new relationship with a total stranger.

Competing pressures

However, the ability to visit antenatally is limited for many health visitors by competing caseload priorities and pressures. For example, only 24 of the 40 interviewed in the Cambridgeshire study (Field et al, 1984) undertook antenatal visiting routinely.

14 health visitors did visit, but felt unable to provide this service for everyone.

One health visitor, on the other hand, made a habit of calling three times in pregnancy. It has been suggested that health visitors might aim for this level of antenatal visiting (Stanton, 1982). If, as it seems, the health visitors in Cambridgeshire find this difficult to put into action, then it is hardly surprising that Jane Schofield (1982), working in an inner city area, would find it quite out of the question!

Antenatal visits to first-time parents were seen as important by the authors of 'Health Visiting in the Eighties' (Health Visitor, 1981). They assigned this aspect of our work higher priority than the routine visiting of all children to school age. As most women work during their first pregnancy, visits during the earlier part may need to be in the evening, in order to fit in with patterns of work.

Uneven take-up

A review of research into antenatal services intended to prepare people for parenthood, showed them to be inadequate (Pugh, 1980, pp. 24–28). The increasing popularity of the National Childbirth Trust and the large number of books on parenting that are now available, give a measure of public demand for, and recognition of, the importance of learning in this phase of life. However, these facilities, both books and antenatal classes, tend to be taken up by the middle classes, people who are likely to face fewer problems overall. Those who may be missing out, such as the very young, the unsupported and couples on low incomes, have a greater need for special initiatives by midwives, health visitors and volunteers.

SPECIAL SCHEMES

Pugh (1980, p. 80) called for professional workers in the field to become more involved on two fronts: firstly, to provide support and encouragement to enable self-help groups to establish themselves fully and to tell parents about them; secondly, it is suggested help should be provided for particu-

larly deprived families who would not normally join in self-help groups.

Collaboration with parents

One such scheme is currently being undertaken and the experiment assiduously monitored and assessed (Child Development Project, 1984, pp. 17–18). It starts with monthly antenatal visiting of primiparae in disadvantaged areas by 'first-parent visitors' and continues for six months after the birth. These health visitors provide a specially designed supportive and collaborative service for which they are given special training.

The aim is to draw out and to develop the dormant potential in parents, rather than to make them dependent on the advice of the health visitor. In the second stage of the project these visitors have been assigned solely to this particular work. The aim is to ensure enough time for preventive and developmental work by removing them from the hurly-burly of responding to urgent calls, pressing clinics and other duties.

Initially six Health Authorities took part. In the event, the first phase has been a considerable success (Barker & Anderson, 1988). The project has shown significant achievements, particularly in raising both the confidence levels of the young parents and their ability to provide a good environment for their children (see also Ch. 5, p. 81).

Creativity and imagination

Sue Dowling (1983) has reported on a very wide range of recent initiatives. She has found that where services are specially modified to have regard for people's particular way of life, contact can be made remarkably easily with most families, even the most socially and economically deprived. Dowling points out that 'creativity' is the basic ingredient needed. She adds, however, that, although there are plenty of imaginative workers in health care, apparently 'in the NHS there is some reluctance to recognise, promote and utilise this creativity for change' (p. 167).

Dr Dowling feels that the current emphasis on scientific management, concern with the evaluation and measurement of current practice, the cuts in budgets and the restructuring of the NHS, all tend to lead to a resistance to new ideas. To the managers feeling vulnerable, the old ways are seen as 'safer'. She says that more ideas and experiences of workers in the lower echelons of the NHS hierarchy need to reach their managers and to be included in health care planning. We return to these issues in Chapter 14. In her book, Dr Dowling describes some health visitors' new initiatives in the community. More are needed.

Even though the importance of preparation is now well recognised (Maternity Services Advisory Committee, 1982; House of Commons Social Services Committee, 1980), health visitors can only take part in antenatal services if they are notified of the pregnancies in their area. Obviously, the earlier these notifications can be received, the better is the opportunity to provide for the needs of the families. Much depends on health authority policy and work practices enabling this contact to be made.

LIAISON

Schemes for informing health visitors about pregnancies vary significantly from place to place. In some cases, the GP or the practice manager will leave messages, or use a notebook to list his pregnant patients. Some hospitals may use a computerised system, a handwritten scheme or send messages through the liaison health visitor. Sometimes local midwives provide the information.

Working together

The health visitor's role during the antenatal period is not always fully understood, interprofessionally, and occasionally rivalries can intervene (Skinner, 1982; Lythgoe, 1982). In order to improve health visitor–midwifery working relationships, the Royal College of Midwives (RCM) and the Health Visitors Association (HVA) produced a joint statement in June, 1982. The document

which provided 'a shared vision of ideal arrangements for antenatal preparation', described succinctly the monitoring, supportive and educative responsibilities of the midwife throughout the pregnancy, birth and post-partum period.

The educative role of the health visitor was outlined in the statement, as was the dual responsibility for antenatal education of both professions. Perhaps both should give extra priority to women attending hospital-based, crowded antenatal clinics, as Field et al (1982a) said that in their study these women found it more difficult to discuss their problems than those cared for by domiciliary midwives.

The RCM and HVA suggested that particular attention be given to antenatal education at home for anyone unlikely to attend antenatal classes and that health visitors make extra visits to women whom they would not be meeting at antenatal classes. Sadly, the 'ideal', as set out in the joint statement, rarely balances with current caseloads.

Others' views

Many people may be involved with a woman in her antenatal preparations. For example,

- general practitioner
- community midwife
- hospital consultant
- junior doctors
- hospital midwives
- friends and family
- National Childbirth Trust counsellor

and, perhaps, other organisations such as Foresight and La Leche League.

It can be very helpful if health visitors are able to meet the professionals and volunteers likely to be involved in the care of several of their families. There can then be discussions about the sort of advice commonly given, for example on:

- breastfeeding
- smoking
- alcohol
- nutrition
- impact on family relationships

and the sort of literature these people tend to

recommend to their patients/clients. Being aware of other advisers' views and working patterns helps to cut down on confusion due to conflicting advice and some repetitiveness of professional questioning.

The best advice

Inevitably, of course, young couples have to face the dilemma of conflicting opinion. Family, friends, voluntary associations, a multitude of books and various professionals each give the advice they feel to be the best. In matters of health, ways of living and child-rearing, cultural variations abound and there is no absolute and indisputable truth. Also, medical views, for example on nutrition or where babies should be born, are vulnerable to change in the light of research findings and further change when these are refined.

Clulow (1982) remarks that health visitors need to be able to live with uncertainty and to cope with it, both in themselves and in the families they visit. An important part of health visiting is to encourage young couples to have the confidence to choose, out of all the views available, those which they themselves feel the most logical and the best suited to their particular circumstances. Books like *Your Body, Your Baby, Your Life* (Philips, 1983) encourage parents to take an active part in their antenatal care and to make their own choices.

THE VISIT

FAMILY HEALTH NEEDS FRAMEWORK

At an antenatal visit, there are, of course, a very wide range of matters a mother or a couple may wish to discuss with their health visitor. In this chapter and the next, the family health needs framework, the second of the three outlined in the introductory chapter, is used to categorise the topics discussed here.

This model is useful in the context of a specific visit, because it concentrates on the particular requirements of a family, many of which may be considered, and some actually discussed, at such a visit. These matters are categorised in these chapters, occasionally rather arbitrarily, under 'environmental', 'physical', 'mental/emotional' and 'social' factors. Box 3.1 lists some of these issues and is expanded in the subsequent text.

It is not proposed to attempt to cover every possible item which might be relevant at antenatal visits. Equally, as in the whole of this book, the range of topics mentioned is not intended to provide an ideal model of what should be discussed. Time at a visit is limited and, anyway, each family will voice a variety of different issues and needs.

Use of this model is demonstrated in two exam-

Box 3.1   Aspects of family health that might need consideration antenatally

General environment	Physical health	Mental/emotional health	Social aspects of health
The community Social mix Infrastructure Employment	*Mother* .... Antenatal checks and education liaison Dental care	*Parental knowledge* Seek information Library: liaison	*Immediate family* Relationships: readjustment
The home Type Surroundings	*... and baby* Life-style influences Nutrition Smoking	*Expectations* Difficult to visualise	*Wider family, and friends* Grandmother Others
Standard of living Rights and benefits		*Adjustment* Mostly for mother Outlook good?	*Community agencies* Antenatal groups and contacts
Working mother	*Discussions about* (Immunisation and infant surveillance scheme)	*Discussion points* Breastfeeding Sex in pregnancy Depression	

ples of a health visitor making an antenatal visit. Many of the issues raised in the examples are discussed in the rest of this section.

EXAMPLES OF ANTENATAL VISITS

The first is to a single parent and the second to a young couple living in the wife's parents' home. Their physical and mental health and some environmental and social aspects of health considered at the visit are described. They are tabulated under these four aspects of family health need in Boxes 3.2 and 3.3. Some readers may prefer to go straight on to the discussions about family health requirements in the rest of the chapter and then return to these examples.

EXAMPLE ONE: NANCY MANNERS

A 20-year-old student nurse, Miss Nancy Manners, had chosen shared hospital and GP antenatal care. The routine in this surgery was for the community midwife to arrange an appointment for Mrs Hannah Van der Haastrecht (HV) to visit the home at around the 28th week. Miss Manners lived alone, self-catering, in rented rooms in an Edwardian terrace house close to the Royal Overhampton Hospital where she was in training. The first thing mentioned after the normal introductory remarks was how grateful she was that her landlady was prepared to break her own rules in order to let her stay on until a council flat became vacant — promised within a year.

Apparently the *Pregnancy Book* (Health Education Council, 1984) was found especially helpful with regard to its overview of maternity rights and benefits. It seems the hospital personnel department had been very supportive and helpful. Miss Manners had heard there was a hospital crèche. The school of nursing had explained with which of the later sets of student nurses she was now likely to qualify. She had been advised to 'eat properly' and to 'keep off baccy and booze'!

When telling people of her intention to breastfeed as long as she could, Miss Manners found she was getting remarkably divergent and confused advice. The health visitor told her that there were in fact quite a number of good ways of setting about it. It was really a question of finding out all one could and then deciding which scheme seemed preferable. The aim then, in health visiting, was to help people achieve their chosen goals. Maire Messenger's (1982) book (probably available from the hospital library) and Garner's (1980) *How to Survive as a Working Mother* were recommended.

Hoping to learn something of Miss Manners' attitudes towards child rearing and her own mother, HV asked 'Now you're to be a mother, how will you bring your baby up? Will it be the same way as your mother did you?' The

Box 3.2 Example one: Nancy Manners

General environment	Physical health	Mental/emotional health	Social aspects of health
Local community Dominated by hospital and a college	*Mother . . .* Antenatal checks regular	*Parental knowledge* Keen to learn	*Immediate family* Lives alone
The home Bedsitter: access to bathroom	*. . . and baby* Life-style: ● Eats at work ● Non-smoker ● Avoiding alcohol	*Expectations* Non-idealistic Pragmatic	*Wider family, friends* G'mother: mainly telephone contact Landlady supportive
Standard of living Employed, low income Claiming benefits		*Adjustment* Early days good relationship with own mother	*Community agencies* Helpful at work
		Discussed: Breastfeeding, books recommended	*Plans* to tell about useful agencies
		Plans to follow up	

response was: 'I shall try to. She may not be perfect, but she did her best.' And with a twinkle, 'I don't suppose I shall be perfect either!' In response to a further question asking in what way she would particularly want to be the same, HV was told that her mother had always been moderately firm but had listened to reason and had tried to be just. She added 'You can't ask for more.' Her mother had accepted her pregnancy and had applauded her spirit of independence. She had promised her support in the normal granny role, and was keeping in telephone contact. This all augured well.

It seemed to HV that some of the problems that so frequently beset single parents of employment and housing were not, in the short term, to be a problem to this pleasant, well-organised young woman. She would, however, be on a marginal income and might well have problems over child care and of loneliness.

The health visitor decided to offer to call again in a month. An appointment was made. She planned to discuss organisations such as the National Council for One Parent Families and Gingerbread, and to back up the midwife's invitation to the antenatal classes. The main aim was to provide potential for social links with other parents, if they were desired.

They parted on first name terms. By the following antenatal visit Nancy had realised that she could not possibly afford full-time crèche fees. Her mother had offered to have the baby for the necessary eight months so she could complete her training. After that she planned to cease work until child care arrangements

became possible. The birth visit is described in the next chapter.

EXAMPLE TWO: THE KIRKS

Notification of pregnancies from the large maternity hospital where 21-year-old Mrs Kirk was attending for antenatal care tends to come to the health visitors very late. Ms Heather Vaughan (HV) called at the home one evening when Mary Kirk was some eight months pregnant. A mistake in the information she had been given had caused her to deliver the note proposing her visit to the house next door. She had been redirected and was therefore unannounced. HV had generally found a poorer introduction than one that was pre-arranged.

Mr and Mrs Kirk were living with Mrs Kirk's parents, the Grahams. After the introductory conversations, Mrs Graham suggested the young couple take HV into the 'front room' in order to have privacy for their discussions. 'It's their baby' she said. She seemed rather tense and was very apologetic because there was no fire alight in the room. The health visitor apologised again that her visit had been unexpected and explained her normal appointment system.

Fire or no, the conversation flowed very warmly. The young couple were obviously looking forward to having their child. Mr Kirk, a packer at a local factory, said they were hoping to buy a small home within about six months. The Grahams had been trying to help them save for a deposit. There were some difficulties with two families living in so small a house, but they

---

Box 3.3 Example two: the Kirks

General environment	Physical health	Mental/emotional health	Social aspects of health
The community Estate, small houses Poor infrastructure — No public halls Industrial area	*Mother* . . . . Antenatal checks regular attender . . . *and baby* Lifestyle: Not discussed	*Parental knowledge* Intend to consult: ● G'mother ● clinic ● library *Expectations* Open-minded *Adjustment* Seems positive	*Immediate family* Warm relationship between parents Father wishes to help with baby *Wider family, friends* Grandparents' support Friends locally *Community agencies* Invitation to mothers' 'Get Together Group'
The home Shared with grandparents *Living standard* Low wages Saving for own home			

felt the grandparents would encourage them to bring up their baby in their own way.

Mrs Kirk said she would be asking her mother's advice if she needed it: she trusted her mother's opinion. She hoped also to attend the mobile child health clinic. A group for first-time mothers in the estate (with especial emphasis on trying to draw in mothers receiving hospital antenatal care only) was newly set up and HV invited Mrs Kirk to come to it, both before and after the birth. The health visitor thought how much better an earlier notification would have been.

Mrs Kirk had heard about the mothers' group from one of her school friends who was already attending and she said that meeting the health visitor gave her the courage to come. The group, meeting above the surgery premises, provided the mothers with somewhere to meet regularly and make themselves a cup of tea. Ms Vaughan supplied health education films, tape-slide presentations and other material on topics chosen by the group. It was becoming quite a debating chamber!

When asked whether there was anything they wanted to ask about, the couple said they were concerned as to whether sexual intercourse would be bad for the baby or the pregnancy in any way. They had been abstaining the few weeks previously 'in case'. At the clinic everyone was so busy, there was no one Mrs Kirk dared ask. The matter was discussed. Because the couple agreed that it might be a good idea to follow up the conversation with some relevant reading, HV gave them a photostat of the Savage and Reader (1984) list of books. Several of the books were generally available in their local library. The baby care section there was recommended. The couple had not been in the habit of getting books out of the library, but thought it a good idea to look. Ms Vaughan was glad they had felt able to raise such a sensitive subject. She left, calling her thanks and goodbye to the Grahams, and expecting to see Mary Kirk again at the mothers' group and subsequently at the birth visit.

This young mother became a lively and regular attender at the group meetings. Eighteen months later a full time hospital liaison health visitor was employed by the Health Authority, enabling earlier and more rationally directed antenatal health visiting.

GENERAL ENVIRONMENT

The community

On their way to a home, health visitors naturally make a mental note of the environment and general social circumstances in which the family lives. This helps their general understanding of the sort of problems, or otherwise, faced by the people they visit. Factors such as those in Figure 3.1, considered together, can give an impression of a probable quality and way of life available to the family.

The home

Approaching the dwelling itself, the architectural design:

- new or old
- multistorey or single dwelling
- access by lift or steps
- clothes drying facilities
- safe play areas
- availability of own garden

adds to this impression. For many there is no problem. However, a Child Development Project (1984, p. 9) photograph showing a mother struggling with steps in a modern housing complex, gives a feel for the sort of problems some families face. It is pointed out that there are large numbers of parents living in distinctly disadvantaged circumstances, even in this affluent country.

Problems

People whose basic pre-occupation and concern is a roof over their heads or the availability of accessible employment, may need guidance and support over these basic matters before they can turn their thoughts more fully towards preparation for the baby. Also, there is mounting evidence of the effect of unemployment on family health (McLellan, 1985; Maternity Alliance, 1985).

All too often unemployment and poor housing seem insurmountable problems. Portwood and Steventon (1984) provided some practical suggestions on how health visitors can help unemployed people. Frequently it is they who call before a

Quality of infrastructure?
- public halls
- health clinics
- libraries
- shopping facilities
- community organisations
- maternity facilities
- pre-school care
- housing
- public transport

Type of community?
- urban
- suburban
- rural

Social mix of community?
- static/mobile
- high/low income
- cultural variations

Employment?
- job prospects
- atmospheric pollution
- special features

Fig. 3.1 Community factors.

crisis develops. This provides an advantage. The authors said that help can be given by disseminating information. Pamphlets and leaflets that explain in simple, straightforward terms, for example how to claim benefits, hunt for a job and keep mentally active and optimistic, would be of particular value. It was suggested that a local college might be encouraged to produce a booklet that lists agencies of particular help to the unemployed. A sample of the sort of thing that can be produced is available and can be sent for through Dr Portwood. Nowadays an even more proactive approach is becoming more common. Michael Proctor (1990) described a scheme in which a health promotion display was taken out to the unemployed — at a local benefits office. Vari Drennan (1988)

has outlined some of the ways these new approaches can be set up.

Some health visitors found that joining an organisation such as their local Radical Health Visitors group meant they met a supportive circle of people concerned with these basic problems and, in addition, found a good source of creative ideas and encouragement as well as useful addresses for people with problems. (Spray, 1988). Now the special interest groups of the Health Visitors' Association (see useful addresses) and locally-based support groups tend to fill this sort of role.

Inner city health visiting is considered in Chapter 13 and we return to unemployment towards the end of Chapter 15.

Rights and benefits

Many people will find very helpful the clearly set out and simply stated 'what', 'who', 'when' and 'how' on grants, allowances and other rights and entitlements which can be found in the Health Education Council's (1984, pp. 35–39) *Pregnancy Book*. It is a book which is widely available and covers many aspects of pregnancy and early child care. People who wish to know more than this book outlines, may find that specific DSS leaflets (Department of Social Security, 1990), the trade unionists' *State Benefits* (Labour Research Department, 1984), *Maternity Rights at Work* (Coussins et al, 1987) or *Maternity Rights for Working Women* (Coussins, 1980) give some guidance. Maternity Alliance have some useful leaflets and an informative book (Evans & Durward, 1984). The Child Poverty Action Group's annually updated benefits handbooks (Chapman et al, 1990; Kennedy et al, 1990), are much used by health visitors.

Working mothers

Coussins provides a table of entitlements under the Employment Protection Act, 1975, and explains in clear and reassuring terms how to make a complaint to a tribunal, should that be necessary.

Some mothers will want just to talk about the fact that they are choosing to continue in employment after their maternity leave. Leslie Garner (1980) has written giving useful tips, telling of helpful organisations and, perhaps most important of all, putting that niggling sense of guilt that some feel in perspective. On these occasions, the listening role of the health visitor can be particularly useful in helping people think through their feelings, their situation and intentions, and come to their own conclusions.

Confidentiality

Many people talk matters over with their family, neighbours or friends. Others feel they cannot, fearing gossip or interference in their affairs, and, when they need to talk about such things, prefer to discuss these sensitive matters with an objective listener who has a professional obligation to respect their confidence.

PHYSICAL ASPECTS OF HEALTH

Mother . . . . .

Antenatal check-ups

Health visitors may, in some cases, find it necessary to encourage mothers to attend for antenatal care. However, for the most part, health visitors will only come to hear about those who are already attending.

Health visitors who have the opportunity to observe at local antenatal clinics and get to know current local practice, will, when on their visits to people's homes, be more able to work in cooperation with these services. Experience in these clinics could provide useful liaison links and also valuable knowledge for some health visitors, as it is no longer compulsory for a health visitor to have a midwifery qualification.

The mothers may ask advice about a very wide range of issues, though most of the mothers' questions specific to antenatal supervision and the birth of the baby are likely to be asked of their midwives or doctors undertaking this care.

Dental care

One matter which health visitors might raise is that of dental care. Dental treatment is available free for all pregnant women and for the first year of motherhood. Draper et al (1983) found many of their interviewees were visiting their dentists. However, only one of them was aware of the increased possibility of gingivitis and the need for good oral hygiene in pregnancy. Besford (1984) explains about the changes that take place. Some of the Cambridgeshire mothers, having never visited a dentist before, said they were intending to take advantage of the free service.

..... and baby

Life-style influences

Nutrition. There are high levels of professional agreement now on the importance of nutrition in the pre-conceptual period and in early pregnancy (Wynn & Wynn, 1979, 1981; Foresight, 1980; Dening, 1983; Margiotta, 1984). However, by the time notification comes through to the health visitor, the pregnancy is generally well established and it is rather too late for there to be much influence on the growing baby. Even so, if expectant parents seek information about what they should eat, a positive and active response could be a sound investment. This is a longterm matter. There is an obvious need for parents with a new baby to be as well nourished as possible, especially if the mother is breastfeeding. Then later comes the stage of preparing for the possibility of another pregnancy.

What advice should be given? Many hospitals supply diet sheets which parents may wish to discuss. The papers recommended by Pat Margiotta, Jervis's (1983) diet plan and the Community Outlook fact sheet (Pickard, 1983) provide good basic advice on diet, although intended mainly for pre-conceptual care. Discussions about weight gain (Pipe, 1983) and coffee drinking (Shai Linn et al, 1982) can now be guided by some scientifically-based evidence. It is likely that there will be further research into the effects of nutrition (Holt, 1982; Morgan, 1980) and it will be interesting to read about the newer theories as they emerge.

It is not always easy to afford a good diet. Some of those recommended by many hospitals could cost up to a third or a half of some mothers' incomes (Durward, 1984). Lyn Durward gives examples of the sort of diets actually eaten by mothers in the lower socio-economic groups. There is much room for improvement. She provides tables which show the stark differential between the social classes in rates of perinatal death, low birthweight and a specific malformation. For example, in 1981 the perinatal death rate for (legitimate) births was 8.2 for social class I and 15.5 for social class V; birth weight under 2.5 kg was between 5 and 6 per hundred births for social classes I to III, compared with 8.4 for social class V. A malformation ratio calculated for 1977–1979,

showed the ratio for anencephalus and/or spina bifida to be four times higher for social class V than for social class I (pp. 3–4).

In general terms, nutritional status tends to improve with income. To what extent are health visitors able to help the poorly nourished? Perhaps the Child Development Project (1984, pp. 41–46, 66) will show one of the ways it could be done: a facilitative approach, helping people gain an insight into nutritional alternatives.

Smoking, alcohol and drugs. Tobacco, alcohol and several drugs can cross the placenta by simple diffusion and, on occasions, harm the fetus. Doctors frequently give advice and, through prescription, have control over the use of much unsafe medication (Drury, 1982). It is another matter with social drugs: advice can be given, but, inevitably, it is a personal decision as to whether or not to give them up prior to or during pregnancy.

It seems there is a great deal of variation in the amount that mothers know about harmful effects of drugs, smoking, alcohol and other matters pertaining to their health. Some appear to receive no information, others only cursory advice (Moore, 1984; Draper et al, 1983). The GP is the first point of contact in pregnancy — sometimes as early as six weeks. Health visitors might suggest that the GPs have available and recommend some of the Health Education Council's (1984, p. 78) free leaflets. Their *Pregnancy Book* (Health Education Council, 1984, pp. 15–16, 40) provides an excellent base from which to stimulate discussion about these, as well as many other, matters in pregnancy. For topics on which suitable pamphlets are not available from any of the normal sources, a local hand-out might be prepared, for example on alcohol if it is felt that people are likely to find it useful.

In order that people have adequate information early enough, it seems likely that health visitors will need to become increasingly more involved in pre-conceptual counselling — with GPs playing an active part or, perhaps for many, a referral role. The school classroom is, of course, the best place to start his teaching.

Reviews of research findings (Sidle, 1983; Edwards, 1983; Hawkins, 1983; Dowdell, 1981) can help keep health visitors abreast of recent thinking. Literature such as the Health Education Council's 'stop smoking packs' for health visitors (Nursing Times, 1983), and Plant's (1983) clearly stated and brief overview of pregnancy and alcohol, may prove useful for helping people understand the issues involved.

The problem is that it is not easy to give up these addictive drugs. A large proportion of women continue to smoke, even though they know it might have harmful effects, although a few may cut down significantly (Moore, 1984; Black, 1984; Draper et al, 1983). In America, there was a phase when coffee was also thought to be potentially harmful to the fetus. It is now disproved, but it seems it was much easier to give up coffee drinking when it was deemed ill advised, than it was to stop smoking (Shai Linn et al, 1982). For this reason, care has to be taken not to act like an over-zealous missionary and cause feelings of guilt which, instead of leading to the intended positive action, could result in anxiety and perhaps resentment.

It has been suggested that counselling at home may produce the best results (King & Eiser, 1981). There are obvious advantages to home-based work. The subject of alcohol is returned to in Chapter 4, under 'medication and lactation'.

Discussions about infant health schemes

Frequently, health visitors on an antenatal visit bring the conversation round to matters such as child immunisation or their local infant surveillance scheme. There is an advantage in being able to introduce these notions prior to, and away from, the emotional confusions and the practical preoccupations involved in having a new baby. This is particularly so with a first baby as there are so many new things to think about. Another advantage is that it provides parents with the opportunity to formulate any questions they might like to raise well in advance of any decision they might need to make, over aspects of immunisation for their baby, or to enquire about postnatal services.

As many health visitors are still unable to provide a full antenatal visiting service, discussion

of these matters has been deferred to Chapters 4 and 5.

MENTAL/EMOTIONAL HEALTH

Parental knowledge

Since the advent of smaller families, relatively fewer people expecting their first baby have had much practical experience in child care since their own childhood. Generally, pregnancy is a time when there is a great desire to learn about parentcraft and health. Some seek word-of-mouth information, whilst others prefer to read. If health visitors call into the local library, they can find out what books are readily available. After liaison with the local midwives, they can also discuss with the librarians which books are the most likely to be recommended.

Sometimes at antenatal classes books such as *Family Feelings* (Rayner, 1977) or *New Baby Growing Up* (Scowen, 1981) might be lent to each member of the group for a week or so. Opinions and questions arising out of this reading can then form the basis of a subsequent meeting. However, certain issues can be felt to be too personal, or the parents are too self-conscious, to mention them within the group. At a home visit, they may feel far freer to raise sensitive and delicate matters. Whether they do or not is likely, at least partly, to depend upon their having a good relationship with the health visitor.

Expectations and adjustment

It is very difficult for people to visualise in advance, and therefore to be prepared for, what it feels like to be a parent. The baby's stages and phases may seem, when it comes to it, to present insuperable difficulties. Parenthood can turn out to be very different from that which was anticipated. It is at this stage that someone known and trusted enough to be turned to, can provide part of an important 'safety net' in child care services.

In classes and in home visiting schemes, valuable attempts are made to give parents a chance to think about the emotional implications of parenthood in realistic, non-glamourised and non-idealistic terms. However, there are no glib and simple solutions to this aspect of health education.

Clulow (1982) studied the effect of the first baby upon marriage relationships. Enormous adjustments are needed — especially by the mother. He invited expectant parents to attend discussion groups to see if foreknowledge of the psychological factors associated with having a first baby would reduce the risk of painful problems. In the event, it seems that it is not until problems arise that people can realise to what extent they have been seeing matters in an idealised light. Descriptions by Ann Oakley (1982) and Liz Walton (1983) show just how surprised and emotionally shaken some women can be by the reality of motherhood. Jayne Price (1988) provides yet another perspective.

The National Childbirth Trust is one of the organisations which tries to provide a service which will help in these adjustment processes. They give antenatal classes and produce some excellent leaflets and a helpful book: *Pregnancy and Parenthood* (Loader, 1980).

Looking ahead. People vary in the extent to which they are able to make the necessary adjustment. Factors such as

- social circumstances
- family circumstances
- baby's behaviour
- levels of confidence
- mother's personality
- her own childhood experiences
- levels of support from
    - partner
    - family
    - friends
    - professionals

can all have an influence. Health visitors sensitive to these factors may, to some extent, be able to make a reasonable guess at which parents are more likely to be in need of extra support once the baby arrives. Ann Gath (1977) suggested a series of questions which she felt to be friendly rather than personal. These questions were intended to help discover the mothers most at risk of emotional problems. They asked:

- how much her partner is able to be with her at this time
- about her relationship with her mother
- what sort of occupation the mother uses for fun and relaxation.

There is, of course a need to be sensitive to how much people wish to be questioned, however well intentioned the questioning may be.

Pugh (1980, p. 75) suggests there should be plans to concentrate help upon vulnerable groups such as

- teenagers
- unemployed young people
- those brought up in care
- late attenders at antenatal clinics
- older middle class women

who may have difficulty in adjusting to parenthood. Care has to be taken that people selected in this way should not be considered 'people with problems'. Through their attitudes some professionals can assign such people a lowered status. The problem, if there is one, is in shared misunderstandings. Health visitors, for example, tend to be middle class and, like everyone else, have a limited knowledge of how other people's lives are led. Also they may use jargon terms and have speech mannerisms strange to many of the people they visit (Pugh, 1980, p. 76). These sorts of limitations to good two-way communication and understanding need to be taken into consideration throughout the practice of health visiting.

Discussion points pertaining to emotional well-being

Some of the sensitive issues affecting emotional health which expectant parents may seek to discuss could be sexual activity during pregnancy, postnatal depression and emotional aspects of breastfeeding.

Coitus in pregnancy. It has been suggested that a large proportion of pregnant women would like advice on sexual activity during pregnancy. Savage and Reader (1984) point out that abstention was commonly advised for about two thirds of pregnancy a few decades ago. Extensive research has now shown there is no association between intercourse during pregnancy and adverse outcome of pregnancy (Klebanoff et al, 1984). The advice given now can be far more reassuring. There are, of course, exceptions. For example, abstinence is advised where there has been some bleeding during this pregnancy and may be suggested in the case of a threatened miscarriage or premature labour.

About half the 218 women interviewed by Savage and Reader (1984) received no advice on the subject. Some 40% read books to get the appropriate information. Savage and Reader said that sex in pregnancy should be discussed routinely. They have listed in their article books on the subject and the relevant page numbers, both for professional education and for recommending to pregnant women.

Postnatal depression. It seems that various researchers have associated a multitude of different factors with that of postnatal depression: high anxiety levels, marital tension, earlier doubts about the pregnancy, for example, and problems in relationships with the mother's parents (Ball, 1982). It is a condition which can manifest itself in a variety of ways. Parents who wish to know how they might be able to recognise it and to find out how to help, should it occur in their own family or amongst their friends, may find the National Childbirth Trust's booklet (Waumsley, 1983) a very good starting point. Several mothers' personal experiences are described in it and guidance is given on further reading and agencies that might prove helpful. Postnatal depression is returned to in Chapter 5 (pp. 89 *and* 98).

Breastfeeding. Three-quarters of the 500 first time mothers interviewed by Hally et al (1984) had already made up their minds about which way they would feed their babies and mostly fed them the way intended.

There are many factors which influence the way people decide whether or not to breastfeed. Solberg (1984) reviewed some of them. Historically, there have been differences between the social classes, and there is a correlation between the experiences of friends and family, for example growing up in an environment where it is commonplace, and breastfeeding.

A positive attitude by the partner means the mother is more likely to breastfeed. Apparently, in a study quoted by Solberg, half the mothers who gave up did so due to objections by the father. It seems that the role of the breast in a couple's sexual activities can be influential. For some people, the sexual and the nurturant roles are felt to be incompatible.

Solberg also says that there is conflicting evidence on the benefits or otherwise of physical preparation of the breasts, but that it can be psychologically beneficial if it makes the mother *feel* better prepared.

It seems that the quality of information given to the couple is the key to successful breastfeeding and that the early experiences in breastfeeding are very influential (Hally et al, 1984). *The Breastfeeding Book* (Messenger, 1982) gives detailed and logically presented information and is likely to be popular.

SOCIAL ASPECTS OF HEALTH

Social support systems are of great importance to the young family — those within the immediate family, the broader family network and close friends, and also certain community agencies. They all play some part in ameliorating the loneliness and the strains and tensions which frequently arise from the care of babies and children. Forethought and action in the antenatal period may pave the way for help to be available later, should it be needed. For example, many new mothers can easily become exhausted. Tiredness is the most common symptom in postnatal depression (Hennessy, 1986), and it is worth thinking ahead and planning for its alleviation.

The immediate family

Many mothers give up work for their first baby and therefore become that much more dependent upon their partner economically, for social contact and as 'sharer of problems'. The father, therefore, becomes a key figure.

If antenatal visiting takes place in the evenings, it is more probable that both parents will be met.

There is then an opportunity to learn not only the mother's view-point and wishes, but her partner's too. An appointment system, where this exists, enables visits to be arranged when both parents are likely to be free.

There is now increasing awareness of the importance of a father's active involvement in care of his children. Verny and Kelly (1982) described how this can begin even before the birth. The father's voice can be heard by the baby, in utero, and recognised after birth. Bonding and an enhanced relationship can begin this soon, it is suggested, by the father talking to his unborn child and using short soothing words.

To encourage involvement, some mothers may give their partner *The Baby Book for Dads* (Little & Ralston, 1980) or get it from the library. It is well written and shows, in a constructive and humorous way, the important social and emotional role of the father. The advice includes some inaccuracies, but parents have plenty of other opportunities to find more up-to-date advice. Antenatally, for example, there may be classes in the locality where fathers are made welcome.

Wider family, friends and neighbours

Most new mothers enjoy and feel the need for social contact outside their immediate nuclear family. A supportive grandparental link can be much appreciated and very helpful. Friends and neighbours may be able to help fill the gap created by the loss of long-standing social networks associated with going out to work. Mothers who have special circumstances such as a poor marriage, frequent house moving or no support from their own mother, may feel a particular need.

Postnatal groups, where friendships become established antenatally, can be invaluable. Clulow (1982) felt that the 'safety net' factor, the availability of sympathetic support, where people could talk through their problems, was a very important aspect of these groups.

Karin Christiani (Nursing Times, 1982) described Swedish antenatal groups where parents came from the same area and stayed together after the birth of their babies. Similarly, the National Childbirth Trust groups which meet in people's homes can lead on to very valuable friendships and mutual support. Their clientele, however, is predominantly middle class.

Health visitors can help by telling expectant parents about groups and schemes in their area and by encouraging and providing support to new groups and, especially, by concentrating effort on provision for the disadvantaged.

As an alternative to group support, a project based at Lisson Grove Health Centre (Wood, 1985; Hills, 1981) fosters links between established parents and expectant parents in the area. Regular contact is maintained between mothers-to-be and their doctor and health visitor during the pregnancy. An introduction to established parents and attendance at antenatal classes which continue through to postnatal sessions, are offered. When the research on the project is completed, it will be interesting to discover whether this project has been successful and to what extent this sort of approach might be applicable elsewhere. Postnatal groups will be considered in the next chapter.

In this section, we have looked at environmental, physical, mental/emotional and social aspects of health which may be considered or discussed during a health visitor's visit to expectant parents.

AFTER THE VISIT

Record making is increasingly being undertaken during the visit. However, if this is not done, the health visitor will need to make a note of pertinent points immediately afterwards. For example, the date of the next appointment should be noted, assuming one was arranged. It will also be necessary to jot down any particular requests the parent or parents might have made. They might have shown an interest in being put in touch with agencies such as the National Childbirth Trust (NCT) or La Leche League. It might have been agreed that the health visitor should discuss some issue with the midwife. Also, the parents may have expressed an interest in certain health education subjects on which the health visitor has promised to provide further information, or has made a mental note to do so.

It is best if a record of the visit is made as soon as possible. A handbag-sized dictating machine can be invaluable for immediate recording (Robertson, 1982). An audio-typist then transcribes the notes in due course. Such records are generally considered to be much more reliable than hand written records made at the end of the day — or some days later! The problem is overcome, of course, when notes are written up on site.

Recalling and reviewing the visit involves a form of evaluation. As described in the previous chapter, it is part of the process of thinking about how to provide an appropriate service at subsequent encounters. The health visitor would tend to mentally run through:

- how parents seem to feel about the visit and the service provided by the health visitor
- their probable environmental, physical, emotional and social health requirements
- to what extent these were met in terms of:
  1. preventing occurrence: for example, through health education on an aspect such as breastfeeding
  2. preventing development: for example, through assessment of special need, perhaps using social factors as criteria for this assessment
  3. preventing deterioration: perhaps by listening whilst the mother-to-be talks through and sorts out her anxieties about her intentions to return to work
- which of the family's health requirements seem now to need most attention and to consider these as tentative objectives for the next visit
- immediate objectives for health visitor action, such as liaison with the NCT or midwife, or to find health education information ready for the next visit.

A note of any particular issue needing immediate attention or action at a subsequent visit can then be added to the records. This next encounter might be at another antenatal visit, at antenatal classes or at the birth visit.

This chapter has considered home visiting for people preparing for parenthood. It has looked at some schemes currently being tried out and at the need to keep in touch with others caring for these parents-to-be. Some possible health needs have been briefly mentioned. Health visiting at this stage gives an opportunity to provide health education and to explain about the purpose and style of health visiting. This helps the development of a good working relationship, which is particularly important once the baby is born.

USEFUL ADDRESSES

HVA Community Development Special Interest Group;
HVA Special Interest Group for Homelessness;
HVA Special Interest Group for Older People;
HVA Training Group;
HVA School Nurses Group;
HVA Overseas Group;

HVA Special Interest group for Health Advisers;
HVA Senior Managers Group
c/o Jill Carter, Executive Committee Secretary, Health Visitors' Association, 50 Southwark Street, London SEI 1UN
Tel 071 378 7255

La Leche League (Great Britain) Breastfeeding Help and Information, BM 3424 London WCIV 6XX
Tel 071 242 1278

National Childbirth Trust, Alexander House, Oldham Terrace, London W3 6NH
Tel 081 992 6762

REFERENCES

Ball J 1982 Stress and the postnatal care of women. Nursing Times 78: 1904–1907
Barker W and Anderson R 1988 The child development programme: an evaluation of process and outcome. Early

Childhood Development Unit, University of Bristol
Besford J 1984 Good mouthkeeping or how to save your children's teeth and your own, too, while you're about it. Oxford University Press, Oxford, p 40–41; 122–124

Black P 1984 Who stops smoking in pregnancy? Nursing Times 80, 19: 59–61

Chapman V, Lakhani B, Read J, Wood P 1990 National welfare benefits handbook, 1990–91, 20th edn. Child Poverty Action Group, London

Child Development Project 1984 Child development programme. Early Childhood Development Unit, Senate House, University of Bristol, Bristol BS8 1TH

Clulow C F 1982 To have and to hold. Marriage, the first baby and preparing couples for parenthood. Aberdeen University Press, Aberdeen, p 105

Coussins J 1980 Maternity rights for working women. National Council for Civil Liberties, London, p 24–25

Coussins J, Durward K, Evans R 1987 Maternity rights at work. National Council for Civil Liberties Women's Rights Unit and Maternity Alliance, London

Dening F 1983 Infant morbidity and preconceptual care. Nursing Times Supplement 79, 29: 3–6

Department of Social Security 1990 Which benefit? Leaflet FB.2 Oct 90. Department of Social Security, London

Dowdell P M 1981 Alcohol and pregnancy. A review of the literature 1968–1980. Nursing Times 77, 43: 1825–1831

Dowling S 1983 Health for a change. The provision of preventive health care in pregnancy and early childhood. Child Poverty Action Group, London

Draper J, Field S, Kerr M, Hare M J 1983 Women's knowledge of health care during pregnancy. Health Visitor 56: 86–88

Drennan V 1988 Ideas for practice. In: Drennan V (ed) Health visitors and groups: politics and practice. Heinemann Nursing, Oxford

Drury V W M 1982 Prescribing in pregnancy. Maternal and Child Health 7: 351–352

Durward L 1984 Poverty in pregnancy: the cost of an adequate diet for expectant mothers. Maternity Alliance, London

Edwards G 1983 Alcohol and advice to the pregnant woman. British Medical Journal 286: 247–248

Evans R, Durward L 1984 Maternity rights handbook. Know your rights: the questions and answers. Penguin Books, London

Field S, Draper J, Kerr M, Hare M J 1982a Interaction with health care personnel Part 1 The antenatal period. Midwife, Health Visitor and Community Nurse 18, 5: 197–198

Field S, Draper J, Kerr M, Hare M J 1982b Interaction with health care personnel Part 3 The postnatal period. Midwife, Health Visitor and Community Nurse 18, 7: 279; 287

Field S, Draper J, Thomas H, Farmer S, Hare M J 1984 The health visitor's view of consumer criticisms. Health Visitor 57: 273–275

Foresight 1980 Guidelines for future parents. The Association for the Promotion of Pre-conceptual Care, Woodhurst, Hydestile, Godalming, Surrey GU8 4AY

Gath A 1977 Emotional needs in a new family. Nursing Mirror 143, 28: 52–54

Garner L 1980 How to survive as a working mother. Jill Norman, p 25–37

Hally M R, Bond J, Crawley J, Gregson B, Philips P, Russell I 1984 What influences a mother's choice of infant feeding method? Nursing Times Occasional Paper No 4 80, 4: 65–68

Hawkins D F 1983 Drugs and pregnancy. Human teratogenesis and related problems. Churchill Livingstone, Edinburgh

Health Education Council 1984 Pregnancy book. A guide to becoming pregnant, being pregnant and caring for your newborn baby. Available through District Health Authority Health Education Units (in telephone directory under name of Health Authority: eg Winchester Health Authority)

Health Visitor 1981 Health visiting in the eighties. Health Visitor 54, 2: centre pages supplement

Hennessy D A 1986 Should health visitors also care for mothers? Proceedings of the Rcn Research Society, 1985 conference. Royal College of Nursing, London

Hills A 1981 Getting it right first time. Health and Social Services Journal XCI: 892

Holt K S 1982 Diets and development. Child: care, health and development 8: 183–201

House of Commons Social Services Committee 1980 Second Report, Session 1979–80 Perinatal and Neonatal Mortality. HMSO, London (Chairman Renee Short)

Jervis R 1983 Planning a balanced diet. In: Foresight Supplementary Chapters to Guidelines for Future Parents. The Association for the Promotion of Preconceptual Care, Godalming, Surrey

Kennedy C, McMullen J, Rowland M 1990 Rights guide to non-means-tested benefits 1990–91, 13th edn. Child Poverty Action Group, London

King J and Eiser J R 1981 A strategy for counselling pregnant smokers. Health Education Journal 40: 66–68

Klebanoff M A, Nugent R P, Rhoads G G 1984 Coitus during pregnancy: is it safe? The Lancet II: 914–917

Labour Research Department 1984 State benefits. A guide for trade unionists. LRD Publications Ltd, London

Little P and Ralston D 1980 The baby book for dads. New English Library

Loader A (editor) 1980 Pregnancy and parenthood. Oxford University Press, Oxford

Lythgoe E J 1982 HVs and antenatal care (letter). Nursing Times 78: 1475

McLellan J 1985 The effect of unemployment on the family. Health Visitor 58: 157–161

Margiotta P 1984 The importance of pre-conceptual nutrition. Nursing Times Health Visitors' Supplement 80, 42: 11–12

Maternity Alliance 1985 Born unequal: perspectives on pregnancy and childbearing in unemployed families. Maternity Alliance, 59–61 Camden High Street, London NW1 7JL

Maternity Services Advisory Committee 1982 Maternity care in action Part 1: antenatal care. DHSS (Leaflets) PO Box 21, Stanmore, Middlesex HA7 1AY. p 17, 19

Messenger M 1982 The breastfeeding book. Century Publishing Co Ltd, London

Moore J 1984 Antenatal ignorance. Nursing Times Community Outlook 80, 19: 147–148

Morgan J B 1980 Nutrition during pregnancy. Nutrition Bulletin 5, 6: 300–308

Nursing Times 1982 Parent groups help in pregnancy. Nursing Times: 78, 37: 1532

Nursing Times 1983 Helping people to stop smoking. Nursing Times 79, 23: 62–65

Oakley A 1982 From here to maternity. Becoming a mother. Penguin Books Ltd, London

Philips A 1983 Your body, your baby, your life. Pandora Press, London

Pickard B 1983 Fact sheet on pre-pregnancy care. Nursing Times Community Outlook 79, 23: 255–258

Pipe N G J 1983 Weight gain in pregnancy. Maternal and Child Health 8: 370–375

Plant M 1983 Alcohol in pregnancy: is it safe? Nursing Mirror Midwifery Forum 157, 14: ii–iv

Portwood D, Steventon B 1984 Health visitors and the unemployed. Health Visitor 57: 17–18

Price J 1988 Motherhood: what it does to your mind. Pandora Press, London

Proctor M 1990 Doling out fitness. Nursing Times 86, 26: 54–55

Pugh G (ed) 1980 Preparation for parenthood. Some current initiatives and thinking. National Childrens' Bureau, London

Rayner C 1977 Family feelings, Understanding your child from 0–5. Arrow Books Ltd, London

Robertson C A 1982 Becoming a health visitor — an obstacle course? Nursing Times 78, 36: 1508–1512

Royal College of Midwives and Health Visitors Association 1982 Joint statement on antenatal preparation. Health Visitors Association, 50 Southwark Street, London SE1 1UN

Savage W, Reader F 1984 Sexual activity during pregnancy. Midwife, Health Visitor and Community Nurse 20: 398–402

Schofield J 1982 Health visiting — quality not quantity (letter). Nursing Mirror 155, 25: 37

Scowen P (editor) 1981 New baby growing up. B Edsall and Co Ltd, London

Shai Linn P H, Schoenbaum S C, Monson R R, Rosner B, Stubblefield P G, Ryan K J 1982 No association between coffee consumption and adverse outcomes of pregnancy. The New England Journal of Medicine 306, 3: 141–145

Sidle N 1983 Smoking in pregnancy — A review. Hera Unit, The Spastics Society, 12 Park Crescent, London W1N 4EQ

Skinner V 1982 HVs, midwives and pregnant women (letter). Nursing Times 78: 1236

Solberg S M 1984 Indicators of successful breast feeding. In: Houston M J (ed) Maternal and infant health care. Churchill Livingstone, Edinburgh

Spray J 1988 The Radical Health Visitors' Group. In: Drennan V (ed) Health visitors and groups: politics and practice. Heinemann Nursing, Oxford

Stanton A 1982 The listening, liaising, counselling HV. Nursing Mirror 155, 22: 57–59

Verny T, Kelly J 1982 The secret life of the unborn child. Sphere Books Ltd, London. p 17–18

Walton L 1983 Thoughts of a new mother. Health Visitor 56: 208–209

Waumsley L 1983 Mothers talking about postnatal depression. National Childbirth Trust, London

Wood T 1985 Formal and informal support systems for mothers with newborn. Midwife, Health Visitor and Community Nurse 21: 42–49

Wynn M, Wynn A 1979 Prevention of handicap and the health of women. Routledge and Kegan Paul, London

Wynn M, Wynn A 1981 The prevention of handicap of early pregnancy origin. Some evidence for the value of good health before conception. Foundation for Education and Research in Childbearing, 27 Walpole Street, London SW3 4QS

Chapter 4 looks at activities in preparation for and associated with the birth visit. It provides another example of how the family health needs framework can be used to systematise matters that pertain to or may be considered or discussed during the call. The classification this time is under physical, emotional and social aspects of health.

4

Birth visit

BEHIND THE SCENES

By tradition and law

The first home visit after the birth usually takes place between the tenth and fourteenth day post-natally. In many places, the day chosen depends on traditional arrangements made between the midwives and the health visitors. In some instances, the 'hand-over' date is decided on an individual basis. If there is a clinical problem, the midwife may maintain contact with the mother up to the 28th day.

Some health visitors have been known to refer to this first visit as their 'statutory visit', but this is a misnomer. The statutory obligation is on the Health Authorities, under the National Health Services Act, Part II, Section 24

to make provision in their area for the visiting of persons in their homes by . . . . . . health visitors for the purpose of giving advice as to the care of young children, persons suffering from illness and expectant or nursing mothers . . . .

There is no compulsion in the visiting. Although the service must be provided, it does not have to be received. The system depends entirely upon these nurses being seen as acceptable and helpful visitors as was discussed in Chapter 2.

INFORMATION GATHERING

The law requiring notification of the birth by the midwife enables this information to be passed on to the health visitor. Parents have six weeks in which to notify the Registrar of Births.

The record card

Normally, with each new birth a health visitor record card is sent through the administrative system to the health visitor's desk. Besides the child's

- surname
- home address
- and date of birth

there may be an indication of its

- sex
- weight
- length
- 'at risk' factors, if any
- congenital malformation, if any
- phenylketonuria test date
- hearing test date
- and other tests.

Regarding the mother, it may show her

- age
- number of previous births
- general practitioner
- midwife
- and where the birth took place.

The amount of information actually recorded on the card varies according to local custom and practice. In some places, for example, the phenylketonuria test may be considered so commonplace as not to be worth recording — unless a problem has been detected.

Liaison

The health visitor may be informed of much of the information mentioned above or alerted to relevant medical or social factors through an obstetric discharge computer print-out or a form filled in by the midwife. These papers may be sent to the health visitor through the administrative system, given to the liaison health visitor or left with the mother to hand on at the visit.

The McClymont (1983, p. 10) working party suggested that useful information might include: type of delivery; Apgar score; the condition of both mother and infant, and several factors that would give an indication of social background. Some of the factors useful in helping to identify the families for whom health visitors should give extra consideration and support, were mentioned in Chapter 3 (p. 48). There is also a need to know the discharge address if it differs from the mother's normal place of residence.

Both early notification of important information and personal liaison between the midwife and the health visitor, mean a better service can be given. The same applies, of course, to liaison with the general practitioner.

It seems that around three-quarters of the health visitors interviewed by Dunnell and Dobbs (1982) and Draper et al (1984) felt they had a very good or good working relationship with the GP. However, it follows that a significant number found communication inadequate.

Ann Bowling (1983) studied primary health care teamwork and reviewed some of the pertinent literature. She mentioned Bruces' report that, like GPs, health visitors could also find it difficult to share information, unless it was especially requested.

Health visitors' and GPs' hesitancy about sharing information could be for the same reasons. In both cases, their work is of an independent nature and, for many, a special effort has to be made to make contact. Many from both professions may feel worried when confronted by seemingly contradictory ideals: on one hand, the ideal of information sharing and on the other, the individual's right to privacy and confidentiality. In some cases there may be a fear that clients would not be helped so much as become 'labelled' — branded as having a problem — and denigrated or patronised. This recedes as an issue when the health visitor and the GP (or any other member of the primary health care team) have witnessed improved care through teamwork and have learned, over time, to trust each other's ability to help the families involved.

However, people's basic right to confidentiality and their assumption that medical and personal details will go no further than the professional person in whom they confide, still remain. The matter is returned to in the last section of Chapter 8.

Frequent and flexible meetings on practical issues as they arise, provide a forum for feedback and discussion. These can help to build up this understanding and trust and to overcome common difficulties in teamwork, such as:

- problems of role definition
- friction and stereotyping
- concerns over status and leadership.

Telephoned and written messages can ensure speedy communication in between meetings.

Pamphlets

Several books and papers are available which may be felt worth having to hand on this visit (see Table 4.1). The choice of matters introduced during the call and, therefore, the supportive literature which would be needed, will be influenced by what topics have been discussed antenatally and, also, whether other opportunities for early contact with the family are anticipated.

If, for example, the health visitor is carrying a double caseload, a great deal will have to be fitted into this first visit after the birth. On the other hand, weekly visiting may be the norm, perhaps until the baby is six weeks or so. In this case, certain papers such as pamphlets on immunisation or information about developmental or hearing tests, might be introduced later, at one of those weekly visits, and organised to suit the parents' wishes.

Table 4.1 Examples of literature the health visitor might have available at a birth visit

Items	Source
Cards, lists and forms to leave with the family	Health visitor visiting card — where can be contacted and tel no Immunisation request and consent form — to be completed and returned	Health Authority admin
Lists of: • child health clinics and out of hours health visitor service • family planning clinics • local mothers' groups • local crying baby telephone and other support services	Health visitor office (need frequent updating)
Green card: infant care guide	Foundation for Sudden Infant Death Syndrome
Leaflets and booklets to lend or leave	Safety: HS2 Keeping pets: ID5 Feeding: NT4; NT5 Childminding: CW30; CW31 'Now You're a Family' CW2 'You Know More Than You Think You Do' CW7 Local specially designed leaflets	District Health Authority Health Education Dept
	'The Book of the Child' Child Health Record Booklet	Scottish Health Education Group Edsall, publishers
Books as visual aid or to lend for a week or so	Leach P 1977 Baby and Child. Penguin Books Jolly H 1981 Book of Child Care. Sphere Books Messenger M 1982 The Breastfeeding Book. Century Pub. Scowen P, editor 1981 New Baby Growing Up. Esdall Richards M 1980 Infancy. Harper and Row Rayner C 1977 Family Feelings. Arrow Books	Usually health visitor's own property

Preparing to call

The mother may well appreciate advance warning of when the health visitor expects to visit, either through a telephone call or through a standard arrangement with the midwife.

It is likely that the agreed visit would be written

into the health visitor's diary, the date of birth, name and address put into the appropriate section of that year's birth book, and the record card filed away in the compartment for current visiting, probably with the record cards for other members of that family, should there be any.

THE VISIT

MEETING THE FAMILY

This call may be on a family already known to the health visitor, perhaps through previous children or through antenatal contact. Where there is a high turnover of staff or it is a first baby, and particularly in inner city areas, it is not unusual for this to be the introductory visit.

Making contact with a family was considered in Chapter 2. We looked at some of the elements of success such as establishing a good relationship, helping people understand the purpose of health visiting and making appropriate response to family health requirements. The 'fact gathering' associated with this visit makes it worth mentioning two further points.

Knowledge kept in the background

Health visitors arrive at these households with a fair amount of information about the circumstances of the birth and the baby. However, it is probable that for reasons of diplomacy, they will not wish to *appear* too knowledgeable. There are several reasons. For one thing, they would prefer to encourage the parent or parents to describe various things, in order to gain an understanding of their perspective.

In some cases, parents may be too hesitant to explain, if they feel they may be repeating something already known to their listener. A second reason is that a 'know-all' health visitor may be resented and (perhaps properly) be labelled as a potential autocrat. Thirdly, some issues can be very delicate and people may be better choosing their own time to mention them, should they wish to.

It may help to give an example of this third

reason — a delicate topic. Let us say a record card shows

previous births: 1 + 0

indicating one previous birth and no miscarriages. The case is one where there is no earlier record card in the files and so the health visitor is not aware of a previous child. Liaison may have enabled forewarning of a previous still birth or adoption. Whether they know the whole story or not, many health visitors would not themselves raise the subject, unless it seemed absolutely necessary.

It is the experience of the author that often a small remark, perhaps when the baby is being looked at, a remark such as, 'You must be very proud of your little girl', will cause people to refer back to an earlier, hurtful experience, as part of an explanation as to why they are so happy now. They can then explain in their own way and at their own pace.

This 'background approach' when visiting has the advantage of enabling positive client participation, but it has the disadvantage that health visitors may appear to 'know nothing'. There are, however, many ways in which they can make suggestions and show themselves to be knowledgeable and useful. Some are described in later sections of this chapter under physical, emotional and social aspects of family health need.

Avoiding implied criticism

Health visitor attitude and visible usefulness seem to be the key to success in the work. It is, therefore, somewhat dismaying to read the McClymont (1983, p. 11) working party's list of factors suggested as needing 'to be observed' by the health visitor during this primary visit. The general tenor might easily be interpreted as critical and health visitor centred. Phrases like

- 'ability of mother to cope'
- 'organisation of household, cleanliness'
- 'maturity of parents'
- 'attitude of mother . . . (and) . . . other relatives to HV'

are used. All these are matters on which the health

visitor's observations must have a strongly subjective bias. Household standards, just as one example, are a distinctly questionable means of measuring either the quality of a family's loving relationships or a person's skills in parenting (Goodwin, 1982).

However, the working party did not claim to have all the answers — in fact the reverse (p. (i)). They published the outcome of their activities because they could *not* provide clear answers to the questions posed and they hoped to encourage further study.

Their list of matters suggested as needing 'to be clarified' during the visit is much more helpful (pp. 11–12). This list includes factors about the baby and the family situation such as:

- feeding method and routine
- sterilisation of equipment
- whether benefits have been claimed
- family planning services
- mother's return to work
- sibling relationships.

Its value lies in its drawing together a range of possible discussion points which the family may wish to raise, or perhaps develop, if they were introduced by the health visitor.

However, as shown in the previous chapter and in the list of factors in Box 4.1 and discussed in the following sections of this chapter, the McClymont list should *not* be taken as providing an ideal model of what should be achieved in the visit. There are limitations on time and every family has differing priorities on what they would like discussed during the visit. Added to this, there will be other matters which might be raised and need to be considered. There is not room in a review of this kind, to mention every possible relevant item.

THE FRAMEWORK IN ACTION

As in the previous chapter, a family health needs framework has been chosen to demonstrate one way of organising a mental checklist of the sort of matters that might be considered during a visit. The model, seen in Box 4.1, emphasises some of the physical, mental/emotional and social aspects of health requirements family members may have at this stage of their life.

A section on environmental factors has not been included in this chapter. This is in order to allow more space for matters specific to the health visitor's first visit to a family with a new baby. Environmental factors were introduced in Chapter 3 (p. 43). Naturally, these become increasingly significant with the arrival of young children in a family and their exclusion is in no way intended to minimise their importance or to belittle their influence on family health.

Box 4.1 Some aspects of family health considered at the first visit after the birth

Physical health	Mental/emotional health	Social aspects of health
Mother General health Postnatal factors: • physical condition • postnatal check • medication	*Parental knowledge* Many possible queries *Expectations, adjustment and emotional well-being*	*Mother and father: family network* Important source of help and support Isolated?
Baby Examination e.g. • general appearance • vision • hearing • weight • CDH • record card Boys: foreskin Hygiene and safety Immunisation Artificial feeding	*Mother: baby* Baby's behaviour Bonding Breastfeeding: support needed *Siblings* Rivalry Special attention	*Mother* Lonely? Advice on local support services for young mothers Child health clinic *Siblings* Playgroup Toddler and mother group.
	Father: mother Attention to baby means less time for each other Sexuality Contraception	

EXAMPLES OF BIRTH VISITS

Once again, two examples are given in order to

show the framework in action. The first is the birth visit to Nancy Manners, who featured in the previous chapter as an example of an antenatal visit. The second is to the Clarks, who already have a three-year-old child. Outlines will be found in Boxes 4.2 and 4.3.

EXAMPLE ONE: NANCY MANNERS

The information on the health visitor birth card delivered to Mrs Hannah Van der Haastrecht's (HV) desk, showed that Nancy Manners had had a girl by caesarian section three days previously. The Apgar score (10 after 10 minutes) and other indicators were satisfactory.

The primary health care team weekly meeting was held six days later, when the baby was 10 days old. The GP reported that Miss Manners had been very disappointed not to have a normal delivery but had adjusted to the circumstances well. He had visited the home that day and had examined the baby fully. Glancing down the list of items on the notes, HV saw no abnormality recorded. The community midwife (CMW) said that breastfeeding, on demand and currently around two hourly, was successful so far. Nancy's mother was staying for a week or so to help. HV and CMW arranged to visit together for the handover.

Box 4.2   Example one: Nancy Manners

Physical health	Mental/emotional health	Social aspects of health
Mother Caesarian stitches Breasts comfortable Not smoking No alcohol Postnatal exam at hospital nearby	*Parental knowledge* Given booklet CW2 Messenger book still useful *Adjustment and emotional well-being*	*Mother* Grandmother supporting Gingerbread contacts NCT discontinued Contact with nursing friends Invited to clinic
Baby Examined by GP including CDH Vision: eye contact Hearing: startles Skin: good colour Fontanelle normal Passing urine; faeces normal Weight: 3 kg	*Mother: baby* Breastfeeding seeks support Baby wakefulness: acceptable 'Bonding' discussed	

On the morning of the fourteenth day, as prearranged, they called. Mrs Manners answered the door and HV was pleased to have a chance to meet her. The baby had just finished being fed. Breastfeeding was progressing very satisfactorily, now generally at three or four hourly intervals. Nancy, who was still taking 'no baccy or booze' very seriously, had told the midwife how much she had appreciated her motherliness and support, especially over breastfeeding. She seemed pleased when HV said she would be able to call weekly for a few weeks.

Baby Pauline was tending to be wakeful in the evenings, but, it seems, Nancy and her mother were making it an opportunity to cuddle and to play with her. Whilst the nappy was being changed, they enjoyed showing HV and CMW the baby's ability to make eye contact and to respond to facial expressions. Pauline startled and blinked in response to a loud hand clap, she looked well, her eyes were clear and HV noted that her umbilicus was dry. The baby was weighed by CMW. She had regained her birthweight of 3 kg and it was recorded on the 50th centile. The doctor had checked her hips four days previously.

When HV asked how the delivery had been, Nancy explained about the breech presentation and the subsequent decisions. She said that in her training, she had heard a good deal about 'bonding'. She was worried in case her relationship with her baby should be inadequate on account of not seeing her immediately after the birth. They discussed current ideas on bonding theory.

When CMW asked if there was anything in her feelings for her baby that made her worry, Nancy said they were a little mixed. As they talked on, particularly about her behaviour with her baby, Nancy realised that she had no real problem. Some pages from a booklet HV had in her bag, 'Now You're a Family', proved useful.

The health visitor described the facilities at the clinic, including those for getting to know other mothers. Nancy said she had met a few mothers at the NCT antenatal classes but felt a closer bond with the people she had met at the Gingerbread meetings. They had made her very welcome and she was grateful to HV for telling her about the local group. Some of the members were babysitting for each other and Nancy planned to join this scheme.

Hannah Van der Haastrecht was glad her caseload was small enough to allow her to keep closely in touch with Nancy. They arranged a date for a morning the following week. As some time was likely to be spent at the mother's home, HV made a note of the telephone numbers, both of this house and of the mother's home.

EXAMPLE TWO: THE CLARK FAMILY

Henrietta Varley (HV), a health visitor in an inner city area, heard of the Clarks, recently moved in, through one of her monthly meetings with the community midwife. The midwife said that Mrs Clark (36 weeks pregnant) did not wish to breastfeed and that they had a three-year-old daughter. A grossly handicapped boy, born five years previously, had lived only four days. An antenatal visit was not possible due to workload pressures: HV was covering the caseload of a colleague on maternity leave.

The baby was born about a fortnight after that meeting and the birth card came through to HV.

Box 4.3 Example two: the Clark family

Physical health	Mental/emotional health	Social aspects of health
Mother Breasts comfortable Painful perineum No medication	*Parental knowledge* Discussion about: • milk formulae • posseting • foreskin care • sexual activity • Pamphlets on immunisation	*Mother* Husband supportive Grandparental homes 200 miles away Newly moved in One friend locally
Father Appears well		
Toddler Alert child	*Adjustment and emotional well-being*	Intends to: • join mothers group • attend clinic
Baby 3–4 hourly feeds = SMA Possetting Sleeping prone Hearing: startles Vision: eye contact CDH test Fontanelles: not depressed	*Parents: baby* Anxious re handicap *Mother: father* Cooperating *Toddler* Involved with care Receiving parental attention	*Toddler* Plans for playgroup

Mr Clark answered the door when she called. He had taken two weeks' leave to look after his wife and daughter. Three-year-old Tracey hung around the living room doorway and HV engaged her in conversation about playschool and about 'her' baby.

Mrs Clark said the discomfort in her breasts had gone; however, an episiotomy wound was proving uncomfortable. She was tired by evening but felt reasonably energetic earlier in the day.

Baby Ian was presenting 'problems'. Mr Clark seemed particularly distressed by the baby's crying each evening. They had 'tried everything'. The baby was posseting and they were considering changing the milk formula. Having explained how to do this in a gradual way, HV went on to describe the minimal differences between the milks. She asked how the feeds were currently being made up.

The baby was asleep, but the couple wanted HV to examine him. She enquired about vision, hearing, whether they had seen the hip test done, remarked on the normality of the fontanelle and mentioned foreskin care. The couple explained that their deepest fear had been that he might be handicapped. In a way, they found it difficult to believe their luck. It sounded as if they would be very active in monitoring his developmental progress in the record booklet which HV gave them.

Ian had regained his birthweight and, for most of the day, was reported as sleeping between three and a half to four hourly feeds. The couple said they would talk later about what had been said about the milk formulae and might wait a while before deciding whether to change it. Having Hugh Jolly's child care book in her bag, HV showed them his reassuring remarks about posseting and they all joked about his (very practical) ideas on placing towels everywhere to protect clothing and floors against the 'overflow'.

The Clarks had involved their daughter in the baby's examination. Later she went to the other side of the room and played quietly.

The forms requesting immunisation were discussed and as the couple wished to 'think about it', HV gave them up-to-date pamphlets and promised to answer their questions next time they met.

Mrs Clark had made a friend through the antenatal clinic. She was very pleased to have the list of local mothers' groups and organisations and also to find it provided addresses of playgroups. The health visitor explained that two retired ladies helped entertain the toddlers at her baby clinic so that the mothers would have a chance to talk and get to know each other.

Towards the end of the visit, HV followed up the earlier remark about the painful episiotomy wound. It transpired that it had been very painful during attempted intercourse. The matter was discussed and HV recommended it should be

mentioned at the six week postnatal check, if it was still painful. She made a mental note to mention it at her next visit.

As she left, the health visitor gave the couple her telephone number. Mrs Clark said she had been a regular attender at the clinic with Tracey and she intended to be with Ian.

PHYSICAL HEALTH

Mother

Liaison with other members of the primary health care team may have alerted the health visitor to a particular problem of general health which the mother may find relevant and wish to discuss. At this visit, matters such as the condition of the breasts, perineum or lochia, dental care and postnatal exercises may be of concern.

Arrangements for the six week postnatal examination and any difficulties likely to arise over attending it, may be discussed. Georgina Ray (1984) discussed and described this visit for parents and reminded mothers to take with them, as appropriate:

- a sample of urine
- their maternal cooperation card

and if attending their GP, their baby's National Health Service registration card, so that, presuming they wish it, the baby can be registered there.

Dr Gunn (1983) describes the physical examination and encourages mothers to ask questions about their labour, their current condition and what they might expect in a subsequent pregnancy. He provides a useful checklist of 20 possible questions about such things as:

- vaginal discharge
- when the next period would be expected
- use of tampons
- discomfort of stitches
- painful intercourse
- lumpy breasts
- how long to breastfeed
- caesarian scar
- likelihood of another caesarian/forceps/episiotomy
- the reason for needing to be induced

- method of contraception
- how to help get figure back.

Medication and lactation

Some drugs are best avoided by breastfeeding mothers. Lewis and Hurden (1983) provide an overview of the subject. They include a list of drugs where deleterious effects have been reported, another of drugs about which there is some doubt and a third list showing those which are probably safe for nursing mothers.

Grant and Golightly (1984) describe how new information from research can mean that reviews can soon be out of date. They outline the Drugs and Breast Milk Information Service (DIBMIS) which is available both to the professions and the public. It has already been made use of by health visitors and breastfeeding counsellors as well as many others.

Canadian researchers looking into postpartum consumption of alcohol (Davidson et al, 1981), were concerned to find that a significant proportion of the 260 women taking part in their study, *started* to drink at this time — on *professional advice*, suggesting that it would aid lactation and relaxation. Only two women had been warned to avoid alcohol both in pregnancy and for the breastfeeding period. The question arises as to whether this hazardous sort of 'medication' is being advised here too — and encouraging the lone drinking discovered in the Canadian study.

Father and siblings

The general health of the father and the baby's siblings is, naturally, also of importance in the family equation. Basic health matters such as safety, nutrition and sleeping patterns might receive consideration. In the current economic climate, the relationship between health and unemployment becomes a significant factor (Fagin & Little, 1984) and is discussed towards the end of Chapter 15. Some relevant men's health topics will be found in the further reading list at the end of this chapter.

Baby

It may not always be convenient to the family for the baby to be disturbed for an examination. A separate appointment may have to be made. Even so, the family are generally very pleased for their visitor to admire their baby in its cot. If there are felt to be any problems, it is not unusual for the parents to be anxious for the health visitor to make a thorough check, even if this means disturbing a peaceful sleep.

The extent to which the baby should be examined will vary according to the local service provided. Awareness of local GP and hospital routines will increase the chance of being able to guess which babies could possibly have fallen through the normal infant screening safety net, and therefore, need greater attention.

A paper by the Department of Health and Social Security (DHSS, 1980a) suggested 6–10 days as one of the key ages for the baby to be examined, and proposed that this examination should be carried out by a doctor trained for this purpose. Health visitors curious to know about likely procedures, will find outlines by Illingworth (1928) and Curtis Jenkins and Newton (1981).

Curtis Jenkins emphasises the effect of the examination on the mother — for better or for worse. He says that appropriate demonstrations and explanations, and a well-performed examination, may make the examining doctor 'a friend for life'. Particularly important is showing the baby's ability to see, hear and, usually, to smile. The author provides pictures which show the doctor demonstrating patterns of infant behaviour. Witnessing these can significantly increase the mother's understanding of her baby's skills and abilities and the baby's need for talk and interaction.

Health visitor examination

What form then, should the health visitor's examination take? The phraseology and listing in the McClymont (1983, p. 12) criteria for the 'examination to be made during the visit' imply that the health visitor *must* undertake an investigation in which every part of the baby should be seen. This would mean stripping the baby — possibly risking irritating parents who feel the baby is currently all right and have, anyway, witnessed a recent and thorough inspection by a doctor.

If the health visitor examination is to be a brief one with the baby dressed, then the health visitor's basic nursing habit of observing general appearance is likely to take note, perhaps without comment, of the baby's

- range of facial expression
- skin colour and condition
- apparent temperature
- fontanelle: depressed?

and certainly, to investigate or enquire after
- eyes discharging?
- mouth: thrush?
- umbilicus: still moist?
- vision (making eye contact)
- hearing (startled by sudden loud noise).

In some locations, a record is made of

- naked weight
- head circumference
- length
- certain reflexes

giving the health visitor a better baseline from which to observe and compare with possible later changes.

Foreskin care

This examination provides an appropriate cue for telling parents of boys about correct foreskin care. Griffiths (1984) found people tended to be poorly advised and says initial 'masterly inaction' followed by routine penile hygiene from the age of three or four, will prevent many childhood circumcisions for phimosis, which is the reason for 80% of the circumcisions currently performed.

Congenital dislocation of the hip

The tests for congenital dislocation of the hip (CDH), ably described by Monk and Dowd (1981), are neither simple nor easy. Fixen (1983) feels that health visitors should be properly trained on how to do it and what to be on the lookout for. Perhaps the best way to become more proficient, is to ask to attend the clinic of a local orthopaedic surgeon, who would probably be delighted to help.

It seems that many CDHs have been missed. The reasons were found, in a study by David et al 1983, to be due to failure:

- to examine the baby's hip
- to follow up abnormalities
- to follow parental observation of problem
- of parents to understand the significance of abnormality.

Clearly the current system has room for improvement.

There has been some debate about the significance of clicking or grating hip (Cunningham et al, 1984a, 1984b; Jones, 1989). It is now generally felt that hip examinations should continue after the first month or two of a baby's life. The matter is, therefore, returned to in Chapter 5 (p. 95).

The modern tendency to advise parents to lay their babies in the prone position, thought also to help prevent development of infantile ideopathic scoliosis (McMaster, 1983), could be particularly beneficial to those babies with an undiscovered tendency towards hip dislocation (Wilkinson, 1983). McMaster remarks, however, that only a quarter of the 568 normal infants in an Edinburgh study were, in fact, nursed prone. It would be interesting to know in what position people elsewhere place their babies and how this correlates with these orthopaedic problems.

Parents' own record

In some places, child health record cards (see Ch. 8, p. 149) for the parents' own record, are made available (Green & Macfarlane, 1985). These are likely to be explained to the parent or parents either during or after the health visitor examination.

General baby care

There are many practical matters which parents may like to discuss. 'Wind', posseting, stools, 'colic' and sleep patterns, for example, are neatly covered in books such as Penelope Leach's (1989) *Baby and Child* and Hugh Jolly's (1981) *Book of Child Care*.

Some health visitors keep a spare copy of their favourite child care book for lending, short term, to parents. They can then take time to think things over and compare the ideas in the book with other views available to them. The book can be picked up at the next visit or when the baby is brought to the clinic.

Hygiene and safety

There is a Community Outlook 'checklist' (Swaffield, 1983) which usefully sets out the major points on how to avoid nappy rash and diarrhoea. The Health Education Council's (198(1)) *Play It Safe* covers the major potential hazards for small babies, through suffocation or choking (p. 7), falls (p. 11) and car travel (p. 29). Cat nets and pram brakes (Scowen, 1984) are also topical at this stage.

A green card outlining infant care guidance on feeding care, crying and the baby's temperature is available to all parents from the Foundation for the Study of Infant Deaths. Situations in which a doctor should be called are described and emergency procedures are listed. It can be hung up in the kitchen for quick and easy reference and for reassurance.

Immunisation

Jenkinson (1982, p. 94) describes the organisation involved in immunisation and provides a table showing the basic programme for children. Since 1988 the mumps, measles and rubella three-in-one immunisation has been added to the repertoire (Cameron, 1988).

Immunisation, since its beginnings, has been a controversial subject and it is still under debate (Jenkinson, 1982; Robertson, 1984; Wells, 1984). It can often be very confusing for parents. It is they who have the responsibility for deciding the relative risks involved — from the disease (Bowler et al, 1988) or from the immunisation — and for deciding what action should be taken for their baby.

Parents need to be fully informed and to have time to consider and raise questions about the matter. Where at all possible, there is much to be said for introducing the subject either antenatally or at a follow-up visit, if one is planned shortly.

Pertussis immunisation has been, in recent years, the main one to suffer from a media scare. The ensuing debate stimulated research, the earlier findings of which have been reported on elsewhere (Robertson, 1984). Some of the important points raised were: the influence of professional opinion, uncertainty about interpretation of contra-indications and inadequacy of records systems. These are outlined below.

Professional advice was found to be such a significant factor in parents' decision-making that, in Calderdale, a special training scheme was offered to professional staff involved in immunisations. It improved professional advice and immunisation procedures and brought good results.

Increasing public awareness of contra-indications for immunisation was made part of the Calderdale programme. Valman (1982) suggested that an appropriate questionnaire, given to parents in the doctors' waiting room, would allow them time to think about possible contra-indications. However, there was another problem. Governmental recommendations on contra-indications were found to be liable to wide variation in interpretation — both within and between the various professional groups whose opinion might be sought. Health visitors may need to seek clarification on local policy and the reasons for the approach adopted.

The National Childhood Encephalopathy Study (NCES) unit which was set up to research the effects of pertussis vaccines found, like some other researchers, that central recording methods could be poor, particularly regarding the details of the vaccine and the date it was given. Some parents were found to have no personal record. Some did not know what immunisations their children had been given. A record in the personal record booklets (Green & Macfarlane, 1985) mentioned above, would provide parents with a useful reference — and a reminder for boosters as the child grows up.

In the event, the results of the NCES and other studies have been reassuring (Bellman et al, 1983; Pollock et al, 1984; Waight et al, 1983) especially for adsorbed preparation of the vaccine.

Current advice is that an interrupted course of immunisation should not be started again. It is now thought the effect of the earlier dose lasts a few years. Also, the frequency of side-effects is liable to increase with the number of injections (Smith, 1983; Waight et al, 1983). A suggested target for pertussis uptake in the community has been put at 80% (Jelley & Nicoll, 1984). Advice available from the Joint Committee on Vaccination and Immunisation (1988) is planned to be updated annually. It is imperative that health visitors undertaking domicilary and opportunistic immunisations have clear legal guidelines and adequate training (Health Visitor, 1989).

Keeping abreast of current thinking and research in this important aspect of health visiting, will need wide reading and support from the health authority, nurse manager, peer group and professional organisation (see Ch. 2, p. 20).

Feeding: artificial

A significant proportion of women are still choosing to bottle feed their babies. There are some clear step-by-step descriptions available for those who need reassurance or instruction on preparing the feed or sterilising equipment (Health Education Council, 1984; Leach, 1979, pp. 64–71). The government has provided guidelines on good feeding practice (DHSS, 1980b; Health Visitor, 1981).

There are several important aspects of artificial feeding in which health visitors may be able to be particularly helpful. For example, they need to explain, in simple terms, the very small differences between milks (Jeffs, 1983). Downing and Howkins (1984) have described the tendency for some people to blame the milk when there are small difficulties for the baby such as skin rashes or wakefulness. They also described common mistakes in making up feeds and parental concern over constipation. All these may need advice and guidance.

In this section we have looked at some of the physical aspects of a family's health that might be considered during a health visitor's first visit after the birth. Breastfeeding, which might have been included in this part, has been held over until the next, in order to highlight, once again, some of its emotional aspects.

MENTAL AND EMOTIONAL HEALTH

Care has to be taken that physical aspects of infant health do not completely overshadow aspects of a family's emotional welfare. Reasons why this might happen could be, for example, that limitations of time at a visit may lure health visitors into giving total priority to, and concentrating on infant care. Also, if this visit is the first time they have met, both sides may hesitate to step into sensitive areas of discussion.

A. Parental knowledge

The sort of issues that parents may wish to raise will depend, primarily, upon the worries currently uppermost in their minds, the extent to which they are encouraged to express them and, of course, just how well they feel they know and trust the health visitor. It will, of course, also depend on what topics have already been covered at previous meetings. Some of the things that might be discussed can be found in this and the previous section, matters such as immunisation, hygiene and safety, infant feeding and developmental progress.

The problem of conflicting advice was mentioned in Chapter 3 (p. 39). Breastfeeding is such an important issue at this stage, that it would seem well worth making special efforts to find out the the sort of advice generally given by the GP and midwives and to keep in touch with changes of policy. In many places, now, there is a locally devised booklet given out at clinics and the hospital.

B. Expectations, adjustment and emotional well-being

Mother

It is fairly common for the mother to feel a degree of fatigue and tension. She, the main carer for the family, needs, herself, to feel cared for. The health visitor, in showing a particular interest in the mother and the way she is feeling can, for many women, provide some part of that support. There is a need for the health visitor to provide opportunities in the conversation for the mother to express her anxieties and how she feels in herself (Fig. 4.1).

Common problems are confused feelings over an unexpected pattern of behaviour in the baby, anxieties about 'bonding' and worries about family and, perhaps, sexual relationships. Breastfeeding mothers are especially in need of support.

Mother: baby

Unexpected behaviour

Mothers, especially of first babies, can feel

Fig. 4.1 Care for the carer.

particularly worried on coming home to what amounts to sole responsibility for the new baby. This is lessened if the baby is readily comforted, sleeps a good deal and feeds well. If the baby does not behave as expected, it can cause great concern and feelings of guilt about ability to care for the baby. Common worries are:

- amount of crying
- amount of sleeping
- bowel movement
- spitting up/posseting
- feeding
- lack of pattern in sleeping and feeding.

One study (Midwife Health Visitor & Community Nurse, 1985) showed a large number of parents are taken by surprise by the amount their babies cry. Some women felt guilty, worrying lest they had failed in some way. It was reported that a large number of the women sought help from health visitors:

. . . who had shown sensitivity to the feelings of the mother and talking out the problem had helped.

Postnatal support groups, the National Childbirth Trust (NCT) and an organisation called 'Cry-sis' were found to be of assistance (see Ch. 5, p. 98).

Bonding

Some mothers hear about bonding and fear that they have missed out in some way (Brown, 1984; Hopkins, 1988). Robson and Powell (1982) discussed the difficulty in clearly defining it and measuring it. They said that, although the initial advantage in early contact has been demonstrated, it is not currently possible to show what the more important long-term effects are.

What seems to be more important is an ongoing sympathetic interaction between mother and baby which is synchronised to suit them both. Enabling a mother to become aware, early, of her baby's skills in communication and perception, can enhance the interactive potential between herself and her baby (see p. 63) — and the baby and the father (Robertson & Robertson, 1982).

Many mothers will find it reassuring to hear that several studies have shown that some 40% of first time mothers feel some indifference towards their newborn babies. Robson and Kumar were reported by Robson and Powell to have found that initial feelings of maternal indifference soon wore off for most mothers.

Breastfeeding

For women who wish to breastfeed, an important key to success seems to lie in the mother's confidence in her ability to do so. It is well known that milk flow is very sensitive to psychological inhibition. Some mothers who originally wished to feed but 'fail' and change to artificial feeding, feel guilty (Houston, 1984a). Women need support in these early days. Pre-arranged, regular visiting seems to help significantly.

Mary Houston (1984a, 1984b) has researched and written on professional support at home for breastfeeding mothers. She found mothers liked to have the same person giving advice and to have appointments made for further visits. This enabled mothers to cope with problems that arose, knowing that help would be coming.

In her small study groups, Dr Houston found Social Class I mothers coped well with or without special support. Social Classes II, III and IV tended to benefit from the extra visiting. This raises the question as to whether health visitors' traditional creed of equal visiting to everyone, should be changed. She suggested it might be better for there to be a bias towards more visits to the social classes less likely to turn to the NCT or La Leche League and towards devoting more time to the encouragement of local self-help groups.

A health visitor, Marion Kelly (1983), compared the duration of breastfeeding of 19 mothers she visited weekly until six weeks and fortnightly to twelve weeks, providing structured practical and emotional support, and a control group who were visited at 11 days, three, six and twelve weeks. A greater number in the study group breastfed for three months, apparently benefiting from the morale boosting and encouragement. The results of a small sample can, of course, provide no more than an indicator.

Books and organisations. The wide range of books available on breastfeeding reflects a large demand by parents feeling the need of support and guidance. Penelope Leach (1979, pp. 48–63) has provided some very practical advice and clear explanatory drawings, which mothers might find helpful. Maire Messenger's (1982) *The Breastfeeding Book* was mentioned in the previous chapter and a book by Celia Worth (1984) may be of interest.

Another response to this need can be seen in the emergence of La Leche League and the National Childbirth Trust and their work in support and counselling in breastfeeding. Health visitors can refer mothers to them. Alison Spiro (1984) describes how NCT counsellors can work together with midwives and health visitors to help give women emotional and practical support. These organisations do tend, however, to have a bias towards catering for the more articulate and middle class mothers.

Enabling, and avoiding discouragement. Caroline Flint (1984) highlights the fact that breastfeeding is an intimate experience between two very individual people and, to a certain extent, one which they will naturally have to work out for themselves. She sees the role of the professional as an 'enabler' — offering a great deal of encouragement — and avoiding the symbols of impending failure: bottles of water or test weighing.

In the community, the 'symbol of failure' might easily be a sample packet of infant milk food. Bergamin et al (1983) studied the effect of giving mothers samples of formula feed. They found this tended to shorten the duration of breastfeeding, especially for first time mothers, the less well educated and mothers who had suffered some small illness postnatally. Complementary 'topping up' feeds at night have been found to tend to undermine breastfeeding and mothers' confidence (Houston & Howie, 1981).

Siblings

The arrival of a new baby necessitates adjustment for everyone within the family circle. There is a need for each family member to be involved with and supportive of the others and this is no less true for the children. Claire Rayner (1977, pp. 44–46) describes how they can feel. She stresses the normality of sibling jealousy and makes practical suggestions for ways in which problems might be prevented or, at least, minimised.

It is interesting to note that in Dunn and Kendrick's (1982) small in-depth study of the relationship between siblings, breastfeeding a second baby did not create jealousy in the first born. For whatever reason, the siblings in this sample were less likely to interfere and irritate when their mothers were breastfeeding the baby than were those whose mothers were bottle feeding.

During visits to a family with a new baby, health visitors tend to give special attention to older brothers or sisters, so that they also feel important and included.

Father: mother

Research on the way fathers can be affected is mentioned by Maureen Laryea (1984). The arrival of a baby, particularly the first, means a significant change in their way of life — changing routines, greater responsibilities and, alongside this, less of their wives' attention devoted entirely to themselves.

The father's active involvement with the children can be an important factor in the support of his wife, as well as in the benefit both he and the children have from it. It is good if the father is at home during the health visitor's call, as he can then be involved in the discussions and explanations.

Parenthood and sexuality

Loss of sexual interest is not at all uncommon amongst women during the first year after the baby is born. Claire Rayner (1977, pp. 14–17) suggests several possible reasons for a woman losing libido at this time:

- current satisfaction
- hormonal changes
- tiredness
- damage creating pain
- fear of pregnancy
- fear of failure
- other psychological problems.

She describes the Masters and Johnson 'sensate focus' exercises, which many couples may find very helpful to know about.

Some practical advice on sexuality and breastfeeding is provided by Maire Messenger (1982) — discussions about feelings whilst feeding, the possibility of breasts leaking whilst love-making and a caution about contraception.

The various methods of family planning have been brought together in *The Which? Guide to Birth Control* (Kane, 1983). Rose Shapiro (1984) provides a brief overview. She reminds nurses that they need to be as aware as possible of the influence in discussions of their own bias and prejudices, and that they need to be sensitive not only to what people know, but also how they feel about various methods of contraception.

These, then, are just some of the mental and emotional factors which a family may wish to discuss with the health visitor. Also, at this stage a health visitor might be thinking of the possibility of a future postnatal depression. It tends to affect a larger number of women some twelve weeks after the birth and is therefore included in Chapter 5 (pp. 89; 98).

SOCIAL ASPECTS OF HEALTH

Families' social needs tie in closely, of course, with their emotional needs for communication and support. Health visitors, as the professional people most closely involved with young families, are in a good position to be able to offer help where it is needed.

Mother and father: family network

Immediate and close family are usually the main sources of help for babysitting, shopping, advice, acting as confidant and all the other aspects of support that are needed when the children are small. Many young parents, however, move a significant distance away from their parents' home. To supplement the help they can give each other, they need assistance from a circle of friends and/or from community organisations.

Mother

Loneliness and isolation can be major problems for young mothers. Some women have no difficulty in finding supportive neighbours and joining friendship groups, whereas others can be more shy and need help to find friends. People with young children and with no one to turn to for support, should be considered an important priority.

Gillian Pugh (1980) suggested that health visitors, on their first call, should take a list of all the locally available schemes and services offering help and support to young families. It is not known how many already do so. She also suggested that lists of services should be clearly displayed in such places as clinics and doctors' waiting rooms.

Mothers may wish to know about organisations and services such as:

- local church groups
- National Childbirth Trust
- National Housewives Register
- mother and baby groups
- keep fit classes
- community centres
- mother and toddler groups
- babysitting services
- out of hours services from health visitors
- telephone contact for worried and stressed parents.

First time mothers and those newly moved in, need to know about the health care facilities at local child health clinics. At this visit, the health visitor can tell them about times, days, alternatives available, whether they are organised with a crèche to entertain the toddlers and if they provide facilities where mothers can meet for a cup of tea and a chat. Many health visitors are involved in setting up mothers' groups in order to help provide both for social and health educational requirements, a matter returned to in the following chapter.

Siblings

If their parents know where to find

- mother and toddler groups
- playgroups
- nurseries

toddlers' social needs, as well as the mothers', can be helped to be satisfied. These facilities should also be included on the listing described above. Keeping the list of mother and toddler groups up to date can sometimes be difficult, but is obviously well worthwhile.

Many pregnant mothers like to see the older children settled into this sort of group well before the arrival of the baby. Others wait until the newness of the baby's arrival has worn off to avoid possible feelings of exclusion.

We have been looking at some of the physical, mental/emotional and social health needs of the members of a family with a new baby and at some of the ways in which a health visitor might be able to help during a first visit after the birth.

ARRANGING FURTHER VISITS

If parents know in advance when the health visitor is likely to call again and at which clinics they will probably be able to talk with 'their' health visitor, they can then prepare questions, knowing when and where help is available, and can plan to use the service in the way that suits them best.

In some areas, a day-time health visiting telephone contact service is provided and, in a few, a seven day health visiting service has been set up. Parents need to have their attention drawn to such services, where they exist, and to be given the telephone numbers involved. Research into an out-of-hours telephone advisory service in Bristol found it to be much needed and well used (Angel et al, 1990). Generally, health visitors have a visiting card with their office telephone number and address on it and, before they leave, inform the parents of the times they can be contacted personally.

Priorities

Where health visitors are unable to visit every family equally, they have to decide who should take precedence in their visiting schedule. Some of the families who would be considered an impor-

tant priority will be met in subsequent chapters, for example, families with a handicapped baby or who have recently immigrated. Some people who would have priority, such as those who have extra difficulty in adjusting to parenthood or who are socially isolated, have already received a mention, though rather briefly, in this and the previous chapter.

Guidance for health visitor priority also comes from the evidence of the Black (1980) Report and other studies which have demonstrated the problem of higher levels of ill-health amongst people from the lower socio-economic groups and yet their lower use of the health services.

It can sometimes be very difficult to respond to this need. The problem is most common in inner city areas and this is where health visitors are more likely to be coping with double caseloads on account of staff shortages and an above average turnover of staff. The problem presents a special challenge. Inner city health visiting and homelessness are the subjects of later chapters where we look at the community perspective in our work.

Sometimes particular circumstances regarding the baby lead the health visitor to give an above average priority to visiting a family. For example, parents of babies recently discharged from the special care baby unit will need extra support. Added to this, the health visitor will need to have assigned time to getting up to date on and becoming familiar with the care of low birth weight babies (Amick, 1984). This becomes less necessary when a specialist community nurse from the unit undertakes home visiting.

Another example of such a priority for more frequent follow-up visiting, would be that of multiple births. Twins occur in about one in eighty pregnancies. They take a great deal of time and ingenuity, particularly in the early days, and there are special problems involved in their care. Parents, especially the mother, need extra help and support (Bryan, 1983; Linney, 1980; Stables, 1980; Haigh, 1989; Sadler, 1989). Books on the care of twins may prove helpful to the parents (Leigh, 1983; Friedrich & Rowland, 1983). The opportunity to be told about such books antenatally, would be preferable, of course.

Choosing priorities for visiting is a complex matter as there are so many factors involved. It is helpful to parents to know to what extent the service is available to them and, for many, to know when to expect the next visit.

In this chapter we have looked at the health visitor's first visit to a family after the birth of their baby. Some behind-the-scenes preparations and considerations were described and some of the matters that may be discussed at a birth visit were classified under physical, mental/emotional and social aspects of family health need.

USEFUL ADDRESSES

Cry-sis, British Monomark Cry-sis,
London WC1N 3XX
Tel 071 404 5011

Foundation for the Study of Infant
Deaths,
5th Floor 4/5 Grosvenor Place,
London SW1X 7HD

La Leche League (Great Britain)
Breastfeeding Help and Information,
BM 3424 London WC1V 6XX
Tel 071 242 1278

National Childbirth Trust,
9 Queensborough Terrace,
London W2 3TB
Tel 071 221 3833

National Housewives Register,
National Office,
245 Warwick Road, Solihull,
West Midlands B92 7AH
Tel 021 706 1101

Scottish Health Education Group,
Woodburn House,
Canaan Lane,
Edinburgh EH10 4SQ

Still Birth and Neonatal Death Society
28 Portland Place
London W1N 3DE
Tel 071 436 5881

Twins Club Association
Mrs D Hoseason (sec) 'Pooh Corner',
54 Broad Lane, Hampton,
Middlesex

Twins and Multiple Births Association
c/o Jenny Smith
41 Fortuna Way
Aylesbury Park
Grimsby
Humberside DN37 9SJ

REFERENCES

Amick J H 1984 Support for parents of babies in special care units. Midwives Chronicle and Nursing Notes 97: 170–175

Angel S, Nicoll J, Amatiello W 1990 Assessing the need for an out-of-hours telephone advisory service. Health Visitor 63, 7: 225–227

Bellman M H, Ross E M, Miller D L 1983 Infantile spasms and pertussis immunisation. The Lancet I: 1031–1034

Bergamin Y, Dougherty C, Kramer M S 1983 Do infant formula samples shorten the duration of feeding? The Lancet I: 1148–1151

Black D 1980 Inequalities in health. Report of a research working party. Department of Health and Social Security, London (chairman Sir Douglas Black)

Bowler I C J, Mandal B K, Schlecht B, Riordan T 1988 Diphtheria, the continuing hazard. Archives of Disease in Childhood 63, 2: 194–195

Bowling A 1983 Teamwork in primary health care. Nursing Times 79, 48: 56–59

Brown J 1984 I can't love my child. Parents 100, 7: 80–81

Bryan E 1983 Twins in the family. Nursing Times 79, 28: 50–52

Cameron J 1988 Countdown to immunity. Nursing Times 84, 37: 20

Cunningham K T, Beningfield S A, Moulton A, Maddock C R 1984a A clicking hip should never be ignored. The Lancet I: 668–670

Cunningham K T, Beningfield S A, Moulton A, Maddock C R 1984b A clicking hip should never be ignored (letter). The Lancet I: 1184–1185

Curtis Jenkins G, Newton R C F 1981 The first year of life. Churchill Livingstone, Edinburgh, pp 36–38; 71–77

David T J, Poynor M U, Simm S A, Parris M R, Hawnaur J M, Rigg E A, McCrae F C 1983 Reasons for late detection of hip dislocation in childhood. The Lancet II: 147–148

Davidson S, Alden L, Davidson P 1981 Changes in alcohol consumption after childbirth. Journal of Advanced Nursing 116: 195–198

DHSS 1980a Prevention in the child health services. Department of Health and Social Security, London

DHSS 1980b Present day practice in infant feeding. HMSO, London

Downing L J and Howkins E J 1984 Infant feeding in practice. Nursing Times 80, 6: 57–60

Draper J, Farmer S, Field S, Thoms H, Hare M J 1984 The working relationship between the general practitioner and the health visitor. Journal of the Royal College of General Practitioners 34: 264–268

Dunn J, Kendrick C 1982 Siblings. Love, envy and understanding. Grant McIntyre, London, p 49–51

Dunnell K, Dobbs J 1982 Nurses working in the community. HMSO, London

Fagin L, Little M 1984 The forsaken families. The effects of unemployment on family life. Penguin Books, Harmondsworth

Fixen J 1983 Congenital dislocation of the hip and club foot in the young child. Health Visitor 56: 281–283

Flint C 1984 Midwives and breastfeeding. Nursing Times 80, 15: 30–31

Friedrich E, Rowland C 1983 The twins handbook. From prebirth to first school days — a parents' guide. Robson Books, London

Goodwin S 1982 HV — by appointment only. Nursing Mirror 155, 2: 19

Grant E, Golightly P W 1984 Providing an information service on drugs and breast milk. Journal of the Royal Society of Health 104: 99–101

Green A, Macfarlane A 1985 Parent-held child health records — a comparison of types. Health Visitor 58: 14–15

Griffiths D M 1984 The health visitor and the foreskin. Health Visitor 57: 275

Gunn A 1983 Why you need a post-natal check. Mother and Baby March: 38–39

Haigh J 1989 Caring for twins. Nursing Times 85, 18: 62

Health Education Council 198(1) Play it safe! A guide to preventing children's accidents. Health Education Council and Scottish Health Education Group in association with BBC

Health Education Council 1984 Pregnancy book. A guide to becoming pregnant, being pregnant and caring for your newborn baby. Health Education Council, London, p 70–72

Health Visitor 1981 Present day practice in infant feeding: 1980 New revised version of 1974 Oppé Report. Health Visitor 54: 179

Health Visitor 1989 Proper training and clear legal guidelines essential. Health Visitor 62: 233

Hopkins J 1988 Problems in bonding: helping parents who do not love their infants. Health Visitor 61: 107

Houston M J 1984a Home support for the breast feeding mother. In: Houston M J (ed) Maternal and infant health care. Churchill Livingstone, Edinburgh

Houston M J 1984b Supporting breast feeding at home. Midwives Chronicle and Nursing Notes 97: 42–44

Houston M J, Howie P W 1981 The importance of support for the breast feeding mother at home. Health Visitor 54: 243–244

Illingworth R S 1982 Basic developmental screening: 0–4 years, 3rd ed. Blackwell Scientific Publications, Oxford, p 38–40

Jeffs J 1983 Happy bottle-feeding. Mother and Baby March: 40–42

Jelley D M, Nicoll A G 1984 Pertussis: what percentage of children can we immunise? British Medical Journal 288: 1582–1584

Jenkinson D 1982 Immunisation. In: Hart C (ed) Child care in general practice. Churchill Livingstone, Edinburgh

Joint Committee on Vaccination and Immunisation 1988 Immunisation against infectious disease. Department of Health and Social Security, Welsh Office and Scottish Home and Health Department. HMSO, London

Jolly H 1981 Baby and Child Care. The complete guide for today's parents, 3rd edn. Allen and Unwin, London

Jones D A 1989 Importance of the clicking hip in screening for congenital dislocation of the hip. The Lancet I, 8638: 599–601

Kane P 1983 The Which? guide to birth control. Consumers Association and Hodder & Stoughton, London

Kelly M 1983 Will mothers breast feed longer if health visitors give more support? Health Visitor 56: 407–409

Laryea M G G 1984 Postnatal care. The midwife's role. Churchill Livingstone, Edinburgh, pp 64–66, 69–71

Leach P 1989 Baby and child. From birth to age five. Penguin Books, Harmondsworth

Leigh G 1983 All about twins. A handbook for parents. Routledge and Kegan Paul, London

Lewis P J and Hurden E L 1983 Drugs and breastfeeding In: Hawkins D F (ed) Drugs and pregnancy. Human teratogenisis and related problems. Churchill Livingstone, Edinburgh, p 217–218

Linney J 1980 The emotional and social aspects of having twins. Nursing Times 76: 276–279

McClymont A 1983 Setting standards in health visiting practice. National Board for Nursing, Midwifery and Health Visiting for Scotland, Edinburgh

McMaster M J 1983 Infantile ideopathic scoliosis: can it be prevented? Journal of Bone and Joint Surgery 65-B: 612–617

Messenger M 1982 The breastfeeding book. Century Publishing Co Ltd, London, p 94–100

Midwife Health Visitor & Community Nurse 1985 Jottings by Janus. Midwife Health Visitor & Community Nurse 21: 149

Monk C J E, Dowd G S E 1981 The problems of early diagnosis and prevention of congenital dislocation of the hip. Journal of Maternal and Child Health 6: 76–85

Pollock T M, Mortimer J Y, Miller E, Smith G 1984 Symptoms after primary immunisation with DPT and with DT vaccine. The Lancet II: 146–149

Pugh G (ed) 1980 Preparation for parenthood. Some current initiatives and thinking. National Children's Bureau, London, p 37

Ray G 1984 Probing postnatal check-ups. Mother April: 42–43

Rayner C 1977 Family feelings. Arrow Books Ltd, London

Robertson C A 1984 Preventive health care for infants. In: Houston M J (ed) Maternal and infant health care. Churchill Livingstone, Edinburgh

Robertson J, Robertson J 1982 A baby in the family. Loved and being loved. Penguin Books, Harmondsworth

Robson K M, Powell E 1982 Early maternal attachment. In: Brockington I F, Kumar R (eds) Motherhood and mental illness. Academic Press, London

Sadler C 1989 Double trouble. Nursing Times 85, 14: 28–31

Scowen P (ed) 1984 New baby. A health visitor's handbook for parents. B Edsall and Co Ltd, London, p 63

Shapiro R 1984 Putting the sex back into contraception. Nursing Times Community Outlook 80, 15: 123–131

Smith J W G 1983 Interrupted immunisation. Archives of Disease in Childhood 58: 167

Spiro A 1984 Counsellors can help. Nursing Times Community Outlook 80, 38: 314–316

Stables J 1980 Breastfeeding twins. Nursing Times 76: 1493–1494

Swaffield L 1983 Clean babies. Nursing Times Community Outlook 79, 51: 369–371

Valman H B 1982 Whooping cough. British Medical Journal 284: 886–887

Waight P A, Pollock T M, Miller E, Coleman E M 1983 Pyrexia after diphtheria/tetanus vaccines. Archives of Disease in Childhood 58: 921–933

Wells N 1984 Childhood vaccination, current controversies. Office of Health Economics, London

Wilkinson J A 1983 Your child's congenital dislocation of the hip: a guide to parents. The author, Southampton General Hospital, Southampton

Worth C 1984 Breastfeeding basics. Unwin Paperback, London

FURTHER READING

Bell I 1990 Testicular self-examination. Nursing Times 86, 9: 38–40 — Men's health.

Darbyshire P 1987 Danger Man. Nursing Times 83, 48: 30–32 — Health consequences of men's lifestyle.

Health Visitors' Association 1988 Guidance to members on vaccination and immunisation. Health Visitors' Association, London

Kohner N 1989 Birth to five. A guide to the first five years of being a parent. Harper and Row, London — Available free for all first-time parents, from the local health education and promotion units.

Price B 1987 What did you do in the home, Daddy? Nursing Times 83, 48: 27–30 — Men's health

Reynolds M W, Hay H S W 1986 Health visiting by appointment. Health Visitor 59, 8: 252–256

Scháufele B 1988 Teaching testicular self-examination. Professional Nurse 3, 10: 409–411 — Men's health.

Sefi S, MacFarlane A 1989 Immunizing children. Oxford University Press, Oxford

Standing Medical Advisory Committee (Chairman M A Wilson) 1989 Drinking problems. A challenge for every doctor. DHSS, London

Swaffield L 1987 Gardening can damage your health. Nursing Times 83, 28: 16–17 — Men's health.

Trevelyan J 1989 Well men. Nursing Times 85, 12: 46–47 — Men's health

Willis A 1988 Singular dads. Nursing Times 84, 29: 47–49 — Men's health.

Chapter 5 looks at the part played by a health visitor in preventive health care for a family with very young children. The work is considered through the perspective of the prevention model. Ways in which help may be given are classified in three groupings: strategies aiming to prevent the occurrence of health problems, those to prevent their development and, thirdly, those to prevent deterioration of established conditions.

5

Families with young children

USING THE PREVENTION MODEL

In these next two chapters, we look at the sort of contribution that the prevention model can make to planning and describing health visiting. This is demonstrated by taking the phase which follows the birth visit, that is, work with families who have children under school age. In this chapter, we look at anticipatory guidance, screening procedures and supportive care for families with babies and children up to about the age of three. Looking at such a wide section of a health visitor's work in only a chapter, means a great deal must be left out. However, it does give an indication of the sort of work entailed and a chance to look briefly at some of the important factors involved.

The prevention framework was the model most fully introduced in Chapter 1 (see pp. 5–8). It will be recalled that facets of the health visitor's role were pigeon-holed into three aspects of prevention:

— *preventing the occurrence* of potential future problems, such as by immunising babies against whooping cough in order to avoid the possibility of unfortunate side-effects of the disease, or, as another example, by promoting good health through health education.
— *preventing the development* of difficulties or handicapping conditions through early discovery and appropriate action. For example, finding deafness in a baby early enables timely use of hearing aids and special teaching and leads to the best

possible development of speech.
— *preventing deterioration* of established conditions or circumstances by helping people cope with and/or overcome, for example, babies' sleep and feeding problems. The aim is that a greater dysfunction does not develop out of the current situation and that, so far as is possible, it is improved.

Table 5.1 Families with very young children: the health visitor's work

Aspect of prevention	Examples of activities	Important considerations
Preventing occurrence of condition (Anticipatory guidance)	*Discussion of:* family diet, smoking safety, breast cancer, immunisation, sleeping, play 'discipline', tooth care, illness, recognition	Parental involvement Promotes self-confidence 'Family visiting' Reach those in need Querying own advice Querying own practice
Preventing development of condition (Surveillance of family health)	*Screening re:* postnatal depression, developmental progress, hearing, vision and speech, weight, length and head circumference, hip dislocation, special schemes	Accessible treatment Early discovery Physical and general welfare Search *and* teach Parental involvement Reach those in need Review monitoring
Preventing deterioration of established condition (Supportive work)	*Sympathetic listening; Information about services; Encouraging self-help groups;* re: common baby and childhood problems, isolation and lack of confidence, postnatal depression, bereavement	Support and teach Availability of service Individual initiative Congeniality of clinic Strategies for problems: • wide-ranging • more rare

This approach, which in essence describes the reasons why the work is undertaken, is particularly useful for looking at our work, both over a range of time and from a case-load-wide perspective.

The family health needs framework of the previous two chapters is rather more useful for looking at what factors need to be considered at a single or at a particular type of visit.

The presentation of the prevention framework in this chapter, shown in Table 5.1, has been modified a little from that in Table 1.2. This is to make space for listing important considerations pertaining to the work, such as availability of the service or parental involvement, whilst still leaving room in the table for lists of the basic health visitor activities.

It may be found helpful if we can start by giving a couple of examples of a health visitor's work with a family and show how this framework can highlight important factors.

EXAMPLES OF WORK WITH FAMILIES WITH VERY YOUNG CHILDREN

The first example outlines some of the work of a health visitor with a couple in their first two years as parents. The other example is of a health visitor in an inner city area, and gives a brief overview of her work with a disadvantaged young family. The factors mentioned are listed in the prevention format, in Tables 5.2 and 5.3.

EXAMPLE ONE: THE FORESTS

Mrs Honor Vincent (HV) had very vivid memories of her early visits to the Forest family. She had just completed her health visitor course and their first baby, Sarah, was the first birth visit on her new caseload. They had had no antenatal visit. In order to give them something of a quick overview of her work with young families, she had shown them the Nelms and Mullens list (see Box 5.2) photostatted for her studies. The Forests had encouraged her to keep it in her bag. It proved, at several of the visits, to be a useful trigger to some pertinent questioning, for example on stimulation and family diet, by the parents and particularly over safety at each phase of development. They enjoyed being able to look, with her, at a phase or two ahead and they said it made them search

Table 5.2 Example one: the Forests

Aspect of prevention	Examples of activities	Important considerations
Preventing occurrence of condition (Anticipatory guidance)	*Discussion of:* immunisation, safety, stimulation family diet	Promote self-confidence Parental involvement 'Family visiting
Preventing development of condition (Surveillance of family health)	*Screening re:* **mother:** postnatal depression **daughter:** hearing, vision, weight developmental progress and head circumference **son:** special scheme	Accessible care Early discovery Search and teach Parental involvement Service reviewed
Preventing deterioration of established condition (Supportive work)	*Sympathetic listening; Information about vol. groups re:* Sleep problem — book lent Postnatal depression — ref. NCT Crying baby service	Support *and* teach Strategy for support service available

things out in the baby manuals they had been given.

The father was usually at home for the visits. He was a night worker, and they chose appointments in the morning so he could join in. Both parents were amused by the lists of hints on whether or not the baby could hear and see, and found them fun to try out. They did not wish to attend the baby clinic and weighed their baby at the chemist, taking a spare set of clothes to weigh in order to be able to deduce the naked weight. They filled in a centile chart themselves and had promised to call into the clinic or ring HV if they were worried. In the event, they did not need to. Also, they did not use the 'crying baby' service, run on a rota basis by some of the health visitors.

There had been a rather worrying patch when, eight weeks postnatally, Mrs Forest's self-assessment questionnaire had shown her, as she had felt, to be depressed. However, both a fortnight and four weeks later, she was seen

to be gradually returning to normal, as she became less restless at night and less despondent and less irritable. She had, however, followed up HV's suggestion and contacted the National Childbirth Trust (NCT) and had said she intended to remain with the group. Mrs Forest was evidently grateful to be able to pour out her feelings, both with the NCT counsellor and with HV. Follow-up assessments showed no problems. The scheme had done what it was intended to do and had alerted the parents and the health visitor to the possibility of postnatal depression. The health visitor was glad that, in this small town environment, her caseload pressures were light enough to enable more frequent visiting, eight times in the first year.

The eighteen month visit had been the most recent one. They had checked Sarah's developmental progress, talked over measles vaccination and the Forests had proudly shown HV their latest safety devices and schemes. They had reported that Sarah's sleeping habits had become unacceptable, and HV had lent them her copy of 'My Child Won't Sleep' which they returned to her through the surgery two weeks later. Mrs Forest had said she was two months pregnant.

Today the practice midwife had told HV that Mrs Forest had had a premature birth and a small baby boy. This baby was likely to qualify as 'high risk' in the newly set up infant surveillance scheme and would be scheduled for weekly weighing until he reached 3 kg or the expected date of delivery, whichever were the later. Mrs Vincent was grateful she now had her own portable baby weighing scales to take with her to the home. She had planned anyway to make extra visits as Mrs Forest had been determined to breastfeed this baby and had previously had postnatal depression. In the event, baby Mark progressed well and Mrs Forest showed no indication of a repeat of the depression.

EXAMPLE TWO: THE LAMBOURNES

The Lambournes were moving to another part of the city and, as Hazel Vickery (HV) glanced through their records before sending them on to the next health visitor, she was reminded of the change of attitude in her client.

At both the antenatal and the birth visit, Mrs Lambourne had been rather deferential and seemed unconfident. The health visitor found herself wishing that she had been trained in the skills employed in the Child Development

Table 5.3 Example two: the Lambournes

Aspect of prevention:	Examples of activities	Important considerations
Preventing occurrence of condition (Anticipatory guidance)	*Discussion of:* Safety, stimulation (Deferential mother) New scheme set up	Promote confidence Parental involvement Querying own practice Reach those in need
Preventing development of condition (Surveillance of family health)	*Screening re:* Weight and head circumference, developmental progress, hearing and speech Vision — re amblyopia: orthoptist seen	Search *and* teach Parental involvement Early discovery Accessible treatment
Preventing deterioration of established condition (Supportive work)	Sympathetic listening; Encouraging self-help groups; re: Loneliness — local women's group Clinic	Strategy for problem Individual initiative Attempt to improve

Projects and knew a few more tips on how to help parents take the initiative in their discussions.

During the next visit HV had shown and discussed the leaflet 'You Know More Than You Think You Do', following up an interest expressed by the mother. She was beginning to suspect the mother could not read, and when at six weeks HV had shown Mrs Lambourne the four aspects of development listed in the stepladder centile charts, she felt pretty sure. She always took care after that, casually, to read aloud things like the phases of development and the lists of 'hints for parents' or any papers they were studying.

Looking together at the developmental centile charts led on to discussions, particularly about stimulation and safety, and gradually Mrs Lambourne gained the confidence to state and expand on her own view. When they went through the nine month assessment tests together and chatted about the next phase of developments, Mrs Lambourne mentioned how much fun her husband was having 'romping' in

the evenings with their baby son. They had bought second-hand gates and a fireguard.

Mrs Lambourne had attended the clinic which was very formally set up, just once. Around that time HV had tried, unsuccessfully, to get the rest of the staff involved in their draughty church hall clinic to agree to a rearrangement to try to make it more welcoming and 'social', and had finally decided she needed to find another solution. She had talked with the GPs in the practice about the isolation and loneliness of women, particularly those such as Mrs Lambourne, on a marginal income and living some distance from their families.

One of the GPs was very sympathetic and persuaded the others to allow the use of an upstairs room once a fortnight for a self-help group, provided HV was prepared to act as background support for it. It was decided it should have a three months trial period. Now, it had been going for a year: the group showed no signs of lack of support and the slow beginnings had been well worth weathering.

The members of the group had picked up issues that caused them concern, and, as they had gained in confidence, had determined together to do something about them. Their latest campaign had been for safety around their blocks of flats, particularly aiming at limiting motor access and in setting up play areas for the young children. They had invited two of their local councillors to come and join them and had shown them a health education film that helped make their point about local safety needs. They had found the road safety officer from the environmental health department very helpful. Mrs Lambourne said she had not realised just how much could be achieved by contacting and talking with such people, and that it was fun working with the other members of the group.

The most recent incident on her card referred to the fact that the Lambournes had been playing with their son and they found he reacted against one of his eyes being covered over. They had been trying out 'helpful hints on vision' and felt he might have a squint. It was in the family. A secondary screening service was available at the orthoptists clinic which meant they would not have to wait on a long waiting list to see the ophthalmologist. Reduced vision in one eye was confirmed, an early case of amblyopia which would need attention. Fortunately the house to which the Lambournes were moving would be within walking distance of the hospital and so trips to visit the orthoptist's clinic would not prove as expensive as bus fares from their current flat.

ANTICIPATORY GUIDANCE

The greater amount of most health visitors' time is taken up with trying to help parents of babies and very young children avoid future potential problems. Health education is undertaken in various ways and is included in work in clinics, in the home and in group work; it is interwoven into screening sessions and supportive care, and provided in special projects.

Many of the topics discussed with parents can be found in well-known manuals and are not repeated here because they could only be covered in a very shallow way. Some of these books are listed in Box 5.1. They are the sort that might be recommended to parents and that some health visitors keep available in their cars to help in giving anticipatory guidance.

In this section we shall look at some of the issues that health visitors need to think about when plan-

ning and undertaking this aspect of their work, such as helping people to know some of the details about aims and intentions, so that the service can be used better; the need to boost morale; discriminatory provision of the service in favour of those with greatest need; and questioning one's day to day advice and practice.

Parental involvement

If parents can have a fair understanding of the way in which the health visitor is aiming to help, then it is much easier for them to make good use of the service. There are some lists available that give an outline of the sort of matters that are of concern in health visiting. Examples will be found on page 80, Box 5.2. Some health visitors find that one or two of these make useful visual aids when they are telling parents about the wide range of topics discussed in the course of their work. The main disadvantage of these papers is that, in them, concern is centred entirely upon the child.

Box 5.1 Books which might be recommended to parents of very young children

Green C
Toddler Taming
A parent's guide to the first four years
Century Publishing, 1984

Scottish Health Education Group
The Book of the Child
Pregnancy to 4 years old
2nd edn
Scottish Health Education Unit, 1980

Rayner C
Family Feelings
Understanding your child from 0 to 5
Arrow Books, 1977

Scowen P (ed)
New Baby Growing Up
Edsall & Co Ltd, 1981

Scarr S & Dunn J
Mother care/other care
Penguin Books, 1988

Leach P
Baby and Child
Penguin Books, 1989

Jolly H
Book of Child Care
The complete guide for today's parents
Sphere Books, 1981

Douglas J & Richman N
My Child Won't Sleep
Penguin Books, 1984

Koch J
Superbaby
Over 300 exercises and games to stimulate your baby's intellectual, physical and emotional development
Orbis Publishing Ltd, 1982

Asher J
Keep your baby safe
Penguin Books, 1988

Box 5.2 Lists showing areas of concern in preventive health care for children under three years

Book	Lists	Indicates
Nelms B C & Mullins R G *Growth and Development* A Primary Health Care Approach Prentice Hall Inc, 1982	pp. 70–73	The sort of background information sought; a range of possible tests; interest in feeding, safety and development; possible anticipatory guidance
Ingalls A J & Salerno M C *Maternal and Child Health Nursing* C V Mosby Company, 1983	pp. 328–341	Physical, motor and language development, listed along with photographs; a range of possible anticipatory guidance; some psychosocial factors
Sheridan M D *The Developmental Progress of Infants and Young Children* HMSO, 1975	Most of booklet	Wide range of developmental stepping-stones listed under: posture and large movements; vision and fine movements; hearing and speech; social behaviour and play
Sheridan M D *Children's Developmental Progress*. From Birth to Five Years: the Stycar Sequences NFER Publishing, 1975	Most of book	Similar information to booklet above with clear line drawings demonstrating attainments and hearing and vision tests
Lee C *The Growth and Development of Children* 3rd edn Longman, 1984	pp.170–183	Child's physical development; his feelings; social behaviour and his needs
	pp. 190–191	Some suggested play materials
Pringle M K *The Needs of Children* Hutchinson, 1974	p. 159	'Ten child care commandments' — aspects of children's needs

Also, by looking at child care so intensely, they may give the impression that health visitors have a vision of and hope for 'ideal parenthood' in the people they visit.

A morale boosting, family visitor!

Excellent antidotes to misconceptions about perfect motherhood or parenting, can be found by referring parents to the booklets 'Now you're a family' and 'You know more than you think you do' (see Table 4.1) and the book by Claire Rayner (1977). Perhaps, even better, is another book for parents called *Toddler Taming* by Dr Christopher Green (1984). It is well presented and amusing, as well as giving very practical advice, and looks fairly and squarely at *parental* needs when confronted with the vagaries of a robust and energetic toddler.

This book covers many matters of importance to health visitors. For example, Dr Green points out that there are no 'right answers' and aims to boost parents' confidence. He tells his readers to beware of books and advisers that set unattainably high goals — and consequently generate feelings of parental inadequacy. A brief history tells how deviant behaviour in the last century was felt to be caused by 'bad breeding', and was later explained, eventually in an extreme form in the 1950s, by 'poor environment'. The doctor explains how, at that time, blame was put on the mothers, consequently giving them enormous feelings of guilt and unhappiness. He warns that some 'helping professionals', still guided by the 'archaic ideas of the 50s', cannot give practical advice without psychoanalysing the parents (Green, 1984, pp. 9, 23–30)! The advice given by Dr Green, in contrast, recognises that some children are more difficult than others and gives parents many useful ideas on how to encourage 'good' and cope with 'bad' behaviour.

Naturally, most health education for families with very young children centres around child care. It tends, therefore, to detract from the image of the health visitor as one concerned with the health of the whole family. The balance is restored a little when subjects are discussed which directly concern other members of the family. An example of this could be asking a mother if she wishes to know about self-examination of the breast (Laurence, 1983; Dening, 1983; Rowden, 1983; Nichols, 1983; Anstoker & Humphreys, 1988). Chapter 4's further reading list included some examples of men's health topics.

Greatest need

An important aspect to be considered is the extent to which the service is provided for those who need it most. Initiatives are necessary to make provision for the people who do not tend to use the standard services. This matter was touched on in Chapter 3 (p. 38). The Child Development Project (1984) was mentioned with regard to antenatal care. In the postnatal period, the specially assigned health visitor calls on each family monthly for six months or so and stays for about an hour at each visit. An assessment is made of recent nutrition, and pamphlets and recipes are available for the parents. The child's health and development are noted. The service is provided in this first, most critical period of parenthood, and is being given to first time parents to get maximum benefit for the family. Good use is made of humour, through cartoons, and the parents are encouraged to contribute to the pool of ideas.

There were 600 'intervention' and 400 control families taking part in this stage of the research project. The work has, of course, been more successful with some families than with others. However, a general pattern is emerging of a greater awareness by 'intervention' mothers of development and good nutrition and of an alertness in their children (Child Development Project, 1984; Barker and Anderson, 1988). Health visitors are very appreciative of these encouraging developments (Cranshaw, 1984; Fairs, 1984; Percy, 1984). Discussions and papers from a national conference of the Child Development Programme provide an up-to-date view (Barker et al, 1987).

The Black (1980, p. 108) Report found evidence that went against the commonly held view that health visitors visit everyone equally without regard to positive discrimination in favour of people in particular need. It seems that looking at 'class' or 'father's occupation' alone gives a distorted view. They describe a study in Glamorgan and in South West England, which found that, when factors such as local social amenities, overcrowding and parental education were taken into consideration, the 'disadvantaged' tended to receive more health visits right through the first three years.

This same Report noted that accidents account for one third of deaths in children, and show a strong class differential (Black, 1980). It is obviously an important matter for preventive health care. The Report suggests that there is much that can be done without great cost to the public to improve the safety of children. Health visitors might try, locally, to 'influence policies affecting health' (CETHV, 1977), perhaps with the help of the Child Accident Prevention Trust, an organisation which undertakes research and is concerned with influencing decision-makers and their policies. Health visitors may know, for example, of low standards of safety in rented accommodation and unsafe areas for children to play, and liaison with environmental health officers, local councillors and voluntary organisations might help instigate improvements. The Trust is keen to hear from health visitors about locally-based activities in relation to child accident prevention (Child Accident Prevention Trust, 1989; Health Visitor, 1989).

Safety should be, of course, an important subject of discussion during health visits and other contacts (Health Education Council, 1981; Moore, 1982; Ray, 1982; Community Outlook, 1982; 1984; Ahamed, 1982; Laidman, 1987), and the effect of poverty on the ability of disadvantaged families to provide a safe environment needs special consideration. Colver and Pearson (1985) showed the value of knowing exactly what grants families on supplementary benefits were entitled to for stairgates, cookers and fire guards, and also where and at what cost safety items could be purchased. Their study showed that a small amount of well-informed, relevant guidance could be very effective. The social security benefits changes abolishing special payments for needy families will have affected this picture (Nursing Times, 1989).

Questioning common practice and advice

A great deal of the sort of advice that health visitors give on child care has not been, and in some cases cannot be, tested properly. Much of that found in the well-known child care manuals varies significantly. For example, there is little agreement between them on views about the use of dummies (Darbyshire, 1985). More 'scientifically'-based advice, such as that founded on 'evidence' about salt in the diet, is still open to controversy (The Economist, 1984; Johnson & Silman, 1985; Stretch, 1983). It seems best for health visitors to try to provide, in their discussions, information about the range of current ideas and to attempt to be as aware as possible of the extent to which these theories have been validated.

In many ways this lack of certainty helps to make it easier to develop a partnership between parent and professional. It also tends to put in perspective what some professionals see as 'non-compliance', where people continue to carry out their own ideas — despite the wonderful advice they have been given! The aim, of course, in health visiting is not to order people's behaviour, but to help them make informed decisions and then to support them in whatever choice they make. Health visitors can learn a great deal from the varied perspectives and the practical experiences of parents. Also, it pays to listen. Offering dogmatic advice which takes no account of the family's views is liable to generate antagonism. Even worse, it can lead to feelings of guilt and inadequacy on account of failure to comply with the instructions. These are very counter-productive and create an atmosphere in which it is most unlikely that there could be open discussion with the health visitor about the true situation.

All common practices need to be examined for their value and for their potential for counter-productivity. Questions are being raised, for example, about the propriety and the effect of health visitors giving out samples on behalf of the infant food manufacturers (Rowe, 1985; Stretch, 1983). The correlation between mothers being given milk samples and lowered rates of breastfeeding was noted in Chapter 4 (p. 68).

Rajan's (1985) small study of the result of giving away samples of babies' weaning foods at clinics, found it correlated with early weaning, again, the reverse of what is being advised as the best policy. There is a clear need for further research. Either way, health visitors do need to be fully aware of the extent to which they are being 'wooed' by baby product firms as a route through to persuading mothers to buy their goods. They need to think carefully, too, about the use of their professional position with regard to their giving that 'preferential consideration' (UKCC, 1984).

These, then, are just some of the issues that health visitors need to consider when planning and thinking about how to prevent the occurrence of problems and conditions, be it through liaison or through anticipatory guidance on matters such as nutrition, safety, and immunisation, for the families they visit.

SCREENING AND SURVEILLANCE

Trying to prevent the development of problems by discovering them early, comes into most aspects of a health visitor's work, both at the clinic and out on home visits. Weighing and measuring babies, searching out vision and hearing defects and surveillance of developmental progress and mothers' emotional health, provide some examples of this sort of work with families with very young children. It involves behind-the-scenes planning and evaluation as well as the more visible practical aspects of screening and surveillance.

BEHIND THE SCENES

There are many questions the primary health care

CONSIDERING WHETHER:
- (i) services available?
- (ii) responds to care?
- (iii) how many benefit?
- (iv) conditions' prevalence?
- (v) potentially disabling?
- (vi) reaches the needy?
- (vii) monitoring informative?

PLANNING SCREENING

Fig. 5.1 Some factors considered in planning screening.

team need to think about when planning and evaluating screening and surveillance programmes (see Fig. 5.1). Time should be set aside for this, to try to ensure that the service provided is the one most appropriate to local circumstances and needs. Some of the questions which may be considered are:

Are services available and accessible?

There is no point in discovering conditions that cannot be improved in any way, once they have been identified. Services may be provided, but there may be problems of geographic inaccessibility or of a long wait for treatment to be made available. Distance from the clinic is, of course, particularly important to the people least able to afford the bus fares and who do not own a car,

especially if they have more than one young child. Health visitor managers and administrators should be informed about clinics affected by travelling difficulties, so that some attempt can be made to provide clinics in the localities where this is known to be a common problem.

If the way cases are referred on to clinics is inadequate or the service is poorly organised, there may be delays in receiving treatment and its effectiveness may be diminished. Health visitors should know about alternative methods of referral and have some idea of the length of the waiting lists. For example, if a squint is discovered, the quickest form of referral is necessary, be it via the GP or straight through to the local eye department/specialist or the local optician. The length of time spent on the waiting list for the orthoptist or/and the consultant, is very important, as very lengthy delays may affect the way the condition responds to treatment. A year between first suspicions of a squint and seeing the specialist, does not seem to be unusual (Johnson, 1984). Where significant delays between discovery and treatment are found, liaison is needed to draw attention to the extent of the problem and to find appropriate solutions.

Will conditions improve with attention?

Consideration needs to be given as to whether problems are likely to be discovered early enough and also whether the degree of improvement is likely to justify the efforts involved. A hearing defect at nine months, for example, can affect the development of speech. The earlier the discovery, the more successful will be the outcome. Encouraging parental involvement in monitoring their children's ability to hear can maximise the chance of discovery (Latham & Haggard, 1980) and takes only a little time to explain (see Fig. 5.6).

Are there problems to justify the service?

Efforts to estimate what the service is likely to bring to light, help to clarify the objectives of the programmes being provided. If research on the epidemiological spread, for example, of vision or hearing defects is available, then this might provide benchmarks against which to plan these aspects of the programme and to compare results (Robertson, 1981). However, looking for medical defects is only one aspect of child surveillance programmes. Health visitors tend to consider a very wide range of features, such as a child's apparent nutritional state and any signs of illness, social aspects of development and indicators of emotional development. They note, for example, a baby's expression and eyes, its apparent relationship with its mother and whether it is alert, withdrawn or subdued (Connolly, 1983). We discuss more specifically the discovery of handicaps in babies and children in Chapter 9, especially on pages 173–174.

Are the problems potentially disabling?

It is only worth seeking to discover and treat problems that are potentially harmful in some way. Many screening programmes aim mainly to discover conditions which threaten life. This is not so in child health surveillance programmes, though such cases have been reported (Powell, 1985). The aim is, rather, to make an early discovery of factors that affect the quality of life, such as hearing and vision defects, developmental delay and social and emotional problems for the various members of the family.

The surveillance programme should also act as a teaching aid and promote parental awareness of the prerequisites for good health. In this way, it should help avoid the occurrence of potentially harmful situations at a later date. For example, assessment of a toddler's developmental progress may bring to light behavioural problems (Hewitt et al, 1989). Discussions at the screening session, and later parents' involvement in monitoring their child's developmental progress, may increase their understanding of the needs and limitations of their child. This, in turn, can help them think of better ways in which they might handle and give attention to their child. Thus the programme should help them avoid behavioural difficulties at a later stage, as well as helping them cope with the current minor problems. Walter Barker (1988)

suggests that health visitors specialise in helping parents develop the socialisation, stimulation and language of their children, which would contribute to overcoming social disability.

Does the programme reach those who need it?

It can be very time consuming to follow up people who either do not wish to, or who are unable to attend clinics. However, it is a very important aspect of surveillance and screening programmes. What is needed is to be able to make contact with these families, in order to explain the purpose of the programmes, offer the tests at home, and/or explain what the parents should be on the look-out for, so that serious problems will be found early. For example, missed vision or hearing defects in babyhood and childhood, can have very serious consequences for a child's ability to learn or to communicate later on. If long-standing problems are not being discovered until the children get to school, then the system is obviously failing.

It has been reported that children can remain unscreened due to shortages of staff, or due to triple duty nursing (health visiting combined with district nursing and midwifery) in which other work is given higher priority (Morris & Hird, 1981). Managers should, of course, be kept up to date on the extent to which inadequate staffing affects the service. However, methods of working out staffing levels such as those in Cheltenham are becoming available (Bell & Moules, 1985). It is important that any such scheme is able to provide indicators of the sort of social problems and the level of 'at risk' factors in the community assigned to each health visitor. The Portsmouth surveillance scheme (Powell, 1985), for example, can provide some indicators. This sort of information can also help managers to be fully aware of the sort of pressures their staff are under, and would, of course, provide some measure of the adequacy of service available to those who most need it.

Not everyone finds the currently provided services to their taste. Where people do not respond to invitations to clinics, it can be a very useful exercise to try to find out what it is that they find difficult or dislike about them. Jane Robinson's (1982) small study of non-attendance found that those who did not come, cared just as much about their children's welfare as those who did. Her study raised some very important questions about, for example, the provision of services, and further research of this sort is needed.

There is the question, too, as to whether health visitors are aware of the whereabouts of all the children in their area. For example, does the Housing Department notify the health visitors of homeless families placed in hostels? Are the children in long-stay hospitals, residential and foster care, receiving the service? Parliament's Social Services Committee (1984) recommended that social services departments should be statutorily obliged to notify the appropriate health authorities of movements of children in their care. In the meantime, it is a matter over which cooperation should be sought between the local services.

Communications can be another barrier. Where lack of a common language leads to a poor service for some families, then efforts should be made to employ staff of the same culture and language. This aspect is returned to in Chapter 10.

Is monitoring informative?

This question is important from several points of view. One is with regard to information on the overall outcome of the programme and how much feedback this information gives to health visitors on what they are achieving. We return to this in Chapter 8. Another is to do with the validity of any screening tests used, that is, the extent to which they bring to light relevant problems. This is a matter which needs urgent attention (HVA, 1985, p. 24). A third aspect concerns to what degree the chosen screening test is informative for parents and is useful in helping to improve their understanding of their children's needs and development. Some valuable attributes of screening tests are listed in Table 5.4.

These then are just a few of the matters that may be raised in appraisals of potential or current screening and surveillance schemes. The Health Visitors' Association's policy statement on the health visitor's role in child health surveillance

Table 5.4 Factors which can help make a test for surveillance of children particularly useful

Factor	Special value	Comment
A minimum of equipment needed	Easier to use in the homes of families not attending clinics or surgery, making service available to all babies whose parents wish it	E.g. Prof Barber's test needs a bell, a rattle, small cubes and brick — and the records
Scheme includes most important and indicative test items only	Leaves time for parental queries and to explain value and purpose of surveillance and screening, so that parents can take an active part in the scheme	Properly researched validation of tests needed
Has spread of test items to accommodate the wide range of variation within normality	Can demonstrate to parents a general picture of development and the individuality of each baby's progress	E.g. Sheridan (1975a), very wide range — very time consuming for health visitor, but can be explained to parents
Simple system of recording, preferably in diagrammatic form	Makes it easier for both examiner and parent to monitor child's progress at a glance, and to compare current attainments with previous and normal performances	E.g. Prof Barber's centile charts (Barber et al, 1976); Bar charts (Bryant, 1980)
Standardised scheme for local use	Enables systematic research and validation of the tests, making it possible to compare different wards and areas	Profesor Barber's scheme allows for computerisation of results

covers several more. For example, it considers health visitor training for screening, the role of the doctor in child health surveillance, the require-

HAD Scale

Name: Date:

Doctors are aware that emotions play an important part in most illnesses. If your doctor knows about these feelings he will be able to help you more.

This questionnaire is designed to help your doctor to know how you feel. Read each item and place a firm tick in the box opposite the reply which comes closest to how you have been feeling in the past week.

Don't take too long over your replies: your immediate reaction to each item will probably be more accurate than a long thought-out response.

Tick only one box in each section

I feel tense or 'wound up':
Most of the time ....
A lot of the time ....
Time to time, Occasionally ....
Not at all ....

I still enjoy the things I used to enjoy:
Definitely as much ....
Not quite so much ....
Only a little ....
Hardly at all ....

I get a sort of frightened feeling as if something awful is about to happen:
Very definitely and quite badly ....
Yes, but not too badly ....
A little, but it doesn't worry me ....
Not at all ....

I can laugh and see the funny side of things:
As much as I always could ....
Not quite so much now ....
Definitely not so much now ....
Not at all ....

Worrying thoughts go through my mind:
A great deal of the time ....
A lot of the time ....
From time to time but not too often ..
Only occasionally ....

I feel cheerful:
Not at all ....
Not often ....
Sometimes ....
Most of the time ....

I can sit at ease and feel relaxed:
Definitely ....
Usually ....
Not often ....
Not at all ....

I feel as if I am slowed down:
Nearly all the time ....
Very often ....
Sometimes ....
Not at all ....

I get a sort of frightened feeling like 'butterflies' in the stomach:
Not at all ....
Occasionally ....
Quite often ....
Very often ....

I have lost interest in my appearance:
Definitely ....
I don't take so much care as I should.....
I may not take quite as much care ....
I take just as much care as ever ....

I feel restless as if I have to be on the move:
Very much indeed ....
Quite a lot ....
Not very much ....
Not at all ....

I look forward with enjoyment to things:
As much as ever I did ....
Rather less than I used to ....
Definitely less than I used to ....
Hardly at all ....

I get sudden feelings of panic:
Very often indeed ....
Quite often ....
Not very often ....
Not at all ....

I can enjoy a good book or radio or TV programme:
Often ....
Sometimes ....
Not often ....
Very seldom ....

Do not write below this line

Printed as a service to medicine by Upjohn

Fig. 5.2 Example of self-assessment questionnaire: Hospital Anxiety and Depression (HAD) scale. Reproduced by kind permission of Dr R P Snaith, Department of Psychiatry, St James University Hospital, Leeds.

FOLD HERE

IDA Scale

[Ref: R. P. Snaith *et al. Brit J Psychiat* (1978). 132. 164–71]

Name: Date:

Instructions for Use

First write your name and date in the space above. This form has been designed so that you can show how you have been feeling in the past few days.

Read each item in turn and then UNDERLINE the response which best shows how you are feeling or have been feeling in the past few days.

Ignore the letters and numbers at the left-hand side and at the end of the questionnaire.

Make sure to complete both sides.

D				I feel cheerful:
0				Yes, definitely
1				Yes, sometimes
2				No, not much
3				No, not at all

	A			I can sit down and relax quite easily:
	0			Yes, definitely
	1			Yes, sometimes
	2			No, not much
	3			No, not at all

D				My appetite is:
3				Very poor
2				Fairly poor
1				Quite good
0				Very good

		O		I lose my temper and shout or snap at others:
		3		Yes, definitely
		2		Yes, sometimes
		1		No, not much
		0		No, not at all

D				I can laugh and feel amused:
0				Yes, definitely
1				Yes, sometimes
2				No, not much
3				No, not at all

		O		I feel I might lose control and hit or hurt someone:
		3		Sometimes
		2		Occasionally
		1		Rarely
		0		Never

	A			I have an uncomfortable feeling like butterflies in the stomach:
	3			Yes, definitely
	2			Yes, sometimes
	1			Not very often
	0			Not at all

			I	The thought of hurting myself occurs to me:
			3	Sometimes
			2	Not very often
			1	Hardly ever
			0	Not at all

PTO

Fig. 5.3a Example of self-assessment questionnaire: Irritability-Depression-Anxiety (IDA) scale. Reproduced by kind permission of Dr R P Snaith, Department of Psychiatry, St James University Hospital, Leeds.

D				I'm awake before I need to get up:
3				For 2 hours or more
2				For about 1 hour
1				For less than an hour
0				Not at all, I sleep until it is time to get up

A

3 Yes, definitely
2 Yes, sometimes
1 No, not much
0 No, not at all

(I feel tense or 'wound up':)

I

3 Yes, definitely
2 Yes, sometimes
1 No, not much
0 No, not at all

(I feel like harming myself:)

D

0 Yes, most of them
1 Yes, some of them
2 No, not many of them
3 No, none of them

(I have kept up my old interests:)

O

0 All the time
1 Most of the time
2 Some of the time
3 Hardly ever

(I am patient with other people:)

A

3 Yes, definitely
2 Yes, sometimes
1 No, not much
0 No, not at all

(I get scared or panicky for no very good reason:)

I

3 Yes, definitely
2 Yes, sometimes
1 Not often
0 No, not at all

(I get angry with myself or call myself names:)

O

3 Yes, often
2 Yes, sometimes
1 Only occasionally
0 Not at all

(People upset me so that I feel like slamming doors or banging about:)

A

0 Yes, always
1 Yes, sometimes
2 No, not often
3 No, I never can

(I can go out on my own without feeling anxious:)

I

3 Very much so
2 Rather a lot
1 Not much
0 Not at all

(Lately I have been getting annoyed with myself:)

FOLD HERE

FOR OFFICE USE ONLY	
D (4–6)	A (6–8) ....
IN. IRR (4–6)	OUT. IRR (5–7) ....
Figures in parentheses denote borderline ranges	

Fig. 5.3b Examples of self-assessment questionnaire: Irritability-Depression-Anxiety (IDA) scale — overleaf. Reproduced by kind permission of Dr R P Snaith, Department of Psychiatry, St James University Hospital, Leeds.

ments of children with special educational needs and the conditions for satisfactory testing of vision and hearing (HVA, 1985). Several other documents also make a useful contribution to the debate (Royal College of Nursing Health Visitors Advisory Group, 1983; 1984; Royal College of General Practitioners, 1982; General Medical Services Committee of the British Medical Association, 1984; see also later this chapter: 'Many schemes inadequate').

THE PROGRAMMES
For the mothers
Postnatal depression

It is logical, when seeking early signs of family ill health, to start with the mother. Her health, particularly her emotional health, is a corner-stone of family welfare. As the main carer, the mother's mental state is likely to be reflected in the way she copes with her responsibilities. Jacqueline Habgood (1985) a former health visitor, has described how postnatal depression affected her and her relationship with her child. She felt and looked ill and drained of strength over a six-year period. Mrs Habgood had shouted at and smacked her little girl, who had needed a great deal of good mothering to compensate, once the depression was overcome.

Some 20–30% of mothers are affected by postnatal depression and it is important to recognise it early. Mrs Habgood says health visitors in Edinburgh use a self-report screening test designed by Professor Cox (1986; Cox et al, 1987; Holden, 1985) to detect postnatal depression and health visitor counselling has proved to be very effective (Holden et al, 1989). There is an obvious advantage if parents can learn something about this problem antenatally as was discussed in Chapter 3.

Self-assessment tests from Leeds University have been available for a while. These are the hospital anxiety and depression (HAD) scale (Zigmond & Snaith, 1983) and the irritability-depression-anxiety (IDA) scale (Snaith et al, 1978), shown in Figures 5.2, 5.3a and 5.3b. The IDA scale, perhaps the more appropriate for the

postnatal period (Snaith, 1984), and its scoring system are very clearly explained by Snaith et al. The HAD scale, which is managed in the same way, may, however, be more acceptable to mothers. Some may be rather sensitive about the questioning on irritability. Both of the scales could be completed, perhaps whilst waiting in a clinic, and, certainly, in the privacy of the mother's own home. They are both readily available (information included with references), the IDA scale with a small charge, the HAD scale free. The Edinburgh postnatal depression scale will be found printed in full in the British Journal of Psychiatry (Cox et al, 1987).

Recognition of the condition is the first important step, and there is an obvious advantage to parents who have had forewarning that it might occur and have learned something about it in the antenatal period. It cannot come as such a shock. There are, however, very many views about postnatal depression and what should be done about it (Kumar, 1982; Atkinson, 1983). The National Childbirth Trust booklet (Waumsley, 1983) points out that merely knowing there is someone who cares and will listen, is of great importance, a subject returned to in the next section (p. 98).

For babies and very young children
Suggested pattern

In 1976, the Court Report (1976) made proposals for child health services. By 1980, the Department of Health and Social Security (DHSS) had issued guidelines for practice. The DHSS (1980) proposed that health visitors should undertake health surveillance on babies and toddlers at six weeks for general welfare and development, and again at seven to eight months but with special attention to sensory problems and to vision and hearing. In a further test at eighteen months, the Department advised that health visitors should undertake a review of development to include vision, hearing and early language, mobility, manipulative skills, social relationships and also to discuss the range of normal growth and behaviour.

In a policy statement, the Health Visitors' Association (HVA) suggested that the six week test could be undertaken, either by a health visitor alone, or jointly by a doctor and a health visitor. Whether it was alone or together would depend on the sort of information received about the previous examinations at or soon after birth and any particular concerns the parents or professionals might have (HVA, 1985, p. 11). The HVA suggested that thereafter babies should be screened at seven to nine months, at eighteen months and at two-and-a-half to three years of age. It proposed that these three tests should be undertaken by the health visitor alone, with doctors providing further assessment as a support service.

Many schemes inadequate

An inquiry in the late '70s and early '80s found a wide variety of tests in use in the, then, Area Health Authorities (Connolly, 1983). Thirteen of the 88 Authorities provided guidelines involving Sheridan, Denver, Griffiths and locally devised tests. In 54, set schemes were issued and for these specially designed record forms were provided. It was found that none of these forms incorporated scales or grading schemes. It was not possible, therefore, to accommodate individual differences in children's progress.

In 1989, a programme for child health surveillance proposed in the report of an eminent working party (Hall, 1989; Potrykus, 1989a) evoked many apprehensions (Bax & Whitmore, 1989; Cupid, 1989; Fry, 1989; Law, 1989; Potrykus, 1989b). In a well-argued defence of the report, Sheila Twinn (1990) shows how it provides the opportunity to develop a more proactive approach to our work. It will be interesting to see if the proposed basic core programme and surrounding activities, fare any better than the existing schemes, either in early discovery and/or as a basis for health education and support.

Stepladder, centile charts

One very good scheme has been devised in Glasgow by Professor Barber et al (1976a; Barber, 1982). The Woodside test is designed for use by health visitors, employing the sort of timing proposed by the DHSS and HVA. When reviewing the

literature on developmental screening, I felt this scheme was the best of all those reported (Robertson, 1984). Stepladder, centile charts have been devised, using specially selected and graded test items for each of the main four aspects of development: gross motor development; speech and language; vision and fine movement; and lastly, social aspects of development. There are four tests for hearing under nine months, and vision is given special attention early on. There is a booklet which describes exactly how the tests should be conducted (Barber et al, 1976b) and a very clear introduction to the test will be found in Barber et al (1976a).

As can be seen from a glance at Figures 5.4 and 5.5, these charts provide immediate visual comparison with previous attainments and allow for continuous comparisons over time, similar to that of weight and height charts. As in other centile charts, the age of the child is marked along the horizontal axis. The vertical axis on this scale starts at the bottom with babyhood attainments, graduating up to pre-school skills. In this scheme, children who are seen outside the standard time, either because they need extra attention or because they were missed at the scheduled time, are able to have a relevant and valid test, recorded appropriately on the graph. A very important plus point is that it would take little explanation to enable parents to understand the scheme and, therefore, to become fully involved and for the charts to be used as a visual aid for discussions about child behaviour and development.

A bar chart

The Denver developmental screening test is another test which uses a visual record, this time a bar chart. It is a system based on the percentages of population able to achieve various activities by a given age and is explained very clearly by Ingalls and Salerno (1983) and Bryant (1980). The latter described how Cardiff health visitors had tested babies aged nine months with a modification of this test, adjusted to match the local population. The scheme was limited as it was undertaken only at nine months.

The Denver test was tried out on 198 pre-term

FAMILIES WITH YOUNG CHILDREN **91**

SOCIAL

1. Able to dress — except laces and back buttons (H).
2. Dry at night (H).

3. Washes hands (H).
4. Pulls pants up and down (H).

5. Drinks and replaces cup (H).
6. Dry by day (H).

7. Drinks from cup without spilling (H).
8. Indicates toilet needs (H).

9. Puts cubes into box after being shown.
10. Finds toy under cup.

11. Rings bell.
12. Chews and swallows biscuit (observed).
    Copes with solid food.

13. Puts objects into mouth (cubes!).
14. Reaches for and shakes rattle.

15. Aware of and responsive to bath (H).
16. Enjoys being handled by mother (H).

17. Smiles when spoken to (H).
18. Some vocal sounds (H).

(H) = History of achievement sufficient

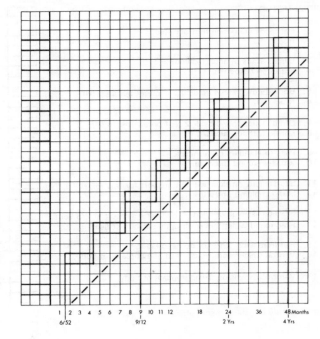

A

HEARING AND LANGUAGE

1. Hears whispers at 0.9 m (3 ft) — R&L (Reed test).
2. Grammatical speech articulated correctly.

3. Says first name.
4. Knows own sex.

5. Simple sentences (H).
6. Plays with miniature cup and saucer.

7. Points to parts of body.
8. Says five or more words (H).

9. Obeys simple commands e.g. clap hands.
10. Says less than 5 words excluding
    "Mama" "Dada" "Baba" (H).

11. "Mama" "Dada" "Baba".
12. Hearing tests above ear level.

13. Unintelligible babble.
14. Hearing tests at ear level.

15. Turns eyes to sound.
16. Looks round meaningfully when spoken to.

17. Stills to bell.
18. Stills to mother's voice.

(H) = History of achievement sufficient.

B

Fig. 5.4 Step-ladder charts for recording pre-school developmental progress: social and hearing and language. Reproduced by kind permission of Professor J H Barber, University of Glasgow Department of General Practice. (Note change in scale after 12 months.)

GROSS MOTOR

1. Descends stairs one foot per step.
2. Hops.

3. Climbs stairs in adult fashion.
4. Walks on tiptoe (H).

5. Up and down stairs holding on, 2 feet per step (H).
6. Kicks ball.

7. Climbs stairs, hand held, 2 feet on each step (H).
8. Kneels without support. (H).

9. Pulls to standing on furniture.
10. 'Cruises' round furniture.

11. Sits steadily on floor without support for few mins. (H).
12. Stands holding on to furniture.

13. Sits against wall or hand — no lateral support — 2/3 secs.
14. Hold round waist, lower abruptly exclude scissoring.

15. Pull from lying. Little or no head lag.
16. Ventral suspension. Holds head above plane of body.

17. Ventral suspension. Head in plane of body.

(H) = History of achievement sufficient.

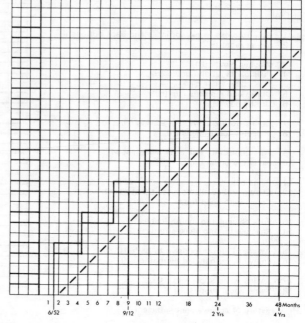

A

VISION AND FINE MOTOR

1. Picks up and replaces very small objects, e.g. pins, with each eye covered separately.
2. Copies a square.

3. Copies a circle.
4. Builds a bridge of three bricks when shown.

5. Makes a vertical line when shown.
6. Makes a tower of six bricks when shown.

7. Makes a scribble on paper.
8. Makes a tower of three bricks when shown.

9. Pincer grasp using a small object e.g. Smartie.
10. Bangs bricks together when shown.

11. Side of finger grasp using a small object e.g. Smartie.
12. Matches cubes.

13. Picks up cube from table or hand.
14. Transfers cube from one hand to another.

15. Holds a pencil briefly.
16. Follows a moving person with eyes.

17. Follows a moving face with eyes.

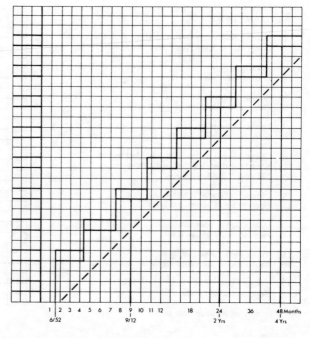

B

Fig. 5.5 Step-ladder charts for recording pre-school developmental gross motor and vision and fine movements. Reproduced by kind permission of Professor J H Barber, University of Glasgow Department of General Practice. (Note change in scale after 12 months.)

children (Elliman et al, 1985). It was found that, when using the test at their actual age, about 40% would be rated as possibly having abnormal development, a significant rate of over-referral for the assessment clinic. The problem was that using an age corrected for the pre-term birth, the test was unable to pick up several who did, in fact, have abnormal progress. It seems some 7% of babies born are pre-term and, therefore, need special consideration. It was concluded that the over-referral rate for more detailed assessment would be small enough to be outweighed, easily, by the advantage of being able to provide early identification and treatment for those who needed it. The advice given was that tests should be undertaken at the true age in order to find need for further assessment, and also at the adjusted age in order to prevent undue anxiety.

Listed attainments

Surrey's (Owen, 1982) structured system of health surveillance provides an example of a scheme without pictorial or graphic feedback. Lists are used with 'yes/no' and 'remarks' columns, for possible topics for discussion and observations at the visit, as well as for the child's skills. These lists do not provide a comparison of the stage at which the individual attainments of this child are achieved in comparison with others, nor do they give a continuous clear picture over time, for both parents and professionals. They are scheduled to be filled in five times in the first year, twice in the second and annually thereafter. It is suggested that the structured visiting promotes professional standards (Owen, 1982). It would be interesting to know if this notion is founded on a proven improved rate of discovering incipient problems.

If a child does not achieve one of the listed items by a given date, there is the question as to whether parents might be unnecessarily worried by the apparent pass/fail status implied in this sort of system. Professor Illingworth (1981) has described how he had heard of health visitors 'failing' 40% in a 6 month test and telling the mothers their babies had failed! Such apocryphal stories do at least draw our attention to the problem, and in a subsequent article he gave excellent advice on how to phrase things both realistically and carefully for parents (Illingworth & Illingworth, 1984).

Health visitors need to explain to parents that in a test of this nature they are looking at only a very limited profile. It could be likened to taking a snapshot as compared with a home movie which could show all aspects and moods! It can sometimes be helpful to have available one or another of the wider ranging descriptions of infant development, in order to show the limited nature of most screening tests. For example, Sheridan's (1975a) book or booklet (Sheridan, 1975b) can help put the matter in perspective. The items listed are presented as a large number of *possible* skills. Each child attains its *own individual* two thirds or three-quarters or so, of the entire range, by each stated age. Where a mother is suspicious about her child's development, health visitors should not be too reassuring (Sheridan, 1975a).

Special programmes

Sudden infant death is receiving more and more attention (Knight, 1983; Golding et al, 1985; Limerick, 1988). Various schemes have been set up. In these, infants thought to be at increased risk of dying unexpectedly from preventable causes, are identified. This is done by comparing all babies against a researched scoring system, at birth and again a month later. Studies have been undertaken in Sheffield and Portsmouth. Increased visiting by health visitors, paying particular attention to the babies' weight gain, feeding, developmental attainments and general health, and allied health education, is given to these families. These areas have seen a significant decrease in the number of unexpected infant deaths (Carpenter et al, 1983; Powell, 1984; 1985).

Jean Powell described how the Portsmouth study was set up. She explains how in her scheme, selection factors differ from those in Sheffield. She also describes a pattern of visiting undertaken by health visitors, according to estimated risk for the baby. A computer is used to help sort out the 46 variables from the midwives' birth information and the scoring factors arising out of a visit at four weeks. Both the GP and the health visitor are informed of whether each baby is low risk, high risk or very high risk. So far, 10% of the babies have been classified as high risk and 1% as very high risk.

The schedule arranges for 19 visits in the first year of life for very high risk babies. Those deemed to be at high risk are programmed to receive 11 visits, which can be compared with the 5 visits planned for low risk babies. The health visitors in one sector of the District have chosen to follow their own judgement about visiting, rather than to stick rigidly to the guidelines. It would be interesting to know to what extent their actual pattern of visiting varies from the guidelines, in what ways they choose to tackle the problem using another approach, for example through group work, and what effect this has on the infant mortality and morbidity rate.

Richard Madeley (1988) has argued cogently for Districts not to set up birth scoring systems. He advocates working on social inequalities and on improving primary health care to make it immediately responsive to parents' requests and worries about their babies. The ideas used in community health development provide one way of enabling this approach. We will be looking at these in Chapter 12.

Weight, length and head circumference

Early discovery of failure to thrive or abnormal weight gain, can be achieved only with accurate methods and adequate recording. Abnormalities of growth can also be found — with the same provisos. Describing weighing in clinics, Davies and Williams (1983) remark on the lack of guidance given on this widely practised procedure. They feel that abnormal weight gain often goes undetected and that, all too often, normal weight gain is misinterpreted as abnormal. The problems are:

- unreliable techniques in weighing
- insufficient use of centile charts
- inadequate understanding of normal patterns in weight gain
- insufficient understanding of nutritional influences on weight.

They describe how centile charts are now widely available and are becoming increasingly used in clinics, and they have provided very good diagrams to show the difference between normal and abnormal patterns on a centile chart. It is interesting to note that in the Portsmouth surveillance scheme, each health visitor has her own portable weighing machine in order to enable adequate and accurate weighing in the home. Hopefully, this idea will spread to become the norm.

Professor Tanner (1985), who has devised height and weight charts for child health clinics (Tanner & Whitehouse, 1973), describes the diagnosis and treatment of various growth disorders which are best treated as early as possible. Harvey and Wallis (1978a, 1978b) have given some very helpful hints, with photographs, on how to measure a baby's length (up to two years of age) and, later, height. They say that the commonest cause of low stature in a Newcastle-upon-Tyne study was social deprivation, and that it accounted for a third of the cases.

The value of head circumference as a measure is explained by Wood and Walker-Smith (1981). Its size relative to length and weight can be a useful measure for indicating stunted growth. Its size relative to chest size can also be an indicator.

Vision, hearing and speech

There seems little doubt that the more parents are involved with monitoring the vision and hearing of their babies, the greater will be the chance of early diagnosis and treatment (Robertson, 1984; Robinson, 1983). A checklist of general signs of ability to hear in the first year of life, and another suggesting some simple tests for vision that parents should know about, will be found in Figure 5.6 and Table 5.5. McCormick (1983) has described the successful outcome, in Nottingham, of improvements in training health visitors to test babies' hearing, and gives good advice for District Health Authorities who may wish to check their policies and procedures on this issue.

Speech and language are said to be the most common developmental problem in young children and Professor R J Robinson (1982) suggests that it should receive attention because it:

CH 31 (COM)

Nottingham Health Authority ——— **Hints for Parents** ————

"Can your baby hear you?"

Here is a checklist of some of the general signs you can look for in your baby's first year:-

YES/NO

Shortly after birth
Your baby should be startled by a sudden loud noise such as a hand clap or a door slamming and should blink or open his eyes widely to such sounds.

By 1 Month
Your baby should be beginning to notice sudden prolonged sounds like the noise of a vacuum cleaner and he should pause and listen to them when they begin.

By 4 Months
He should quieten or smile to the sound of your voice even when he cannot see you. He may also turn his head or eyes toward you if you come up from behind and speak to him from the side.

By 7 Months
He should turn immediately to your voice across the room or to very quiet noises made on each side if he is not too occupied with other things.

By 9 Months
He should listen attentively to familiar everyday sounds and search for very quiet sounds made out of sight. He should also show pleasure in babbling loudly and tunefully.

By 12 Months
He should show some response to his own name and to other familiar words. He may also respond when you say 'no' and 'bye bye' even when he cannot see any accompanying gesture.

> Your health visitor will perform a routine hearing screening test on your baby between seven and nine months of age. She will be able to help and advise you at any time before or after this test if you are concerned about your baby and his development. If you suspect that your baby is not hearing normally, either because you cannot answer yes to the items above or for some other reason, then seek advice from your health visitor.

Fig. 5.6 Hints for parents on testing their children's hearing. Reproduced by kind permission of Dr Barry McCormick, Children's Hearing Assessment Centre, Nottingham Health Authority.

Table 5.5 Indicators of a baby's ability to see

	Does the baby:	Comments
Early weeks	Have eye-to-eye contact with the mother Fixate on the mother's face? Follow a moving object?	Seek mother's opinion, but may be observed May be observed or reported Early test: follows a dangling object 30 cm (12 in) away, through a quarter of a circle
Early months	Recognise familiar sights? Follow a moving person with his eyes?	Seek mother's opinion May be observed during screening
Later months	Object to having one of his eyes covered when playing games?	Parental opinion should be sought, as this could indicate quite a marked loss of vision in the uncovered eye

- may be a sign of deafness or another underlying condition
- commonly leads to emotional and behavioural problems
- has a strong association with later difficulties in reading, writing and spelling
- is likely to improve with skilled intervention.

The professor says there should be concern about a child not using words with meaning by 21 months or constructing simple sentences by 3 years, but cautions us against the unthinking use of arbitrary cut-off points of this nature. Understanding statements is particularly important, and it is suggested that a child who does not understand simple commands at eighteen months should also be referred for assessment. Dr Barker (1989) describes how considerations of language environment and health visitors' sensitive and intuitive appraisal are key factors.

Congenital dislocation of the hip

Some cases of hip dislocation (see Ch. 4, p. 64 cannot be detected at birth. In half the 'missed' cases looked at by David et al (1983) there had been no routine hip checks after three months. They advised follow-up of babies with transient instability or clicking hips at birth, at six weeks,

three months, six months and twelve months, and at six monthly intervals until they walk normally. Babies at high risk, such as breech deliveries or where there is a family tendency, should receive special attention. In a quarter of the cases studied, there was no record of the test having been undertaken at birth. Health visitors should check on this to see if it was, in fact, undertaken, and to find out the result.

Again, it helps if parents are aware of the need for vigilance. Stephen Ware (1984) describes how he gives parents an outline of the mechanics of the disease and suggests they gently abduct their babies' hips each time the nappy is changed and report any asymmetry immediately to the health visitor or the GP. He tells the parents, too, that abduction normally becomes more limited as the baby gets older. A Northern Ireland study showed that mothers tended to be the first to notice that something was wrong. However, their views were often overlooked or ignored. Post-hospital support services were poor (Nugent, 1987). Self-help groups, such as STEPS and HIPS can offer help and guidance (Young, 1987; see useful addresses).

In this section on screening and surveillance, we have looked at planning and monitoring screening programmes, at assessment of mothers' emotional health and at a variety of tests available for use with babies and very young children.

GIVING SUPPORT

Supportive aspects of the work can range from helping couples who are experiencing the day-to-day anxieties associated with early parenthood, through to helping young families who have come up against a major problem, or even a tragedy. The aim in either case is to ameliorate the position, in order to prevent greater dysfunction growing out of the current difficulties.

Common problems

Although sympathetic listening is an important therapeutic aspect of the service they can give, health visitors would wish to provide other practical help too, where this is possible. Some will not only keep available books they can lend people (see Table 4.1), but also their copy of well-written, reassuring and helpful articles on common problems. These might be, for example, infantile colic (Jones, 1984), unacceptable sleeping habits (Richman, 1983; Kitzinger, 1985) and 'hyperactivity' (Delvin, 1984). Such articles can be found through the HVA *Current Awareness Bulletin*.

It seems probable that discussions on how to cope are more successful, particularly in the longer term, if they are backed up by background information which helps the parents understand more about the mechanics of what is happening. Health education is intertwined with supportive aspects of health visiting, just as it is in screening and surveillance. Being able to give information about relevant voluntary and statutory agencies is also very important (Webb, 1985), a matter discussed in earlier chapters.

It is important to plan how to help people facing these common problems. They can be very distressing. Crying babies can serve as an example. It is common for babies to cry a great deal (Lyall, 1989). In a study reported by Sheila Kitzinger (1985), a quarter of the mothers who had responded to the questionnaire had felt like smacking their crying baby, one in ten had actually done so. This was a self-selective, non-random sample, but it does give an indication of how distraught people can become.
Sheila Kitzinger's advice to mothers was:

- find a 'support network' before baby's birth
- there is no need to fear asking for help
- arrange for a break away from the baby
- the excessive crying generally stops by six months of age
- get partner to help
- talk to someone about the crying
- note some useful addresses of relevant organisations.

Four out of five of the mothers in the study had talked with their health visitor and this was found to be very helpful.

Availability

Access to our service is important. Field et al (1983) said that parents facing decisions as to whether or not their child is ill, particularly those living alone, can feel very confused and delay seeking help. Besides needing to know and be confident about normal behaviour and common illnesses, Field et al said that parents need also to have both GP and health visitor services available at unsocial hours when they require it.

Health visitors in Richmond (Beech, 1981) and Plymouth (Bogie, 1981) have written about how they have organised out-of-hours service for parents with crying babies. More recently, a seven day health visiting service has been set up in Peterborough (Rawdon-Smith, 1984). The telephone number of the service is given routinely to new mothers. The service has been particularly helpful to parents with very young babies. It has been found to be very well used and inexpensive to run.

Mothers can also routinely be told of voluntary organisations in the locality interested in supporting mothers. There may be nearby groups from, for example, the National Childbirth Trust, Meet-a-Mum Association or Parents Anonymous. Laura Swaffield (1984) has described how Cry-sis, a voluntary group which aims to help distraught mothers, is seeking to make itself known to, and to work in cooperation with, people like health visitors.

Work with groups

The importance of mothers' need for each other's company, mutual support and guidance they can give one another, is well recognised by many health visitors who have set up groups (Wood, 1985; Moulds et al, 1983; Hennessy et al, 1978). Deborah Hennessy (1983) has provided practical advice on planning and setting up support groups, making suggestions for matters such as:

- leadership arrangements
- length of meetings
- number of meetings
- size of group

- supervision of children
- drawing meetings to a close.

Vari Drennan (1988) has drawn together many aspects of health visitor groupwork as a guide for future initiatives. Two health visitors have described their work with self-help groups. Diana Balter (1985) was approached by a group of women who organised themselves a course on health topics. She ordered films and acted generally as a background resource. It is interesting to note that the group were able to obtain grant aid to pay for their accommodation through a special social services fund. Nina Trick (1985) discussed the problem of first time mothers' loneliness with the doctors in the rural practice to which she was attached. They offered a room in the surgery for a weekly meeting. This team venture has been successful and has resulted in increased confidence for the mothers.

Child health clinics which are appropriately geared for it can make an excellent place for mothers to meet and give each other sympathetic support and encouragement. Formal clinics where mothers have to queue in row upon row of chairs make it less easy to foster friendships or mutual support. However, the less formal ones with

- a clear welcome for newcomers
- chairs grouped in small circles
- toys for the children
- a volunteer who can
  — help with the children
  — make mothers a cup of tea

and where mothers are encouraged to tell each other of their experiences, are more likely to be successful in this direction.

The clinic, on the other hand, often lacks privacy and therefore does not provide a good place for health visitors to offer support over some of the greater problems parents can face. These are usually followed up in the home. In the long term, the mutual support offered in self-help groupwork is for many people the best solution. In planning their work, health visitors need to have thought out how they will help parents who have particular problems, be they quite common or a rare occurrence. Parents whose baby has died suddenly and

unexpectedly and mothers suffering from postnatal depression are given as two examples.

Postnatal depression

It is quite a challenge to plan to arrange supportive care for mothers with postnatal depression. It tends to manifest itself six weeks postnatally, by which time the health visitor is generally calling less frequently. Also it is thought to be very common and to involve at least one in ten mothers. Besides helping parents become aware of its existence (Ch. 3, p. 49) and discovering it early (see above, p. 89), health visitors need to know about all the relevant helping agencies in the locality (Waumsley, 1983, pp. 30–31) and to have thought about what approach might best help the mother. There are no simple solutions, but just raising the issue by suggesting the self-assessment questionnaire shows the health visitor wishes to help in this direction. The same can be achieved, of course, by simply asking the mother how she feels and helping her express this.

Waumsley (1983, pp. 32–33, 35–36) has described how the supportive gestures of volunteers have helped depressed mothers, and she lists some suggestions for dealing with the feelings of anger and stress that people experience at this time. Jenifer Holden (1985) has described a study in which some health visitors have been given special training in non-directive counselling techniques. They visit for eight, weekly half-hour sessions, which the mothers spend talking about their feelings. It is evident that the scheme is being appreciated.

In order to alleviate loneliness and depression, a 'walk-in unit' was set up by health visitors in Hertfordshire in which small children could come and play, with or without their parents. They are now planning to extend its facilities and its hours of opening. Group counselling sessions of six to eight weeks duration, to help mothers with emotional problems, were set up by three health visitors in Hampshire. Their success led them to recommend others to do something similar (Hennessy et al, 1978).

Sudden infant death

Cot death affects around two per thousand live births. Some of the difficulties parents face, such as feelings of guilt, considerable stress, sometimes involving problems within the marriage and with the surviving children, and the practical aspects of the death, are described by Luben (1986), Woodward et al (1985) and Audrey Heycock (1984). They also suggest ways that health visitors can help. The Foundation for the Study of Infant Death is an organisation which supplies information to parents and professionals; it raises funds for research, and formerly bereaved parents, Friends of the Foundation, are able to give personal support to the grieving parents. The process of grief and bereavement visiting are discussed in Chapter 7 (pp. 130–131).

Health visitors can themselves need support (see Ch. 2, p. 20). In an attempt to 'help the helpers', a psychiatrist, Michael Clarke (1980), held a series of fortnightly seminars in which health visitors presented problematic cases. The psychological consequences for parents following the death of a child, was one of the four areas that health visitors found particularly difficult. Clarke remarked on the important role for health visitors in identifying distortions in parents' mourning and in aiming to prevent further complications.

This chapter has given an overview of work with families with babies and very young children, especially with regard to certain aspects of planning. By artificially dividing the work into guidance, surveillance and supportive care, we have been able to look more closely at some of the particular issues and schemes and at a few of the dilemmas that are involved. We have discussed the need to make special efforts for the underprivileged, to work in partnership with parents and to help them understand so that they can be actively involved in health care decisions.

USEFUL ADDRESSES

Child Accident Prevention Trust
75 Portland Place,
London W1N 3AL
Tel 071 636 2545

Cry-sis, British Monomark Cry-sis,
London WC1N 3XX
Tel 071 404 5011

The Foundation for Sudden Infant Deaths,
5th Floor, 4/5 Grosvenor Place,
London SW1X 7HD
Tel 071 235 1721 or 071 245 9421

HIPS c/o Belinda Young,
22 Claudius Gardens,
Chandlers Ford SO5 2NY
Tel 0703 268223

Meet-A-Mum Association
3 Woodside Avenue, South Norwood,
London SE25 5DW.
Please enclose a stamped self addressed envelope

National Childbirth Trust
9 Queensborough Terrace,
London W2 3TB
Tel 071 221 3833

Parents Anonymous
6–9 Manor Gardens,
London N7
Tel 071 263 5672 (office),
071 263 8918 (Lifeline)

STEPS
8 Princess Road,
Urmston,
Manchester M31 3SS

REFERENCES

Ahamed M 1982 A research project. Nursing Times Community Outlook 78: 223

Anstoker J, Humphreys J 1988 Breast cancer screening. A practical guide. Oxford University Press, Oxford

Atkinson D 1983 Postnatal depression (letter). Health Visitor 56: 116

Balter D 1985 Working with a women's self-help group. Health Visitor 58: 260

Barber J H 1982 Preschool developmental screening — the results of a four year period. Health Bulletin 40: 170–178

Barber J H, Boothman R, Stanfield J P 1976a A new visual chart for preschool developmental screening. Health Bulletin 34: 80–91

Barber J H, Department of General Practice, University of Glasgow with assistance from the Department of Child Health, University of Glasgow 1976b The Woodside system pre-school developmental screening: description of the tests. Econoprint, Edinburgh

Barker W 1988 The value of developmental tests. Health Visitor 61: 373–374

Barker W 1989 Once again on child surveillance. Health Visitor 62: 174

Barker W, Anderson R 1988 The child development programme: an evaluation of process and outcome. Early Childhood Development Unit, University of Bristol

Barker W, Rowe G and Sutcliffe D (Eds) 1987 Community Health and the Child Development Programme. Early Childhood Development Unit, University of Bristol.

Bax M, Witmore K 1989 (letter) Identifying disabilities. Health Visitor 62: 106.

Beech C P 1981 A new service for parents with crying babies. Nursing Times 77: 245–246

Bell A, Moules E 1985 The demographic factor. Nursing Times 81, 31: 28–30

Black D 1980 Inequalities in health. Report of a research working party, Department of Health and Social Security, London. p 328–329 (Chairman Sir Douglas Black)

Bogie A 1981 A crying baby advisory service. Health Visitor 54: 535–537

Bryant G M 1980 Use of Denver developmental screening test by health visitors. Health Visitor 53: 2–5

Carpenter R G, Gardner A, Jepson M, Taylor E M, Salvin A, Sunderland R, Emery J L, Pursall E, Roe J, Sheffield Health Visitors 1983 Prevention of unexpected infant death. The Lancet I: 723–727

CETHV 1977 An investigation into the principles of health visiting. Council for the Education and Training of Health Visitors, London

Child Accident Prevention Trust 1989 Basic principles of child accident prevention: a guide to action. Child Accident Prevention Trust, London

Child Development Project 1984 Child development programme. Early Childhood Development Unit, Senate House, University of Bristol, Bristol BS8 ITH. p 12

Clarke M G 1980 Psychiatric liaison with health visitors. Health Trends 12: 98–100

Community Outlook 1982 Fact sheet. Nursing Times Community Outlook 78, 32: 220–221

Community Outlook 1984 Which should you choose? Nursing Times Community Outlook 80, 27: 250–253

Colver A, Pearson P 1985 Safety in the home: how are we doing? Health Visitor 58: 41–42

Connolly P 1983 The health visitor's contribution. Nursing Times 79, 38: 30–32

Court Report 1976 Report of the Committee on Child Health Services, Fit for the future. Cmnd 6684. HMSO, London

Cox J 1986 Postnatal depression. A guide for health professionals. Churchill Livingstone, Edinburgh

Cox J L, Holden J M, Sagovsky R 1987 Detection of postnatal depression. Development of the 10-item Edinburgh postnatal depression scale. British Journal of Psychiatry 150: 782–786 — A copy of their depression scale and instructions for users can be seen on the final page of the article.

Cranshaw S 1984 Remarkable changes in parents' competence. Nursing Times Supplement 80, 42: 8

Cupid A 1989 (letter) Changes in surveillance. Health Visitor 62: 288

Darbyshire P 1985 Thumbs up for dummies. Nursing Times 81, 38: 40–42

David T J, Parris M R, Poynor M U, Hawnaur J M, Simm S A, Rigg E A, McCrae F C 1983 Reasons for late detection of hip dislocation in childhood. The Lancet II: 147–149

Davies D P, Williams T 1983 Is weighing babies in clinics worth while? British Medical Journal 286: 860–863

Dening F 1983 Tackling breast cancer. Nursing Times 79, 34: 13

DHSS 1980 Prevention in the child health services. Department of Health and Social Security, London

Delvin D 1984 Is he really hyperactive? Mother and Baby December: 61–62

Drennan V (ed) 1988 Health visitors and groups: politics and practice. Heinemann Nursing, Oxford

The Economist 1984 Some doctors still eat salt. The Economist 292, 7355: 67–68

Elliman A M, Bryan E M, Elliman A D, Palmer P, Dubowitz L 1985 Denver developmental screening test and preterm infants. Archives of Disease in Childhood 60: 20–24

Fairs J M 1984 A more caring family approach. Nursing Times Supplement 80, 42: 8

Field S, Draper J, Kerr M, Hare M J 1983 Babies' illnesses from the parents' point of view. Maternal and Child Health 8: 252–256

Fry T 1989 Wrong on growth. Health Visitor 62: 257

General Medical Services Committee of the British Medical Association 1984 Handbook of preventive care for pre-school children. General Medical Services Defence Fund Ltd and the Royal College of General Practitioners, London

Golding J, Limerick S, Macfarlane A 1985 Sudden infant death. Patterns, puzzles and problems. Open Books Publishing Ltd, Shepton Mallet, Somerset

Green C 1984 Toddler taming. A parents' guide to the first four years. Century Publishing Co Ltd, London

Habgood J 1985 Exposing the blues . . . Nursing Times Community Outlook 81, 33: 4–6

Hall D M B (ed) 1989 Health for all children. A programme for child health surveillance. The report of the joint working party on child health surveillance. Oxford University Press, Oxford.

Harris G 1987 Screening: progress and pitfalls. Nursing Times 83, 11: 18

Harvey D, Wallis S 1978a Children of short stature: part 1. Midwife Health Visitor and Community Nurse 14: 136–139

Harvey D, Wallis S 1978b Children of short stature: part 2. Midwife Health Visitor and Community Nurse 14: 177–178

Health Education Council 1981 Play it safe! A guide to preventing children's accidents. Health Education Council and Scottish Health Education Group in association with the BBC

Health Visitor 1989 Books. Health Visitor 62, 10: 300

Hennessy D 1983 Parents support groups. Nursing 2, 19: 552–554

Hennessy D, Holgate B, Marr J 1978 With a little help from my friends. Nursing Times Community Outlook 74: 103–106

Hewitt K, Powell I, Tait V 1989 The behaviour of nine-month and two-year olds as assessed by health visitors and parents. Health Visitor 62: 52–55

Heycock A 1984 Coping with a cot death. Nursing Mirror 158, 4: iii-viii

Holden J 1985 Talking it out. Nursing Times Community Outlook 81, 41: 6,10

Holden J M, Sagovsky R, Cox J L 1989 Counselling in a general practice setting: controlled study of health visitor intervention in treatment of postnatal depression. British Medical Journal 298: 223 — Non-directive counselling methods taught and applied.

HVA 1985 The health visitor's role in child health surveillance: a policy statement. Health Visitors Association, 50 Southwark St, London SE1

Illingworth R S 1981 The importance of knowing what is normal. Public Health, London 95: 66–68

Illingworth R S, Illingworth C M 1984 Mothers are easily worried. Archives of Disease in Childhood 59: 380–384

Ingalls A J, Salerno M C 1983 Maternal and child health nursing, 5th edn. Mosby, St Louis, p 328–360

Johnson A M 1984 Visual problems in children: detection and referral. Journal of the Royal College of General Practitioners 34: 32–35

Johnson L, Silman A 1985 Ready salted. Nursing Times 81, 32: 34–35

Jones I H 1984 Colic enough to make you scream. Mother July: 30

Kitzinger S 1985 Why do babies cry? Parents March: 37–38

Knight B 1983 Sudden death in infancy. The 'cot death' syndrome. Faber and Faber, London

Kumar R 1982 Neurotic disorders in childbearing women. In: Brockington I F, Kumar R (eds) Motherhood and mental illness. Academic Press, London

Laidman P 1987 Health visiting and preventing accidents to children. The role of the health visitor in the prevention of accidents to children in the period between ante-natal contact and the child's entry to school. Research Report No 12. Health Education Authority/Child Accident Prevention Trust, London — Recommended reading

Latham A D, Haggard M P 1980 A pilot study to detect hearing impairment in the young. Midwife, Health Visitor and Community Nurse 16: 370–374

Laurence V 1983 An alternative approach. Nursing Times 79, 12: 14

Law J 1989 Surveillance — shifting priorities. Health Visitor 62: 155

Limerick S 1988 Sudden infant deaths: cause for concern. Health Visitor 61: 233–234

Luben J 1986 Cot deaths. Coping with sudden infant death syndrome. Thorsens, Wellingborough

Lyall J 1989 Crying with confidence. Nursing Times 85, 42: 20

McCormick B 1983 Hearing screening by health visitors: a critical appraisal of the distraction test. Health Visitor 56: 449–451

Madeley R 1988 Preventing sudden infant death syndrome: future strategies. Health Visitor 61: 241–243

Moore J 1982 Can they be prevented? Nursing Times, Community Outlook 78, 32: 212–214

Morris J B, Hird M D 1981 A neurodevelopmental infant screening programme undertaken by health visitors — preliminary report. Health Bulletin 39: 236–250

Moulds V, Hennessy D, Crack P 1983 Innovations by a primary health care team. 2. A postnatal group for first-time mothers. Health Visitor 56: 296–297

Nichols S 1983 The Southampton breast study — implications for nurses. Nursing Times 79, 50: 24–29

Nugent G 1987 Parental understanding of congenital hip dislocation. Nursing Times 83, 28: 28–31

Nursing Times 1989 Down . . . . and out. Nursing Times 85, 6: 24

Owen C M 1982 How Surrey implemented the Court Report. Nursing Times 78: 673–675

Percy P 1984 Disturbingly poor levels of nutrition. Nursing Times Supplement 80, 42: 9

Potrykus C 1989a Ringing the changes in child health. Health Visitor 62: 239–241

Potrykus C 1989b Health for all children. A threat to effective child health surveillance? Health Visitor 62: 207–209

Powell J 1984 Cot deaths — can they be prevented? Journal of the Royal Society of Health 104: 203–205

Powell J 1985 Keeping watch. Nursing Times Community Outlook 81, 2: 15–19

Rajan L 1985 Time to avoid the clinic? Nursing Times 81, 32: 24–26

Rawdon-Smith J 1984 Introduction of seven-day health visiting cover in Peterborough. Health Visitor 57: 53–54

Ray G 1982 At risk. Nursing Times Community Outlook 78, 32: 217–218

Rayner C 1977 Family feelings. Understanding your child from 0 to 5. Hutchinson & Co Ltd, London

Richman N 1983 Management of sleep problems. Maternal and Child Health 8: 227–233

Robertson C A 1981 Evaluation of screening: an epidemiological approach. 1: Measuring the effectiveness of health visitors. Health Visitor 54: 20–21

Robertson C A 1984 Preventive health care for infants. In: Houston M J (ed) Maternal and Infant Health Care. Churchill Livingstone, London

Robinson J 1982 An evaluation of health visiting. Council for the Education and Training of Health Visitors, London

Robinson K 1983 The scandal of late diagnosis of deafness in children. Health Visitor 56: 452–453

Robinson R J 1982 The child who is slow to talk. British Medical Journal 285: 671–672

Rowden R 1983 Talking about taboos. Nursing Times 79, 50: 12

Rowe J 1985 Supply and demand. Nursing Times 81, 4: 52

Royal College of General Practitioners 1982 Healthier children — thinking prevention. Royal College of General Practitioners, London

Royal College of Nursing Health Visitors' Advisory Group 1983 Thinking about health visiting. Royal College of Nursing of the United Kingdom Society of Primary Health Care Nursing, London

Royal College of Nursing Health Visitors' Advisory Group 1984 Further thinking about health visiting. Royal College of Nursing of the United Kingdom Society of Primary Health Care Nursing, London

Sheridan M D 1975a Children's developmental progress from birth to five years: the Stycar sequences. NFER Publishing Company Ltd, Windsor

Sheridan M D 1975b The developmental progress of infants and young children. HMSO, London

Snaith R P 1984 Birth of the first child (letter). British Medical Journal 288: 2000–2001

Snaith R P, Constantopoulos A A, Jardine M Y. McGuffin P A 1978 A clinical scale for the self-assessment of irritability, depression and anxiety. British Journal of Psychiatry 132: 164–171 (These questionnaires are available, with a charge for postage and printing, from Leeds University through R P Snaith, Senior Lecturer in Psychiatry, Department of Psychiatry, St James

University Hospital, Leeds LS9 7TF Tel 0532 433144)

Social Services Committee 1984 Children in care. Second report from the Social Services Committee, 1983–84 Vol I. House of Commons Paper 360–1, London (Chairman: Renée Short)

Stretch C 1983 Does mother know best? Nursing Times 79, 10: 14

Swaffield L 1984 Cry babies. Nursing Times 80, 31: 16–17

Tanner J M 1985 Catching them early. Nursing Times Community Outlook 81, 15: 19–22

Tanner J M, Whitehouse R H 1973 Height and weight charts from birth to 5 years allowing for length of gestation. Archives of Disease in Childhood 48: 786–789

Trick N 1985 Forming a new baby group. Health Visitor 58: 78

Twinn S 1990 Nothing to fear. Health Visitor 63, 7: 230–231

UKCC 1984 Code of professional conduct. United Kingdom Central Council for Nursing, Midwifery and Health Visiting, 23 Portland Place London WlN 3AF. paragraphs 13, 14

Ware S 1984 A clicking hip in a newborn baby should never be ignored (letter). The Lancet I: 1184–1185

Waumsley L 1983 Mothers talking about postnatal depression. National Childbirth Trust, London

Webb P 1985 Someone to talk to directory 1985. A directory of self help and community support agencies in the UK and Republic of Ireland. Mental Health Foundation, London

Wood C B S, Walker-Smith J A 1981 MacKeith's infant feeding and feeding difficulties, 6th edn. Churchill Livingstone, Edinburgh. p 15

Wood T 1985 Formal and informal support systems for mothers with newborn. Midwife Health Visitor and Community Nurse 21: 42–49

Woodward S, Pope A, Robson W J, Hagan O 1985 Bereavement counselling after sudden infant death. British Medical Journal 290: 363–365

Young B 1987 (letter) Support groups for CDH sufferers. Nursing Times 83, 50: 12

Zigmond A S, Snaith R P 1983 The hospital anxiety and depression (HAD) scale. Acta Psychiatrica Scandinavica 67: 361–370 (These questionnaires are available, free, through Mr D d'E Panrucker, Professional Communications Manager, Upjohn Ltd, Fleming Way, Crawley, West Sussex RH10 2NJ Tel 0293 31133)

FURTHER READING

Balfour A M 1988 Group for parents. Health Visitor 61, 10: 316–318 — Sleep problems.

Coates C, Godwin B, Grove T, Lazzell C, Stengelhofen J, Zee M (1980) Talking is child's play, part one. Infant gossip. College of Speech Therapists, Harold Poster House, 6 Lechmere Road, London NW2 5BU Tel: 081 459 8521 — Useful for parents.

Coates C, Godwin B, Grove T, Lazzell C, Stengelhofen J (1980) Talking is child's play, part two. Into the world of word. College of Speech Therapists, Harold Poster House, 6 Lechmere Road, London NW2 5BU Tel: 081 459 8521 — Useful for parents.

Crawford W, Bennet R, Hewitt K 1989 Sleep problems in pre-school children. Health Visitor 62, 3: 79–81

De'ath E, Pugh G 1986 Working with parents. A training resource pack. National Children's Bureau, London

De'ath E, Pugh G 1989 Working towards partnership in the early years. National Children's Bureau, London

De'ath E, Webster G 1989 Families and self-help. A resource pack. National Children's Bureau, London

Elfer P, Gatiss S 1990 Charting child health. A survey of community child health services provided by health authorities in England and Wales. National Children's Bureau, London, Section Three — Recommended reading.

Gilbert R G, Fleming P J, Azaz Y, Rudd P T 1990 Signs of illness preceding sudden unexpected death in infants. British Medical Journal 300, 6734: 1237–1239

Kay E 1989 'Accidents will happen.' Nursing Times 85, 3: 26–29

Strategy Group 1990 Action on accidents. The unique role of the Health Service. Report of a NAHA/RoSPA strategy group. National Association of Health Authorities, Birmingham

Wier I K, Dinnick S 1988 Behaviour modification. Child Care Health and Development 14, 5: 355–367 — Sleep problems.

Chapter 6 gives a second and more simple example of the use of the prevention model. Again, it provides a way of thinking about the role of the health visitor, this time with regard to families with children of around the age of three onwards. In this phase, thought is given to preparing the child for his/her school years and to continued surveillance and support for the family.

6

Pre-school visiting

CONTINUING EDUCATION, SCREENING AND SUPPORT

In the two years immediately prior to school entry, the aim is to continue to prevent the occurrence, development and deterioration of problems (see Table 6.1). This is done by encouraging parents to think ahead and prepare their children for their experiences and needs at school, by continuing the search for early signs of health problems and by offering support and/or referral to appropriate services where problems are already established.

A health visitor with a normal caseload would probably expect to visit most families only once or twice in this time. In Portsmouth, for example, they plan for one visit during the third year and then another between three and a half to four and a half years (Powell, 1985). In general, visiting from eighteen months onwards is much less frequent than that during the first year.

It was found by Mayall and Grossmith (1985) to be important that mothers should feel their health visitor was still accessible. They were sure a flying visit was not the answer: to some mothers it could be more irritating than helpful. Mayall and Grossmith suggested that during these years, when the health visitor calls less frequently, families should be sent a regular letter, letting them know or reminding them of where their health visitor can be contacted. They also felt that when their health visitor leaves the post, parents should be notified in writing. This sort of measure becomes much more important in areas of underprivilege where there tends to be a high turnover of staff.

Table 6.1 Pre-school visiting: the work of the health visitor

Aspect of prevention	Examples of activities
Preventing occurrence of condition (Anticipatory guidance)	*Discussion of:* booster immunisation, diet, sleep and stimulation, footwear, ability to dress, creative and social play, head lice, dental care and safety
Preventing development of condition (Surveillance of family health)	*Screening re:* gross motor and fine movements social attainments speech: sentence at 3, articulation at 4 hearing: especially after otitis media vision: especially re amblyopia height: on centile chart
Preventing deterioration of established condition (Supportive work)	*Sympathetic listening Information about services Encouraging self-help groups* re: childhood problem behaviour, marital stress e.g. sex problem, divorce, finance, housing, unemployment, alcoholism in the family, maternal incontinence

EXAMPLES OF PRE-SCHOOL VISITING

The first example follows up Nancy Manners, introduced earlier in the chapters on antenatal and birth visits. She has moved house and has managed to return to work. The second concerns Helen Voisey's work with Mrs Prince, who attended a 'pre-school preparation group' and also a self-help group which Helen had told her about. Outlines of the examples will be found in Tables 6.2 and 6.3.

EXAMPLE ONE: THE MANNERS FAMILY

Mrs Hannah Van der Haastrecht (HV) was planning the priorities in her caseload and, at the same time, attempting to evaluate what had been achieved in recent years amongst the families with children soon to be going to school.

She came to the Manners family's cards and found it difficult to believe that Pauline was now nearly five years old.

Miss Nancy Manners had a very difficult time in getting new accommodation. In the end, when Pauline was two and a half, she had been given a council flat. Three months later she had been able to return to work because she had found, living in the same block of flats, another nurse with a child who wanted to work. Mrs Smith, her husband and Nancy were able to work between them a scheme which allowed them all to work full time. They had checked with the Social Services Department about whether they were obliged to register as a babysitter, and all was well.

When HV had called at the flat for the three year visit, Nancy had shown her how much easier it was now to maintain a safe environment than in the large-roomed bedsitter with an open plan kitchen. They had discussed preparation for school. Pauline was attending the same playgroup as the Smith's son, Eric. Mrs Manners was paying the playgroup fees. Head lice was mentioned and Nancy was very amused by HV's nit in a bottle. It seems that they had had 'trouble' at the nursery but that they had not been given good instructions on how to deal with, or how to avoid, infestation. The health visitor made a mental note to mention to her colleague attached to that playgroup, that they needed some guidance.

At the next visit, when Pauline was four and a half years, Nancy had reported that the

Table 6.2 Example one: the Manners family

Aspect of prevention	Examples of activities
Preventing occurrence of condition (Anticipatory guidance)	Booster immunisation mentioned Safety mentioned Head lice discussed in depth Creative and social play discussed
Preventing development of condition (Surveillance of family health)	*Screening re:* gross motor and fine movements social attainments speech hearing vision, referred to orthoptists height on centile chart
Preventing deterioration of established condition (Supportive work)	*Encouraging self-help groups Information about services Sympathetic listening* None needed

nursery's new approach had been successful and that they now had only a minimal and occasional problem with head lice. Booster immunisations were discussed at that visit, as were the exercises that Pauline had to do for her squint.

The squint had been brought to light at the three and a half year clinic assessment session for height, weight, hearing, vision and developmental attainments. Nancy had said she was not happy about the way Pauline responded to games entailing covering up her right eye. The child was referred to the orthoptists' secondary screening clinic, where she was confirmed to be an early case of straight-eyed amblyopia. Having been caught in good time, the problem was already beginning to be resolved.

Nancy had brought to that clinic her HMSO Sheridan (1975) booklet, marked with all of the attainments at each stage over the years. It had evidently caused both grandmother and mother a great deal of amusement and, HV gathered, a fair amount of effort to cover the full test each time. They had been fascinated to see how consistently Pauline attained about three quarters of each stage in total, but sometimes more heavily in one of the four sectors and sometimes in another at each stage. The centile charts were completed as planned.

During these past two years, Nancy had been in no need of 'supportive' work. She had always known where to contact HV when she wished to. Nancy's accommodation, child care and occupation problems had been solved. Her general outlook and her very clear understanding of her daughter's developmental needs and potential, meant she had been able to cope competently with the normal child behaviour problems. The health visitor felt pleased that deficiencies in Pauline's vision, like several other possible problems, had been prevented from developing (or occurring) on account of the surveillance and information service she had offered. It had seemed relevant to the mother and had been used by her.

EXAMPLE TWO: THE PRINCE FAMILY

Miss Helen Voisey (HV) was looking through the health visitor records of the families who had a child due to attend the pre-school medical examination for the spring term. She was making a special note of children whose developmental surveillance had shown any unusual pattern, in order to bring it to the attention of the school nurse and the doctor.

On looking through the notes of the Prince family, she was reminded of how Daniel had 'faltered' in a social assessment test at three years. He had not needed to be referred, either at that stage or later. Christine had been aged one when Daniel had attended that clinic assessment session. Vera Prince had reported that he was not yet washing his hands, nor was he pulling his pants up and down. He had, until then, always attained either one or two of the items at each stage of the (Barber) developmental centile chart. There had not been much time for discussion at the time, as other people were waiting for their appointments.

Miss Voisey made an appointment to call on the Princes the following week, in order, sensitively, to make sure that Vera was in no way worried by the absence of a mark on the chart, and also to discuss stimulation and play for Daniel. At that visit they had discussed the sort of social behaviour, play and fine movements that Daniel would be likely to be capable of and what he might be able to do by the age of four and by five years of age. Vera said later that she had realised then that she had been leaving Daniel to his own devices whilst she was so busy with the new baby. He had consequently benefited from the attention that both she and her husband had given and they had been very proud of his ability, particularly to draw, at the four years test.

Table 6.3 Example two: the Prince family

Aspect of prevention	Examples of activities
Preventing occurrence of condition (Anticipatory guidance)	*Group discussion of*: safety and discipline preparation for independence head lice creative and social play dental care
Preventing occurrence of condition (Surveillance of family health)	*Screening re*: hearing and language vision height, on centile chart gross motor movements fine movements social skills Discussion e.g. stimulation, safety
Preventing deterioration of established condition (Supportive work)	*Sympathetic listening* *Information about services* *Encouraging self-help groups* } re: occasional incontinence: informed about I.I. group, reported as successful

Also, the health visitor suggested Vera and the children attend the mothers' pre-school preparation group held at the health centre. She was pleased to be invited: one of her friends had attended an earlier course and had evidently enjoyed it. It had been a lively group.

Always at the first meeting of the pre-school preparation course there was discussion about which topics should be covered, and a plan for the six sessions was drawn up. This group had included two other mothers from the same multi-storey block as the Prince family and they were all very keen to discuss what to do about the lack of safe play areas in their locality. Their local councillor was now attempting to have one created. Besides safety, the group had chosen to discuss preparation for independence, head lice, tooth care, creative play and, in the final session, discipline. Vera Prince had made very confident contributions, particularly at these later meetings. Some retired ladies from a nearby church came in and looked after the children and made tea for the mothers.

The most significant feature of the most recent home visit was, in response to the question 'Do you ever lose urine when you don't intend to?', Mrs Prince said that she did, but only occasionally and did not need a pad. She had requested complete confidentiality about the issue. She was very sensitive about it and had not told anyone before. Being busy with the new baby meant her postnatal exercises had been given low priority and she attributed her problem to this.

Helen Voisey had told the young mother about a group she and another health visitor had helped set up which was now self-sustaining. It was whimsically referred to as 'Incontinence Inonymous', met fortnightly and all the members aimed to encourage each other to do the necessary exercises. The local incontinence adviser attended when requested to do so. When HV had met Vera in the street four months later, Vera had indicated that after some hesitation she had attended the group and was very pleased with the outcome.

The health visitor thought about what had been achieved. Developmental assessment had played only one, though an important, part in her preventive work. The groups and the clinics had been very valuable, but she felt that it was at home that the instigatory enabling work was done.

THINKING AHEAD

Anticipatory guidance for families preparing a child for school can cover an enormous number of topics; a few, such as safety, dental care and head lice, are mentioned here as examples.

In these few pages it is not possible to present many subjects. Equally, it is not possible to talk over many items in a 20 minute or half-hour call. A large number of health educational matters can only be fitted in when the health visitor 'switches into automatic', rattles off a well-rehearsed speech and checklists queries and items of advice. This leaves very little time to take account of parental views, and the disadvantages of this sort of autocratic approach have already been touched on in earlier chapters. It seems likely that a two-way discussion of a few points, which are chosen and seen as relevant by the parents, will be more acceptable and more educational overall. This is, of course, provided they know what is 'permissible' (Robinson, 1983).

Time is at a premium, but health visitors may be able to give extra help to disadvantaged people by setting up a discussion group over a few weeks to which mothers are invited to exchange ideas on aspects of preparing young children for their schooling. Some of the issues that may be discussed, both at home visits or at group meetings, might be:

- pre-school immunisations
- diet
- footwear
- stimulation and creative play
- play with other children and playgroups
- toilet training
- ability to dress and undress
- head lice
- teaching small children about sex
- dental care and first visit to dentist
- safety, particularly road drill

and any special queries raised by any of the mothers.

Learning independence and sharing

The practical knowledge that children need in preparation for school includes, for example, experience of being away from their mother, sharing things and putting them away where they belong when not in use, taking care of their clothes, knowing left from right shoes and also recognising their name on their coat, wellingtons and other clothing.

This sort of experience is gained by children whose parents choose to and are able to send them to playgroups or nursery classes. A health visitor's knowledge of criteria for admission, waiting lists for places and any subsidised places that may be available, is invaluable, as is personal contact with local groups and classes. An ex-health visitor, Jeanette Clifton (1983), has described her work as chairman of a playgroup committee and has shown how, in a good playgroup, parents can be involved in practical and pleasant ways.

Safety

Home safety was discussed in the previous chapter (p. 81). As children grow more inquisitive, mobile, venturesome and independent, a very wide variety of safety factors needs to be considered. By this stage road safety is particularly important. Parents need, now, to be teaching by example and by showing their children the Green Cross Code (Health Education Council, 1981).

It seems that there has been a worldwide increase in fatal traffic accidents for children, so marked that it has hidden what have, in fact, been declines in other unnatural causes of child death. Dr Sunderland (1984) studied the child traffic accident figures in Sheffield. He has shown that readily available information can be used for planning for prevention and suggests that programmes should start prior to school age.

A significantly greater proportion of deaths were among underprivileged children living in 'accident prone' areas, those with crowded dwellings and often near to main roads. Dr Sunderland made a plea for attractive and safe play areas to be built in high risk zones and says these are now being provided in Sheffield. He says other studies have shown

the main difference between areas with a high accident rate and other areas was the lack of safe play areas.

Perhaps this is a matter over which health visitors would be able to 'influence policies affecting health' (CETHV, 1977; Phillips, 1986) in their locality. They might do this by liaising with voluntary and any statutory agencies involved in such interests. A pre-school mums' discussion group, of the sort described above, might have some constructive suggestions and be prepared to help.

Teaching children about sex

Pre-school children benefit enormously from being told stories and being read to, from being encouraged to talk about what they feel, do, see and hear and, of course, having their questions answered. Parents sometimes wonder how to respond to 'where do babies come from?' The Health Education Council (HEC) have some very helpful little booklets. One, 'Answering a child's questions' (L13), provides general guidance on what approach to take at the various stages of a child's development. It has a list of relevant inexpensive booklets and information about where further literature can be obtained.

Under four years of age it is suggested that parents give simple answers with small amounts of information which is repeated from time to time. The HEC booklet, 'How we grow up' (SE2), makes quite a useful visual aid to explanations as the child gets a little older, for example, how the baby grows and the abdomen expands. There are some colourful and well-presented, but rather more expensive, books. These, such as Claire Rayner's (1978) 'Body Book', could be borrowed from the library. Group discussion might be particularly helpful to mothers unsure of how to discuss sex with their children. If the group is sympathetic and supportive, sexual problems that the parents have, might also be raised.

Head lice

As young children begin to find other young children to play with, to attend playgroup and later go to school, there is an increased risk that they will come into contact with head lice. This problem has grown in recent years, particularly in middle class communities. Young children work and play with their heads very closely together. It can be very useful, therefore, in these pre-school years to draw parents' attention to the situation and to the simple preventive measures they and their children can take.

Silky-looking hair these days is achieved by using a shampoo. In the past, middle class parents tended to encourage their children to brush their hair until it shone, thereby injuring any louse that might be there. This regular habit, particularly last thing at night, prevented egg laying and colonisation. It seems to have been a significant factor in causing the lower levels of infection amongst the wealthier sections of society, and not, as they might have thought, their being 'rich' or 'clean'. Careful attention, therefore, to brushing and combing and the occasional check to see if there is any evidence of the louse, is the best approach to prevention (Wickenden, 1982).

Head lice and their eggs are very difficult to see. Head inspections reveal only very advanced cases, generally of some four months' duration (Wickenden, 1982). John Maunder (1983) described how the distance of the nits from the scalp can give an indication of the length of an infection and, equally, of the duration of the cure. He provided a list of the publications which can be sent for. They are those associated with the regular courses on head louse control held at the London School of Hygiene and Tropical Medicine.

A fairly common problem is that little white hair muffs brought about by a skin condition, can be mistaken for nits. Professor Maunder pointed out that a hand lens makes it easy to distinguish between them. Showing parents photographs (Wickenden, 1982; Maunder, 1983) can give them at least an idea of what they are looking for. However, a specimen louse and nit in a bottle give a truer picture and have been found, when used in group discussions, to help overcome the taboo associated with this subject (Moore, 1982).

Treatment is simple but care has to be taken over the use of carbaryl and malathion shampoos and lotions to prevent a resistance developing (Maunder, 1981). The louse has already become resistant to two insecticides. Adrienne de Mont (1985) explains about and lists preparations currently available. She says the district pharmacist will be able to provide details of current recommendations on the policy of rotation of the use of these insecticides. The health visitor is in a good position to be able to back up the community health physician's communications by keeping in touch with local chemists over this issue.

In a more proactive approach, school nurses in Bradford took a head lice display into a supermarket. Over 250 parents were able to discover and discuss the basic issues involved (Nursing Times, 1989). John Maunder's positive approach has also been paying off. His courses educating more than 500 senior NHS managers have been instrumental in achieving the significant decrease in the infection rate in the last few years (Nursing Times, 1988).

Dental care

In the pre-school and early school years, children become increasingly receptive to health advice, including that of preventive dental care. Their parents will be the best educators that they could have. However, most of the public and many health professionals fatalistically accept dental disease as inevitable and neglect opportunities for prevention. Health visitors, throughout their contact with the family, are in a good position to help improve parental understanding of the essential elements of dental health.

A Community Outlook (1981) 'teeth sheet' may make a useful visual aid. Very practical advice has been provided by Hadley and Sheiham (1984, 1985). They have given clear accounts of how a low sugar diet allows remineralisation of the teeth and can arrest decay, and how fluoride helps in this process. Dosages of fluoride supplements are stated according to different ages and the amount of fluoride in the drinking water. It is suggested that the water authority should be contacted to find out local fluoride levels. Good literature is suggested, and advice is given on tooth brushing techniques and keeping free of plaque.

Hadley and Sheiham say that dental disease is the third most costly aspect of health care and recommend regular contact between health visitors and community dental officers. These officers can be encouraged to come to talk to local groups. Haringey's community dental clinics have taken on and been very successful with a preventive strategy for dental care (Haringey dental officers, 1984). Let us hope the tide is beginning to turn.

In this section we have looked at some aspects of anticipatory guidance for families in the pre-school period, and particularly at road safety, head lice, sex instruction and dental care, and the need for parents to feel that their health visitors are still accessible.

CONTINUING THE SEARCH

The part the health visitor plays in child health screening differs significantly from place to place. There is a great deal of variation between Health Districts as to who is responsible for child health clinics and surveillance: in East Suffolk, for example, it is mostly health visitors; in some other places it is GPs or clinical medical officers (Macfarlane & Pillay, 1984).

In many child health schemes, for example Professor Barber's (1982; Robertson, 1984), the screening is shared between the health visitor and the GP. This fits in well with the Health Visitors Association (1985) (HVA) proposals. The HVA suggestions for the pre-school years are that for the test at about three years of age the health visitor undertakes it alone, and that at the screening prior to school entry it is undertaken by the health visitor and/or the school nurse and the doctor together.

Close cooperation between the health visitor and the GP is required in Somerset in both their urban and their rural schemes. They achieve very high attendance levels at the pre-school test by making it a prerequisite for school entry and by using computerised administration (Bowie & Jones, 1984).

There are many screening and surveillance schemes available. Validated examples range between the time consuming, in-depth Sheridan (1975) approach and the neat, centile chart scheme by Barber et al (1976) discussed in Chapter 5 (pp. 90–92). There is a booklet for use with the Barber scheme which provides a clear description of how it is intended the tests should be undertaken (Barber & Glasgow University Department of Child Health, 1976). Each item is individually explained with the exception of the 'whisper' hearing test at four years of age.

Hearing

The explanation about this item is to be found in the introduction of the Reed hearing test booklet used in the test. This booklet is published by the Royal National Institute for the Deaf (RNID), whose addresses are given at the end of the chapter.

Deafness is liable to be a problem in the aftermath of recurrent ear infections. These infections are fairly common in young children and it therefore seems worth discussing with parents whether their child tends to suffer from them. Barritt and Darbyshire (1984) suggested that GPs examine children's ears six weeks after an attack of otitis media, as they found that children with abnormal eardrums at that stage were more likely to have a problem with deafness and warranted audiological testing. In their small study they found the appearance of the eardrum to be a more reliable indicator than parental opinion about their child's deafness. However, this should not deter health visitors from treating very seriously any concern expressed by parents.

Sight

Vision testing at four years in the Barber scheme uses very simple equipment. Some very small objects such as threads, small beads and pins are put on the table and, with each eye covered separately, the child is asked to pick some up, one at a time. This is likely to be an easier test in the home than the Stycar five letter test, which can present problems when space and light are inadequate (Robertson, 1981).

However, Hall et al (1982) studied various vision screening tests and found that their 'hundreds and thousands' test on older, more reliable six-year olds was able only to discover fairly severe reduction in visual acuity. Regarding squints they found that parents and other non-professionals were generally the people to notice the squint first. Also, it did not tend to be a cover test or corneal reflections but careful observation that led professionals to discover squints. Hall et al felt that earlier referral from the community was encouraged by the reduced ophthalmic outpatient waiting list due to the community orthoptist's secondary screening role. It is important to keep the wait between detection and diagnosis as short as reasonably possible and National Health Service opticians can also be very helpful in this.

A study of school entrants in London by Ismail and Lall (1981) found that two thirds of the children with visual defects had not been detected prior to going to school. However, this is not as bad as it might seem, as all the children with a severe impairment had been diagnosed. Their research led them to feel that the problem was lack of suitable visual screening techniques rather than lack of expertise. They recommended that screening should continue using currently available procedures, but that there should be further investigation and a thorough search for more objective techniques for pre-school vision screening.

Minor and/or recently developed hearing and vision defects were discovered in some school entrants in Gwent. Lambert et al (1984) found some of the children with vision defects had not been tested at the three and a half year medical. They noted that health visitors need a reliable system to inform them of non-attendance. One child had been uncooperative at the test, which it is pointed out can be a sign of a possible problem. Ounsted et al (1983) felt that non-cooperation at the preschool assessment should always be followed up.

Speech

The expectation that a child at three years of age would be able to use three word sentences was mentioned in the previous chapter (p. 95). At four years, a child with poor articulation, perhaps omitting or substituting consonants, would also need to be referred on for investigation by a speech therapist, and by a doctor if necessary. Normally, health visitors can refer clients directly to the speech therapist (Aspinall, 1987; Wiseman, 1987). Margaret Pollak (1984) felt that speech problems are not taken seriously and not dealt with early enough. She explained causes of speech problems, described diagnosis and treatment and demonstrated the value of early referral.

Physical measurements

Parents will be interested to see, as the years have passed, the sort of picture that has emerged on the centile height, weight and head circumference charts (see Ch. 5, p. 94). It is easier to measure the weight and height of children attending a clinic equipped for these procedures. Measuring children who do not attend needs a little more ingenuity.

Height can be measured in the home against a doorway (or a wall) where there is no skirting board, so the child can stand absolutely upright. A carpenter's/DIY collapsible wooden rule or a metal expansible tape could be used. The RNID hearing test booklet or a block of wood could be used to ensure a right angle with the doorway (see Fig. 6.1). Accuracy also depends on the child standing with heels together, touching the ground and against the doorway. The head should be looking straight forward, eyes on a level with the tops of the ears, and, perhaps, with a very gentle upward pressure on the back of the jaw, as shown by Harvey and Wallis (1978). Parents may feel it is worth noting the child's weight at regular intervals at the chemist, and would be particularly encouraged to do so, should there be any concern.

A school nurse in Oxford, Jill Moss (1985), described how she measured children in primary schools and found a number of cases with unidentified growth problems. She used Whitehouse and Castlemead Publications' portable wall chart. Routine measuring in schools was later discontinued there, as it was undertaken in the pre-school period by health visitors at child health

Fig. 6.1   Tape measuring, at home.

clinics, though in many places this measuring is continued into the school years.

The last visit or clinic session before school entry is a good time to check with the parents that they have a complete personal record, not only of immunisations, including the pre-school booster, but also of centile height and weight charts for future reference should they ever be needed.

Maintaining contact and continuity

One of the problems in child health screening and surveillance can be that children sometimes remain unscreened because it is difficult to make contact with the family. A large number of mothers with pre-school children go out to work and their children are minded. Sue Owen (1984) surveyed Area Health Authorities to find out if they had special liaison arrangements between health visitors and social services regarding child-minders and the children who were minded. She asked, too, whether there were special arrangements for health visitors to meet the minders and whether evening child health clinics were available for working mothers.

It was found that most social service departments sent lists of child-minders, but did not state which children were placed with them. However, in three areas health visitors were notified about where children were being minded, one of them very helpfully on a weekly basis. This service depends on the local authority having a scheme which requires weekly returns from the child-minders.

Health visitor contact with child-minders varied. Sue Owen found that geographic patch-based health visitors tended to be in contact with and visit child-minders in their patch. In some health authorities, child-minders were being visited by the health visitor from the practice of the minder's own GP. The health visitor then notified colleagues about the children being minded there. Evening clinics were held in only six health authorities, others relying on evening visits by health visitors and/or assuming parents would ask the minder to take their child to the clinic.

An improvement in health visitor contact with child-minders and the children they care for is much needed. Liaison with the social services department and explanations about the potential benefits to the health of the children being minded, might trigger the appropriate cooperation between a larger number of social service and health departments.

Government advice (DHSS, 1980) is that the results of early childhood surveillance should be made known to those responsible for screening in the school years. Systems of notification and liaison arrangements will vary from place to place. There is an obvious advantage if the height and weight charts can be passed on to and continue through the school medical notes.

Parents who want to know about school medicals, will find a brief outline in Elizabeth Forsythe's (1981) *Preparation for School. A Medical Guide for Parents*. It could also be useful for explaining about some of the common health problems that might be found at these examinations or encountered during the schooldays.

In this section we have looked at some aspects of screening and surveillance in the immediate pre-school years, in particular hearing, vision and speech, and we have looked at the need for liaison with social service departments in order to keep in contact with children who spend their day with a child-minder.

CONTINUED SUPPORT

Supportive work where problems are already established can be very important. By giving people a chance to talk out their problems and by telling them of help and services available, health visitors may be able to help prevent greater difficulties arising out of the current situation. Examples given here of this supportive work are child behavioural difficulties, marital difficulties such as sexual problems and impending separation and divorce, and young women's urinary incontinence. These types of problems might, of course, be encountered at earlier visits too.

Problem behaviour

Studies of children's behaviour up to school age have found that there is far more problem behaviour in the two years prior to school than in babyhood, most occurring at around the age of three. These problems were found to be often associated with mental health problems of the mother (Bax & Hart, 1976). They were also discovered to correlate with speech and language delay (Jenkins et al, 1980). They could easily be overlooked because it was found that mothers did not tend to take problems of the children's behaviour to the doctor, nor were they attending the clinic regularly as they had done.

Assessment

Early attention is warranted, not only to help the mothers' mental state but also on account of the association between speech and language delay with slow attainments in reading and writing and this, in turn, with deviant behaviour later on. The studies found that around a fifth or more of the children seen had behavioural problems in these pre-school years, half of the problems being classed as moderate or severe.

A chart has been provided by Ruth Brink (1982) which can assist in assessing whether or not a child's problem is serious. Some parents might find it a reassuring document. Parent counselling

was discussed by Peter Tucker (1985a, 1985b). He stressed the importance of being able to see the problem from the parents' viewpoint and of having counselling skills that include effective listening.

What can be done

The most disruptive problems for the family and the most difficult to deal with in South Glamorgan research were found to be sleep problems and hyperactivity. A study of the records of eleven health visitors showed that the families with this problem had received more visits than other families, but that over a year little improvement had been achieved. Behavioural techniques developed by South Glamorgan psychologists had been used very successfully, achieving improvements in just a few weeks. It was therefore felt that health visitors should have the opportunity to train in these methods. To use them health visitors would need to change their visiting pattern a little, as the programme needs two or three weekly contacts initially (Thomas et al, 1982).

Practical guidance has been provided by a clinical psychologist, Hewitt (1981a, 1981b), on what help health visitors can give to families with pre-school children who have sleeping problems and those whose children are over-active. Bowler & Watson (1984) described the outcome of a workshop set up to help health visitors gain a better understanding of behavioural techniques. It was very successful. This course and lunchtime follow-up group discussions, enabled more help to be given to families with problems, without referral to the psychology department. Of course, consultation with Child Guidance is always a possible option.

One health visitor, Mavis Maureen Raper (1985a, 1985b, 1985c), made a special study of hyperactive children. She described common characteristics of these children and, by providing a case history, demonstrated the way play therapy is planned. Nicky Milligan (1984) put forward the particular case of 'gifted children'. Both of these writers gave the addresses of support groups. Frieda Painter (1984) has written a parents' guide to *Living with a Gifted Child*, which some parents may find helpful as it offers guidance on a range of problems, ways of coping and of assessing the child.

There is much greater understanding now of the correlation between stress in the mother and preschool childhood behaviour and illness problems. Parental emotional status is therefore an important priority (Bax et al, 1980).

Marital stress and problems

It is generally felt that one of the advantages for areas where health visitors remain with the same caseload and the same families for a long time, is that very delicate issues which trouble the family may more easily be brought into discussions. This is because trust has been built up over the years. However, a health visitor with the appropriate manner, training and skills should be able to establish a good counselling relationship relatively quickly.

Jack Dominian (1982) saw the health visitor as being in a good position to be able to help couples in the early, vulnerable years of their marriage. He said that when a problem is identified, the couple should be persuaded to seek expert help, but that this is not always acceptable to them. In this case, he suggested the health visitor should try to help them 'as best she can'. He provided some helpful tips on counselling style and approach. Further well-written guidance is available from Tony Lake and Fran Acheson (1988). Health visitors can also turn to people such as family planning or marriage guidance counsellors for consultation on the general principles of how to help.

Sexuality

Health visitors sometimes feel inadequately educated for helping a couple with sexual difficulties. Those finding themselves the confidant of couples with problems who are unable or unwilling to seek expert advice, may feel the need to attend a course on psycho-sexual counselling like the one described by Jennett Caldwell (1982). It may be very helpful to consult with and/or involve the GP with a couple's problem, if they wish this.

Sometimes couples can find that a book provides the answers. One that is intended to enable people to help themselves is David Mace's (1972) *Sexual Difficulties in Marriage*. Another approach which can be helpful is to invite several couples facing problems to come to the clinic one evening to see the film, 'Sexuality and Communication'. The film demonstrates the important part played by communication and gives a clear explanation, often demonstrated through role play, of common difficulties. It is very useful as a trigger film or video to encourage discussion. It can be hired for about £13.00 from Concorde (address at end of chapter), or may be available from your local health promotion and education unit.

Divorce

Marital problems may have got to such a pitch that the parents are considering separation and divorce. They will be facing all the feelings associated with grief, so well described by Tony Lake (1984), and have the same need to talk about their problems and feelings. The Divorce Conciliation and Advisory Service (Health Visitor, 1983; Harris, 1983) or the Marriage Guidance Council may be able to offer help. Self-help groups, such as Gingerbread and Families Need Fathers, tend to be turned to later (Richards, 1982).

Dr Richards and Ann Mitchell (1985) both studied the effect of separation and divorce on children and found that they tend to fare better if they are able to talk about it, if they have the family situation explained to them and are able to keep in touch with both parents from very early on. Ann Mitchell feels her book might help parents contemplating divorce, and members of the wider family associated with it, to see how other people's children have felt, and to understand better the problems of their own children. Dr Richards saw support for parents and children as important preventive work for health visitors. He said simple counselling can be very effective and felt discussion might help parents to see their children's needs as separate from their own.

Incontinence

Urinary incontinence has been shown to be a very common problem. Jennifer Sleep (1984) in her study of the effects of episiotomy on around a thousand women found that three months after the birth of a baby 22% of the multiparae and 15% of the primiparae suffered from it. Some 6% were needing to wear a pad. Perhaps it is something health visitors should routinely ask about, very sensitively, as part of their surveillance of mothers' health. It has been suggested that asking if they ever leak when coughing or sneezing is a good way of discovering the sufferers (General Practitioner, 1988).

In explaining about assessment and the promotion of continence, Christine Norton (1984) said that it is still not generally believed that most sufferers can regain continence. A physiotherapist, Sheila Harrison (1984), has described how weakened muscles can be re-educated by regular practice and how assessment and instruction are an essential feature of treatment. Pelvic floor exercises have been compared with other non-operative treatments and were found to be very successful (Henalla et al, 1989).

Feneley and Blannin's (1984) well-written book gives a short, optimistic and clear account of the problem and is very much to be recommended. It is likely to improve the quality of many people's lives. However, a group of mothers may find it particularly helpful to see the tape/slide presentation, 'The management of incontinence' by Camera Talks Ltd (1982), with a health visitor explaining, as necessary, some of the more tech-

nical jargon. They might also find useful some of the literature from the Paddington and North Kensington Health Education Departments with Victoria Health Education Department (1986) catalogue, 'Health Education Resources on Women's Health'. A self-help pamphlet, 'Regaining bladder control. A step-by-step guide to overcoming a very common problem', is available free of charge from the Coloplast Advisory Service (see Useful Addresses). It is not always easy to maintain the necessary level of exercises by oneself, and a small self-help group may be the best answer.

Although the main thrust of health visiting is generally aimed towards preventing the occurrence and the development of problems, supportive work can be an important feature. We have looked at examples such as marital problems of a sexual nature and of impending separation and divorce. Incontinence may occur more widely and also be more amenable to treatment than is generally thought.

This chapter on pre-school visiting provided another example of the way the role of the health visitor can be thought about and described. As before, it has been done by artificially dividing the work into three aspects of the prevention of health problems. Examples were provided of preventing the occurrence and the development of conditions and of preventing deterioration in the case of known problems.

USEFUL ADDRESSES

The Coloplast Advisory Service
Freepost
Peterborough Business Park
Peterborough PE2 0BR
Tel 0733 239898

Concorde Video and Films
201 Felixstowe Road,
Ipswich IP3 9BJ
Tel 0473 715754

Royal National Institute for the Deaf
9a Clairmont Gardens, Glasgow
Tel 041 332 0343
105 Gower Street,
London WC1E 6AH
Tel 071 387 8033

REFERENCES

Aspinwall N R 1987 (letter) Speech therapy referrals. Health Visitor 60, 9: 288
Barber J H 1982 Preschool developmental screening — the results of a four year period. Health Bulletin 40: 170–178

Barber J H, Boothman R, Stanfield J P 1976 A new visual chart for preschool developmental screening. Health Bulletin 34: 80–91
Barber J H, Department of General Practice, University of

Glasgow with assistance from the Department of Child Health, University of Glasgow 1976 The Woodside system of preschool developmental screening: description of the tests. Econoprint, Edinburgh

Barritt P W, Darbyshire P J 1984 Deafness after otitis media in general practice. Journal of the Royal College of General Practitioners 34: 92–94

Bax M, Hart H 1976 Health needs of preschool children. Archives of Disease in Childhood 51: 848–852

Bax M, Hart H, Jenkins S 1980 The health needs of preschool children. Thomas Coram Research Unit, University of London, London

Bowie C, Jones A P 1984 Court come true — for better for worse? British Medical Journal 289: 1322–1324

Bowler J F, Watson P L 1984 A child behaviour workshop. Health Visitor 57: 302–303

Brink R E 1982 How serious is the child's behaviour problem? American Journal of Maternal and Child Nursing 7: 33–36

Caldwell J 1982 On the right course. Nursing Times 78: 58

Camera Talks Ltd 1982 The management of incontinence. Tape/slide: two parts. Camera Talks Ltd, London

Clifton J 1983 What's your view of a playgroup? Health Visitor 56: 342–343

Community Outlook 1981 Teeth sheet. Nursing Times Community Outlook 77, 33: 272–273

CETHV 1977 An investigation into the principles of health visiting. Council for the Education and Training of Health Visitors, London

DHSS 1980 Prevention in the child health services. Department of Health and Social Security, London

Dominian J 1982 Marital stress in the early years. Health Visitor 55: 146–149

Feneley R C L, Blannin J P 1984 incontinence. Help for an unmentionable problem. Churchill Livingstone, Edinburgh

Forsythe E 1981 Preparation for school. A medical guide for parents. Faber and Faber, London

General Practitioner 1988 Ask subtly about leaking. General Practitioner 25th March: 17

Hadley A, Sheiham A 1984 Smile please! Nursing Times 80, 27: 28–31

Hadley A, Sheiham A 1985 Guidelines for promoting better dental health in children. Health Visitor 58: 133–134

Hall S M, Pugh A G, Hall D M B 1982 Vision screening in the under-5s. British Medical Journal 285: 1096–1098

Haringey dental officers 1984 Making sure the children don't have a caries in the world. Health and Social Services Journal XCIV: 322–323

Harris P M 1983 Coping with divorce. Health Visitor 56: 98–99

Harrison S M 1984 Re-education of pelvic floor muscles. Nursing Times Supplement 80, 14: 13–14

Harvey D, Wallis S 1978 Children of short stature: part 1. Midwife, Health Visitor and Community Nurse 14: 136–139

Health Education Council 1981 Play it safe! A guide to preventing children's accidents. Health Education Council and Scottish Health Education Group in Association with the BBC

Health Visitor 1983 The Divorce Conciliation and Advisory Service. Health Visitor 56: 97

Health Visitors Association 1985 The health visitor's role in child health surveillance: a policy statement. Health Visitors Association, London

Henalla S M, Hutchins C J, Robinson P, MacVicar J 1989 Non-operative methods in the treatment of female genuine stress incontinence of urine. Journal of Obstetrics and Gynaecology 9, 3: 222–225

Hewitt K E 1981a Sleeping problems in pre-school children: what to ask and what to do. Health Visitor 54: 100–101

Hewitt K E 1981b Overactivity in young children: how health visitors can help. Health Visitor 54: 276–277

lsmail H, Lall P 1981 Visual acuity of school entrants. Child: Care, Health and Development 7: 127–134

Jenkins S, Bax M, Hart H 1980 Behaviour problems in pre-school children. Journal of Child Psychology and Psychiatry 21: 5–17

Lambert C, Miers M, Edwards J, Farrow 1984 Hearing and vision screening in preschool children. Health Visitor 57: 329–331

Lake T 1984 Living with grief. Sheldon Press, London

Lake T, Acheson F 1988 Room to listen, room to talk. National Council for Voluntary Organisations, Bedford Square Press, London

Mace D 1972 Sexual difficulties in marriage. The National Guidance Council, Rugby

Macfarlane J A, Pillay U 1984 Who does what, and how much in the preschool child health services in England. British Medical Journal 289: 851–852

Maunder J W 1981 Treatment for head lice (letter). Nursing Times 77: 995

Maunder J W 1983 The head louse resurgence. Maternal and Child Health 8: 51–56

Mayall B, Grossmith C 1985 The health visitor and the provision of services. Health Visitor 58: 349–352

Milligan N 1984 Gifted children — how to help in the preschool years. Health Visitor 57: 22–23

Mitchell A 1985 Children in the middle. Living through divorce. Tavistock Publications, London

de Mont A 1985 Don't let your hair down. Nursing Times Community Outlook 81, 37: 16–17

Moore P M 1982 Message-in-a-bottle (letter). Health Visitor 55: 629

Moss J 1985 Measuring up. Nursing Times Community Outlook 81, 15: 24–26

Norton C 1984 The promotion of continence. Nursing Times Supplement 80, 14: 4–10

Nursing Times 1988 Educating parents helped fight against head lice. Nursing Times 84, 13: 10

Nursing Times 1989 Lice advice. Nursing Times 85, 46: 9

Ounsted M, Cockburn J, Moar V A 1983 Developmental assessment at four years: are there any differences between children who do, or do not, cooperate? Archives of Disease in Childhood 58: 286–289

Owen S 1984 Childminders' contact with health visitors: results of a nationwide survey. Health Visitor 57: 171–172

Paddington and North Kensington Health Education Departments with Victoria Health Education Department 1986 Health education resources on women's health. Victoria Health Education Department, 1a Thorndite Close, London SW10

Painter F 1984 Living with a gifted child. Souvenir Press Ltd, London

Phillips S 1986 A centre for change. Nursing Times Community Outlook 82, 7: 15–17

Pollak M 1984 Speech problems in childhood. Health Visitor 57: 334–335

Powell J 1985 Keeping watch. Nursing Times Community Outlook 81, 2: 15–19

Raper M M 1985a In perpetual motion. Nursing Mirror 160, 10: 16–17

Raper M M 1985b Food — the unknown enemy. Nursing Mirror 160, 11: 35–37

Raper M M 1985c Play therapy. Nursing Mirror 160, 12: 19–21

Rayner C 1978 Body book. Deutsch, London

Richards M 1982 Do broken marriages affect children? Health Visitor 55: 152–153

Robertson C A 1981 A review of vision screening in pre-school children. Health Visitor 54: 52–57

Robertson C A 1984 Preventive health care for infants. In: Houston M J (ed) Maternal and Infant Health. Churchill Livingstone, Edinburgh

Robinson K 1983 Talking with clients. In: Clark J, Henderson J (eds) Community health. Churchill Livingstone, Edinburgh

Sheridan M D 1975 The developmental progress of infants and young children. HMSO, London

Sleep J 1984 Management of the perineum. Nursing Times 80, 48: 51–54

Sunderland R 1984 Dying young in traffic. Archives of Disease in Childhood 59: 754–757

Thomas J A, Bidder R T, Hewitt K, Gray O P 1982 Health visiting and pre-school children with behavioural problems in the County of South Glamorgan: an exploratory study. Child: Care, Health and Development 8: 93–103

Tucker P 1985a The scope and practice of parent counselling: part 1. Midwife Health Visitor and Community Nurse 21: 282–286

Tucker P 1985b The scope and practice of parent counselling: part 2. Midwife Health Visitor and Community Nurse 21: 310–313

Wickenden J 1982 'Nurse, why are the kids always getting nits?' Health Visitor 55: 469–476

Wiseman D J C 1987 (letter) Speech therapy referrals. Health Visitor 60, 11: 358

FURTHER READING

Webb C 1985 Sexuality, nursing and health. Scutari Press, Harrow, Middx

Both the prevention and the family health needs frameworks are used in this chapter to describe health visitors' work in preventive health care for the elderly. The chapter ends with two visits given as examples of these activities.

7

Work with the elderly

THE FRAMEWORKS

In this chapter both of the perspectives demonstrated in the previous four chapters are used. In the first three sections we use the prevention model to describe ways in which the health visitor can help prevent the occurrence and the development of problems and a deterioration in established conditions.

The fourth section takes a brief look at an old person's requirements in daily living, using a form of the family health needs model which includes physical, emotional, environmental and social aspects of health. Two examples are given in this format, but running through them are also concepts from the prevention framework of the earlier sections.

The three aspects of prevention

Attachment to general practice has brought health visitors into closer contact with the elderly, but for most this is only once a crisis has occurred. A good preventive service, however, depends on making contact early. For example, increasing people's awareness of health needs in retirement is best undertaken much earlier in life. To be effective, a screening programme needs to bring to light potentially incapacitating problems well before they reach serious proportions. Also, where a crisis such as bereavement has occurred, care should be offered in good time. The prevention framework can draw attention to each of these three aspects of the role of the health visitor in this field.

Preventive health care for the elderly is becoming more and more necessary, but there are many constraints (Robertson, 1984a). For example, care of the elderly has traditionally been given low priority. Also, a special approach is needed, especially with regard to screening. Here the aim is to maximise on an old person's ability to overcome and minimise socio-functional problems rather than to cure disease.

Many examples of activities with the elderly are given in these first three sections. It is *not* the intention to draw up an 'ideal model' of health visiting practice in this field. The aim is to discuss its potential and to present possibilities by looking at a range of schemes currently undertaken. However, a health visitor working only with the elderly may be able to cover quite a number of the points raised.

EDUCATION AND ACTION

Work aimed at avoiding the occurrence of problems and at promoting the health of old people, as shown in Figure 7.1, can involve health visitors in a variety of activities. This might be in clinics and teaching sessions both before and during retirement, in individual and general discussions and sometimes in negotiations in the community to try to improve the environment and local facilities.

EDUCATION **ACTION**

HEALTH IN MIDDLE AGE

Influencing life-style

Attention to problems

'PLANNED' RETIREMENT

Many social factors

ENVIRONMENTAL INFLUENCES

Adequate and appropriate facilities

EARLY EDUCATION

In schools and to women's groups

SELECTIVE IMMUNISATION

e.g. against influenza

Fig. 7.1 Aspects of primary preventive care — to prevent problems occurring in retirement.

EDUCATION

Health education in schools

It could be argued that really effective health education in preparation for old age should be started in the school years. Many significant diseases are affected by life-style, for example, obesity, pulmonary and cardiovascular. Habits established in youth, like eating habits, smoking and exercise, can set patterns for health in later years. Health visitors may be able to help young people become aware of these factors by giving talks in schools or, alternatively, by acting as advisers to teachers.

Health education and screening in the middle years

In the middle years problems can emerge which may be troublesome in old age (Burkitt, 1977). This may also be the best time to start thinking, more specifically, about retirement. Health visitors may be able to become involved at well women or well men clinics like those described by Kerr (1975), Pike (1975) and Antrobus (1981). It seems that the health visitor at the Antrobus clinic covers the more emotional and social aspects of care, whilst the district nurse and the SEN concentrate upon the physical aspects of screening like urinalysis, blood pressure and breast palpation. They back up the examination with health education, using leaflets provided by the local health education department. Mrs Antrobus says the aim is to detect and overcome hidden disease at an early stage and to encourage people to adopt a suitable lifestyle, over the control of obesity for example. The health visitor at Dr Pike's clinic interviews and discusses retirement plans with the middle-aged people who come (Dodsworth, 1976).

Pre-retirement talks and discussions

A happy retirement involves many factors such as those shown in Box 7.5 in the fourth section: adequate finance and housing, friendship, interesting things to do and satisfactory health, both physical and emotional. Retirement can, however, bring the need for enormous, and often sudden, adjustments to accustomed patterns of daily activity and companionship. Early planning and preparation is a great advantage.

Health visitors may have the opportunity to conduct pre-retirement courses or, alternatively, to encourage local employers to undertake them. The Pre-Retirement Association and the Workers Educational Association help employers organise the classes in various parts of the country. It seems that only 6% of those about to retire receive formal pre-retirement preparation (DHSS, 1981).

Stott (1982) and Clapham (1980) have shown how a health visitor with a normal caseload can undertake classes. Denise Stott describes how high levels of redundancy inspired her to start a '50-plus club', eight week pre-retirement course for the over-50s. She used films and other visual aids, tape recordings and visiting speakers to help cover the following topics:

- adjustment to retirement
- bereavement
- diet
- finance
- accommodation
- accidents
- leisure and
- exercise.

A questionnaire completed by the participants at the end of the course proved very useful in helping to plan subsequent sessions. Stott listed the books, films and organisations found to be particularly helpful.

Joyce Clapham found that in addition to teaching on topics such as:

- diet
- constipation
- teeth
- sleeping
- keeping warm
- care of the feet
- influenza and
- home nursing,

she was able to help participants increase their mobility by introducing them to gentle exercises in her 'Keeping Fit in Retirement' classes. After a very disappointing beginning (only one person came to the first session) there was a gradual increase in numbers, levelling out at attendances of around 17 at each session.

There is widespread ignorance about the financial and support services available to people in need (Equal Opportunities Commission, 1980). Knowing how to get this help and awareness of the value of seeking it early may help to avoid potential crises and to enable people to maintain an independent style of life. Health visitors who are asked to give talks to groups such as the Women's Institute, Townswomen's Guild, Ladies' Circle and old people's luncheon clubs, may be able to draw attention to these benefits and find this a useful approach to increasing local understanding of health and social needs retirement. We take a further look at health promotion for older people in the later chapters, especially in Example One in Chapter 12 and Example Two in Chapter 14. Health visitors interested in modern approaches to health promotion for the elderly and the latest schemes, will find much food for thought at the quarterly meetings of the Health Visitors' Association Special Interest Group for Older People (see useful addresses). Vari Drennan's (1988) work also makes a good starting point.

ACTION

Immunisation

Shukla (1981) has suggested that some measure of illness amongst old people could be prevented if those who were particularly vulnerable were given influenza vaccine. Special attention might be given to people over 75 years, those living in old people's homes and those with chronic chest complaints, and health visitors might become involved in this activity by explaining the scheme to those who would qualify for it.

Provision of facilities

Individual preparation for retirement is nullified for some people by their poverty, by lack of local meeting places and by traditional attitudes.

Townsend (1963) has drawn a very sad picture of working class men in their late 60s and early 70s. They showed considerable apprehension about retirement as, once they ceased to work, their status would be lowered in the eyes of their family and they would have little or no spare money for hobbies. After a lifetime where friendships were formed through work or the pub, the prospect of retirement appeared particularly bleak.

Such people need help of a practical nature once retirement has begun. Townsend suggested the need for occupational provision for the retired, a sentiment vaguely reflected in a DHSS (1981) White Paper. This mentioned a range of voluntary occupations, the need for clubs, recreational facilities, low cost holidays, libraries and adult education.

Health visitors may need to step outside their day-to-day visiting role in order to use their influence over the provision of suitable facilities. Liz Day (1981) is a health visitor who is gradually achieving an effect in this way (Day & Mogridge, 1981). At her suggestion, a local vicar incorporated a workshop for the elderly into his community centre and she had plans to set up meeting places which would bring the isolated together as well as providing services such as health education, keep fit and screening. Her appointment is as a specialist health visitor. It is unlikely that a generalist appointment would leave much time for going out and helping to organise community facilities.

In this section, we have looked at health visitors' primary preventive work for the elderly, which tends mostly to be through health education: helping to make people aware of risks to health in old age. The aim is to try to encourage people to pursue suitable life-styles and to organise their environment and their social relationships in order to minimise health risks and to promote good mental and physical health. Activities such as screening for physical, social and emotional difficulties in the middle years and schemes to improve local facilities, can also play an important part.

SCREENING THE ELDERLY

A socio-functional approach

Effective health visitor screening for the elderly is

aimed, not at a search for specific medical conditions, but at discovering *functional disabilities*, basically the *effects* of disease and of social circumstances. Health visitors seek, in particular, the factors which influence people's *ability to cope* (see Fig. 7.2). It is hoped these can be attended early and old people helped to maintain the independence and mobility they desire — despite the presence of disease.

Questions similar to those considered in Chapter 5, such as those about monitoring the programme, the availability of services (in this case mostly social services) and those whom the screening might not be reaching, need to be covered in both planning and evaluation of the programmes. These questions, along with an early example of health visitor geriatric screening, have been discussed

elsewhere. They have, of course, a range of different answers (Robertson, 1984b).

Designing programmes

Every Health District will have a different and particular health and welfare profile of its elderly and ought, therefore, to have a specially designed programme to meet those needs. For this reason I have not put forward a prescribed format. Instead, some illustrations and references are provided, so that health visitors can investigate further and map out a scheme which suits their special circumstances.

A variety of methods have been described in the professional journals and Figure 7.3 shows the elements of the basic framework which the good

Fig. 7.2 The main concern in health visitor screening for the elderly.

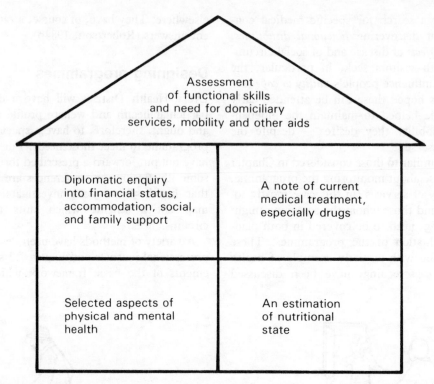

Assessment
of functional skills
and need for domiciliary
services, mobility and other aids

Diplomatic enquiry
into financial status,
accommodation, social,
and family support

A note of current
medical treatment,
especially drugs

Selected aspects of
physical and mental
health

An estimation
of nutritional
state

Fig. 7.3 Screening programmes for the elderly: a basic framework.

ones tend to have. Two screening programmes designed specifically for health visitors are given here as examples. The first used a postal questionnaire and the second was an experimental study. Other programmes and schemes which may provide useful pointers are mentioned briefly.

Example one
Using a postal questionnaire

In Glasgow, a system was designed for use by health visitors (Barber, 1981). A postal questionnaire was used as a basis for screening. It asked whether:

- the person lives alone
- is without a relative to help in time of need
- there are days when the person has no hot meal
- they are concerned about, or suffering from, a problem with
  — general health

— hearing
— vision
- they were in hospital within the previous twelve months.

An affirmative answer to any of the questions on the form, or failure to return it, was taken to indicate a need for comprehensive assessment. Professor Barber says this identified nine tenths of the old people in his study with a problem which needed more investigation.

An assessment interview

The assessment, which took the health visitor about an hour, was in three parts: medico-social problems; social service needs; and questions on physical health. A sample of each of the three assessment record cards used is shown in Professor Barber's article. A checklist format was used. The health visitor referred people with previously undisclosed medical symptoms to the GP and other problems to appropriate members of the health care team. Averaged over a year, it was estimated that it took the health visitor some four and a half hours a week to undertake the scheme, including the associated administrative work.

Example two
An experimental study

The most fully reported screening format is the one undertaken by Karen Luker (1982), who studied the effect of health visiting-intervention in the context of care for the elderly. A problem-oriented format was used for recording, with a separate sheet to show changes in the situation. The interview schedule (pp. 73–88) included:

- a life satisfaction index
- a mental impairment measure
- housing
- finances
- children and social contacts
- health
- cooking and dietary history
- shopping and housework
- mobility
- bathing and dressing
- dentition
- weight
- heating
- sleep
- medication
- vision
- hearing
- balance.

Also listed (pp. 89–94) were the health visitor's responses to some of the problems that were found.

Other programmes and schemes

The Kilsyth Questionnaire (Powell & Crombie, 1974) is an early example of a scheme devised for health visitors to screen old people in their own homes. It included assessment of ability to do everyday tasks, physical and mental health, a nutrition test and an investigation of current drug therapy.

Screening programmes for use by the primary health care team have been described by Williams (1979, Ch. 8), Dodsworth (1976) and Douglas-Jones (1980). Neil (1982) has reported on one undertaken by a health visitor and SEN.

The Williams programme was explained in great detail and many useful ideas were included. One was the checklist for assessment by Barlow and Matthews (pp. 45–46) to help discover old people's need for domiciliary services and is outlined in Table 7.1. Another was the way some old people were selected for regular contact by someone from the primary health care team because they were considered to be 'at risk'. Williams' (pp. 114–115) criteria and some suggested by Stanton (1979) include people:

- living alone
- housebound
- recently bereaved
- liable to hypothermia
- vulnerable to poor nutrition
- liable to fall

Table 7.1 Checklists for assessment of old people's functional ability and need for domiciliary services

Aspect	Examples
Personal	
Involving the whole body	Cutting toe nails; climbing stairs and using public transport
Mobility in the home	Getting around the house; getting in and out of bed and getting to the lavatory
Manipulation of the hands	Shaving, combing the hair, washing and being able to feed self
Mobility outside	Ability to get out of doors
Domestic	
Heavier tasks	Decorating, cleaning windows on the outside and undertaking minor household repairs
Moderate tasks	Cleaning windows inside, washing floors and washing clothes
Lighter tasks	Sewing, cooking, unscrewing jars, using a frying pan and making a cup of tea

(From Williams, 1979, pp. 45–46 (Barlow and Matthews))

N.B A person experiencing difficulty with one task is likely to have difficulty with others in the same group. The list of domestic tasks needs to be used with care as some tasks will not be undertaken, more for reasons of the traditional male and female roles than of functional inability (Williams, 1979, p. 79)

- with locomotor difficulties (whatever the cause)
- showing signs of mental impairment
- recently discharged from hospital (especially if showing signs of self-neglect on admission)
- socially isolated.

Health visitors may find helpful the questionnaire which Dodsworth published. It aimed to cover the more important systems of body function and bring out difficulties often met with in the middle and later years. McCabe (1985) described simple tests to discover old people at greatest risk of falling.

Harwin (1975) described the assessment of old people's mental health and included two questionnaires which, he suggested, GPs might use to find out whether or not an old person is suffering from dementia or depression. The test for dementia amounts to a few simple questions to check on memory and orientation and uses a scoring system. The presence or otherwise of anxiety or depression is gauged by noting the old person's replies to a specially designed series of questions. Harwin found that with a sympathetic approach the questioning had been acceptable to his patients. Other tests are also available (Gilleard, 1984, p. 109; Wilcock, 1982).

Assessment of old people's nutritional status, based on Louise Davies' (1981, p. 135) ten 'at risk' factors, is shown in Box 7.1. A questionnaire for estimating need for meals on wheels and other relevant services incorporating these factors is now available (Davies et al, 1982).

Box 7.1 Inadequate diet — ten 'at risk' factors (from Louise Davies (1981, p. 135))

'At risk' factors

  (i) Less than eight main meals, whether hot or cold, that are eaten in a week
 (ii) Less than half a pint of milk each day
(iii) Almost no fruit or vegetables
 (iv) Food wasted, e.g. uneaten meals on wheels
  (v) Lengthy spells in a day without food
 (vi) Loneliness and depression
(vii) Unexpected and significant weight gain or loss
(viii) Problems with shopping
 (ix) Low income
  (x) Other difficulties or disabilities, including alcohol consumption

---

RESULTS

The results of several studies have been reported. Some researchers have been more concerned with validation of health visitors' ability to discover medical and social conditions, whilst others have concentrated on trying to ascertain the extent to which old people have problems and how they might benefit from screening.

a. Validation

The researchers generally agree that there are a large number of unreported functional, social and medical problems amongst the elderly which are amenable to 'treatment', and that health visitors are competent to discover them. Several studies have compared the health visitors' assessments with those of medical and other specialists in the field (Williamson et al, 1966; Player et al, 1971; Powell & Crombie, 1974) and showed high levels of agreement in functional, social and physical conditions, but a little less so with regard to mental health. Williamson et al pointed out that the health visitors in the study were given no practical instruction for the screening programme and that, like many other medical personnel, they would benefit from specific guidance in psychogeriatrics.

One small study used psychologists and psychiatrists to check health visitors' assessments and showed that out of a sample of 40 people they were able to recognise the four with moderate disability. The health visitors failed to identify mild cases, which is, anyway, an area in which disagreement is not unusual (Player et al, 1971). Perhaps much depends on the quality of the guidance notes and the questionnaire itself.

Using the Kilsyth Questionnaire and guidance notes, health visitors were able to identify 83 old people said to be at risk with regard to mental ill-health. In five of these cases, the health visitors' diagnoses differed from those of the psychiatrists'. As Powell and Crombie point out, this is not important. Health visitors aim, in screening, to identify the need for further investigation or care, not to provide a medical diagnosis.

b. Outcome

Some research reports on the benefits of screening have looked not only at the number of problems discovered and attended to, but also at the morale boosting effect the programme had for some old people.

Barber (1981) studied long-term effectiveness by reassessing 100 old people nine months after the original appraisal. Of the 641 functional, social and medical problems discovered in the first assessment, he found improvements in a third. The reassessment brought to light a further 79 previously unknown problems that would become the object of further attention.

Williams (1974) grouped his sample of 297 old people according to their 'effective health': those coping well (60%); those with restricted movements but managing to deal with their problems (36%) and a small number (4%) who were unable to care for themselves. He followed up his original sample a year later. 75% were revisited. Most of those thought to have needed social services had been able to receive them. Of the original 297 old people, 27% were said to have improved. The percentages in the broad categories according to ability to cope had remained largely unchanged, even though, over time, a decline might have been expected.

These studies had no matched control group against which to compare results, a necessity for more reliable evaluation. There are, however, some difficulties in using control groups in this sort of research. For example, it is difficult to explain to a large number of people that they are to be denied a service and are to be used merely for comparison. Karen Luker's cross-over experiment (see Ch. 2, p. 30) shows one way of avoiding that problem.

Dr Luker (1981a) was able to compare the state of 60 old ladies' problems after six months when no health visitor had come, against 60 where the health visitor had visited. Table 7.2 shows the results. With no health visitor intervention, the problems remained very much the same. There was a significant degree of improvement where the health visitor had called, just as there was in the control group when it crossed to become the experimental group and received health visitor

attention. The group that received no visits in the second six months showed that the effect of the health visitor's intervention lasted after the withdrawal of the service — indicating that such intensive visiting need not be maintained indefinitely.

Table 7.2 Karen Luker's experiment: Assessment of elderly women

	After 1st 6 months	After 2nd 6 months
1st group of 60 elderly women	*Health visitor visiting* Improvement	*No visits* Improvement maintained
2nd group of 60 elderly women	*No visits* No particular change	*Health visitor visiting* Improvement

Effect upon morale

Karen Luker (1981b) also attempted to estimate the old people's opinions about the visits and their degree of satisfaction. Most, though not all, felt the visits to be beneficial and many positively looked forward to them: 'therapeutic anticipation'. Remarks were made such as:

. . . it was nice to think people were taking an interest in you . . .
. . . you knew that somebody was paying attention to how you were and they would be there if you needed them.
It helped. It gave me something to look forward to . . .
. . . and knowing that she is coming it does something for you — it gives you a lift.

Dr Luker feels this may encourage health visitors to adopt the habit of making appointments, the basic message in Figure 7.4.

Williamson says that the effect upon morale is an aspect of assessment which is often neglected. He suggested the type of questions asked by Karen Luker and shown in Box 7.2 could be incorporated into the assessment of screening programmes. Williams (1974) felt that his survey itself had a beneficial effect upon some of the people seen, making them more outgoing and better able to cope. Neil (1982) was aware of a psycho-

The health visitor suggested that I visit the optician and told me about the luncheon club. She is coming again a week on Thursday

You're lucky. I never know when mine will come. No time to tidy up. I feel awful. I wish she'd tell me when!

ANTICIPATION   **APPREHENSION**

Fig. 7.4 Appointments and 'therapeutic anticipation'.

Box 7.2 Assessing satisfaction with the service (Karen Luker (1981a))

Elderly women's opinions

Ask whether or not they:
● enjoyed the health visitor visiting
● thought it helped them
● thought it a good idea
● had previously met health visitors
● would like the visits to continue
Then probe with 'how', 'what', 'why', 'where' and 'when' to encourage a full report

---

logical benefit for some of the old people in her screening programme.

To summarise, outlines and references have been given for a variety of screening programmes. These schemes are designed to find old people's socio-functional disabilities so that timely help can

be given, the aim being to maintain or improve these people's ability to cope, to maintain their independence and to improve their quality of life. We have looked, too, at some reports of results: at the way some researchers have concentrated on validating the health visitors' contribution whilst others have tried to discover the benefits of screening.

SUPPORTIVE WORK

The aim in this aspect of the work, is to avoid deterioration in known problems and to try to bring about an improvement. It is quite often a crisis in the old person's life which precipitates his/her referral for this supportive care. Health visitors are notified through a variety of sources (Robertson, 1984a), for example from GPs, fellow nurses, social workers or the local hospital.

In preparing for the first visit following the referral, just as in any other aspect of their work, health visitors are at a distinct advantage if they can consult any previous notes (e.g. GPs' and/or social workers'), previous health visiting documentation, and find out as much as they can from the person referring the case. During the visit, health visitors are then able to add their own impressions of the practical home situation. More importantly, they can listen carefully to the old person's own view of his/her circumstances, the crucial factor in an assessment of the situation and for decisions on how to help.

Sometimes people merely need some information on appropriate facilities and entitlements. In other cases, follow-up and liaison with other health and welfare services is beneficial. For some people, a listening supportive approach is more appropriate, especially in bereavement. We shall look at each of these three in turn.

REFERRAL TO SERVICES

One of the more difficult things for health visitors is the problem of keeping sufficiently knowledgeable and up to date on the enormous range of health and welfare services which exists in the community. Trying to find out if any particular service is available can be very time consuming, unless there is some local scheme for getting reliable information quickly. Mostly, there is none and health visitors are left to devise their individual ways of coping.

It is, naturally, those taking up a new post who face the greatest problem. There is so much to be learned in so short a time. One health visitor (Neil, 1982) used a notebook to list all the agencies which had been of help to the elderly. Local addresses and telephone numbers might usefully include:

- the Department of Social Security
- local authority officers for rent arrears and homelessness
- luncheon clubs
- meals on wheels

- home helps
- good neighbour schemes
- day centres
- chiropodists
- dentists
- opticians
- Gas and Electricity Services' customer service departments
- Citizens Advice Bureau
- Legal Aid Committee secretary
- Age Concern
- Red Cross Society.

These addresses tend to stay the same over time. However, many health visitors find, like Louise Davies (1981, p. 137), that much of the information they get is incomplete or out of date. Details on groups such as:

- Darby and Joan Clubs
- local church facilities
- delivery services
- shopping assistance schemes

listed in good faith in the local town hall, public library or Citizens Advice Bureau, go quickly out of date. It took the Davies team several days to visit or telephone these local services in order to find out the basic information they needed, i.e.

- costs
- hours of opening
- provision of transport
- organisers' names and addresses and telephone numbers

before they could get on with their study!

Keeping up to date

Good record keeping includes making a note of which services have been recommended to individual retired and elderly people. It provides a reminder to ask how, or whether, the old people found them. Health visitors and social workers might be able to help each other keep up to date by meeting at lunchtime from time to time, to tell each other about changes they have heard of and new and useful self-help groups that are emerging.

The Wessex Library-based service, funded by

the NHS, which provides an up-to-date and wide-ranging information service was mentioned in Chapter 2 (p. 20). Anyone can ring or contact them. Help for Health need only to know what service is sought and they can give details on what is available. Health visitors are saved hours of work on the telephone and following up false starts.

Use of the services

Not all people will want to follow up health visitors' suggestions, however accurate and up to date, and it is difficult to discover what deters them from using the services. To some extent, health visitors are caught in a cleft stick. They hope to disseminate knowledge — not to try to lead people's lives for them. On the other hand, some individuals may feel shy about venturing into a luncheon club where they know no one. They may intend to go to an optician, but not get round to it. Should health visitors make the first appointment? Should they arrange for someone from the luncheon club to come and offer to take them? Maintaining the delicate balance between being as helpful as possible and yet respecting old people's right to make no use of the service needs great sensitivity.

The growing popularity of the idea of self-help groups for the retired and elderly has already been mentioned. But enthusiasm should be tempered with caution. Self-help services can vary in quality. They depend upon the particular skills that the volunteers happen to have. Opportunities for selection and training are sometimes minimal. However, when old people come across a scheme which does not seem to give them what they need, they can, for the most part, simply stop attending. The same does not necessarily apply to old people whose problems are of an emotional nature. They may be in no position to differentiate between good and bad. For example, a bereaved person visited by a volunteer who misuses these visits to work out his/her own personal emotional problems (Milne, 1982) is less likely to see exactly what is happening.

Health visitors trying to discover more about the quality of the service provided by self-help groups and other agencies, may find information from the elderly people referred to them the most useful source. There may also be opportunities to meet some of the personalities involved or, better still, to attend one or two of their meetings. Judgement, however, is necessarily subjective and is always difficult.

LIAISON

There is a large measure of overlap between workers in the community care of the retired and elderly, particularly between health visitors and social workers, district nurses, GPs and some people from voluntary agencies. Personal contact can be very important. It is one way to get to know the particular emphasis, style and approach of other workers. It can help to cut down duplication of services or, at the other extreme, to minimise the number of people who are missed altogether.

Health visitors who are new to a Health District have many people to meet, but it is a sound investment in time. The understanding established between workers means that on many subsequent occasions even the briefest of telephone calls can be very helpful.

Voluntary agencies

Most contacts are with other professional workers. However, it is important to keep in touch with the voluntary agencies, to find out what they do, to tell them of people who would benefit from their service and for feedback on how those people are faring. But there is another side to it. These agencies need encouragement; they face many difficulties, sometimes working on very limited funds. Their workers give their time for little more reward than the satisfaction of seeing things turn out well. Health visitors may be able to offer background support from time to time — if an agency requests it.

Social workers

The work of health visitors and social workers frequently overlaps in supportive, preventive care:

trying to help people through problems. There are disadvantages in this overlap, but it can certainly be used to advantage if the work is taken up in a logical way.

Whether it is the primary health care team or social services who deal with an old person's problem mostly depends on which agency has been contacted. When problems come to the attention of GPs, they sometimes deal with the matter themselves; they may notify the health visitor or the geriatric visitor or, rarely, a social worker attached to the practice. When the matter is brought to the attention of the social services department, it is likely to be taken on by an assistant social worker. Liaison with the health visitor may be of benefit where health considerations put limitations on what their client can do. Conversely, health visitors or geriatric assistants often need to know to what extent local authority services are likely to be available. They may like to talk about the relative priority which might be given to certain needy cases.

If it is possible to meet key workers such as the home help supervisor and the meals-on-wheels administrator, and get to know each other's problems, it can simplify future communications on the allocation of these services. Furthermore, should old people find themselves facing further difficulties once a service is being provided, these key workers are likely to be the first to hear of it when the workers actually delivering the service report in. They would find it much easier to alert the health visitor to what is going on, once good liaison is established.

District nurses

The main overlap between district nurses and health visitors in supportive preventive care is in their listening role and in the information they give their patients about services and facilities that will be useful to them. Some district nurses prefer to take on the bereavement counselling of the families they have been visiting. Some like to take, from the beginning, hospital discharge referrals when, in the long run, it looks as if there is likely to be a need for home nursing. It makes for continuity of care. In many cases the old people are

referred directly to the district nurse. Sometimes both the nurse and the health visitor visit the home (Wilson, 1970). With good liaison, a scheme can be worked out which suits each of their particular skills and circumstances and, more importantly, which benefits the old people they care for.

The changing structure of the ageing population is making people wonder how district nurses and health visitors are going to be able to cope. In *A Happier Old Age* (DHSS, 1978), it is pointed out that 50% of district nurses' cases are elderly, against 15% of health visitors'. The question is raised as to whether there is scope for adjusting community nursing roles. This, it was suggested, could be done by providing auxiliary staff within the district nursing service. The discussion document has provided health visitors and district nurses with a stimulus to think about their role in the future.

One new approach has been piloted in Manchester. A geriatric team has been set up within the health visiting service. The aim is to maintain the health and independence of old people in their own homes. A health visitor helped by two staff nurses and two nursing auxiliaries follow up hospital discharges and bereaved spouses. They help with screening, give support and advice to families with elderly relatives and visit some old people living alone (Halladay, 1981). Working in concert like this in the field of prevention may have great potential.

Liaison health visitor

A very useful link between hospital and the community can be forged by a liaison health visitor who has opportunities for regular meetings and detailed discussions, both with staff in the hospital and with community colleagues.

Sometimes health visitors with a normal caseload can spend half a day a week in the geriatric day hospital, for example, whilst another visits outpatients or the wards. Wallis (1982) describes a full-time liaison post which included opportunities to establish relationships with staff in the hospital and in the community, to contact consultants about queries, to encourage health visitors to send information to the hospital, to talk to relatives and to devise appropriate forms for conveying information. Several of the activities are summarised in Box 7.3.

Telephone calls can be made when information is complex or needs to be conveyed speedily. Where one health visitor undertakes this go-between work, it makes it easier for health visitors and district nurses in the field to identify and use the service.

Box 7.3 The liaison health visitor

Aspects of hospital liaison work
Convey information
• in person
• by phone
• written message
Devise appropriate forms
Explain role of health visitor
Regular meetings in community
Establish relationships
Contacting consultants
Meet relatives
Encourage community staff to give information to hospital

Parnell (1982a, 1982b) reported that hospitals had greater contact with district nurses than health visitors. A liaison health visitor has the opportunity to explain the health visitors' role and encourage their involvement in appropriate cases.

In general terms, however, liaison can often be difficult to achieve. Pressures of work, the distance between offices and the inevitable elusiveness of people working out in the community, make communication difficult. Often even telephone contact is hard to make. It may not be easy, but it is well worth trying to get to know other workers in the field. When health visitors, district nurses, social workers, voluntary agencies and GPs work closely together, they are much more likely to provide a rational and effective service for the retired and elderly.

SUPPORTIVE LISTENING

As in other aspects of their work, health visitors will sometimes find that by listening they can enable old people to talk through their problems, to sort out their thoughts and feelings and to adjust to their circumstances. They may, alternatively, decide on another line of action.

Some old people can benefit from reminiscing. Through reminiscence they may be able to come to terms with their past and find a new equilibrium (Rowlings, 1981). Few generalist health visitors with a busy caseload feel able to become involved in this sort of work. This would be much more likely to be undertaken in casework by a social worker.

Health visitors sometimes meet very lonely elderly people with a great need to talk. The health visitor's role in the case of someone whose problem is basically loneliness, is to act as a referral agent, sensitively arranging for a volunteer visitor or a relevant service to be contacted — if this is acceptable to the old person.

Bereavement visiting

There is one aspect of this supportive role in which health visitors are becoming increasingly involved. This is bereavement visiting. There is now sufficient evidence of high rates of mental and physical illness during or due to bereavement (Grindel, 1981; Godber, 1980) to convince many health visitors that they should be involved at an early stage, to enable people to work through the normal mourning process, especially those people lacking the support of relatives and friends. The aim is to prevent people from becoming locked into one of the earlier stages of grief and, therefore, from being able to arrive at eventual full adjustment.

Bereavement can, of course, affect any group. It is because it is so much more likely to affect the retired and elderly that a description of the sort of commitment and visiting schedule it can involve is included in this chapter.

Prerequisites

Firstly, in order to be of any help the health visitors need to have come to terms with the idea of their own death. Those who have, themselves, suffered a bereavement, need to have achieved readjustment. These people offer a bonus. They can empathise: they have a fuller understanding of how the bereaved person is feeling.

It is also necessary to have studied and understood the complex processes and components of grief: shock, searching, disorganisation, denial, depression, guilt, anxiety, aggression, and, finally, resolution, acceptance and reintegration (Parkes, 1972; Hodgkinson, 1980; Nuttall, 1980; Parkes & Weiss, 1983; Cook & Phillips, 1988).

Thirdly, what is needed is the ability to show acceptance of bereaved people's need to pour out their anguish and grief. This also applies to the bitter anger which may, on occasions, be directed against the health visitor or some other member of the primary health care team.

When should visits begin?

Dr Parkes (1972, Ch. 10) suggests that this may be best in the week after the funeral because this often coincides with the greatest intensity of grief. By this time, the supporting relatives have mainly dispersed. Sometimes bereaved people are more able to pour out their feelings to an 'outsider' than to relatives who are themselves involved.

A health visitor described how she arranged to visit cases of known terminal illness during the course of the disease (Wilson, 1970). As the district nurse where she worked stopped visiting when the patient died, this scheme provided continuity of care. She felt she had a much better opportunity in the early stages to encourage the relatives to let the old people show their grief as they felt inclined.

What should be said?

It is not easy to find the right thing to say when visiting a bereaved person. Parkes says that pity is unwanted and that there is no 'proper thing to say'. It is bound to be painful for both the visitor and the bereaved: neither is able to give what the other wants. The visitor cannot bring back the person who has died. The bereaved person cannot give the visitor the satisfaction of appearing to be helped.

The important thing is to let bereaved people express their feelings in their own way and in their own time. Interpersonal skills (see Ch. 2, pp. 26–28) are crucial in this context.

Practical advice may be requested. A DHSS (1979) leaflet *What to do after a death* is a useful source of information on the more immediate problems following a death. The addresses of several very helpful and supportive organisations such as Cruse, The Compassionate Friends and Age Concern are included. Some members of the St Christopher's Hospice Bereavement service have brought out an excellent book (Dyne, 1981) as a guide for other people thinking of undertaking this sort of work.

Where health visitors know of reliable bereavement counselling services locally, such as through the church or the bodies mentioned above, they may tend to refer people on to them, if it is wished, and play a rather more background role themselves.

Indicators of vulnerability

In a very useful and succinct article, Paddy Yorkstone (1981) lists risk factors in bereavement, the factors that make people more likely to face problems later on if they are unsupported in the critical, early stages. Included are bereaved people where there has been an unexpected death, especially of a young person, child or still birth; those who have no supportive family; people who

Box 7.4 Some trigger signals in bereavement visiting (from Parkes (1972) and Yorkstone (1981))

People needing action or attention

1. Extra *vulnerable* if:
    death unexpected
    • young person
    • child
    • still birth
    have demanding dependants
    no supportive family
    at home all day
    financial difficulties
    housing problems
    history of inadequate personality
2. Extra *help* needed if:
    serious contemplation of suicide
    excessive guilt or anger
    no grief shown when expected
    intense grief, abnormally long time

spend all day at home; and those with financial and housing difficulties. These and the factors below are listed in Box 7.4 as trigger signals for action by the health visitor.

It has been suggested (Parkes, 1972, p. 165) that the visitor should not be afraid to ask direct questions about suicide. People seriously contemplating it tend to admit it. Psychiatric help is needed in such cases.

Other people who need special help are those who suffer from excessive guilt or anger; those who show no grief when it would be expected, or, at the other end of the scale, suffer from intense grief for an abnormally long time. These people need to be brought to the attention of their GP.

When should visiting stop?

Bereavement usually lasts from 6–18 months. Visits generally stop when the health visitors feel they have fulfilled their part in helping a person through to the stage of acceptance and reintegration into society. The anniversary of the death is an important date for a bereaved person. A visit on this day is found to be helpful by many people.

In these three sections, we have looked at work with the elderly from the viewpoint of the sort of activities health visitors might undertake in order to provide a preventive health service. This can involve education and work in the community. Screening programmes were discussed in the second section. Work which involves informing old people about available services, liaising as necessary with other agencies and listening, especially in bereavement, were covered in this last part. We return to bereavement in Chapter 9. In the next section the perspective is changed towards the individual old person's health needs from the standpoint of his/her daily life.

ENVIRONMENTAL, HEALTH AND SOCIAL NEEDS IN RETIREMENT

There is now a wide range of practical and sensitive guidance written for the elderly and those who care for old people (Skeet, 1982; Hooker, 1981; Gray & McKenzie, 1980), though some is written more specifically for the carers (Dartington, 1980; Brown, 1982). It is not possible or necessary, here, to repeat all this information already available to health visitors.

In this section we use a derivative of the family health needs model to provide a way of categorising basic requirements in retirement, in order to help in the mental planning for individual care. The model is later demonstrated in two examples of visits, through which also run themes from the earlier sections.

The suggested categorisation of day-to-day needs in retirement is shown in essence in Figure 7.5. The six factors are expanded into the tabular format in Box 7.5 and classified under environmental, health and social needs, some of which are considered below. The Box is not intended to provide an ideal model: health visitors' experience and individual reading will enable them each to develop their own mental listings of matters affecting old people which might require attention or discussion.

ENVIRONMENTAL FACTORS
Housing

Research shows just how important a part housing plays in the provision of old people's welfare (Tinker, 1984). It is the key to the highly-treasured independence and, like all needs for old people, is best planned for prior to retirement. Warmth and accident hazards can be a problem to many old people.

Falls constitute a large proportion of accidents in the elderly (Abrams, 1985), and there is a growing interest in alarm call systems (Geriatric Medicine, 1981; Butler, 1982). Wild et al (1981; Isaacs, 1981) said the greatest risk factors associated with falling are:

- being female
- over 75 years
- having fallen previously
- difficulties in mobility and gait
- impaired balance

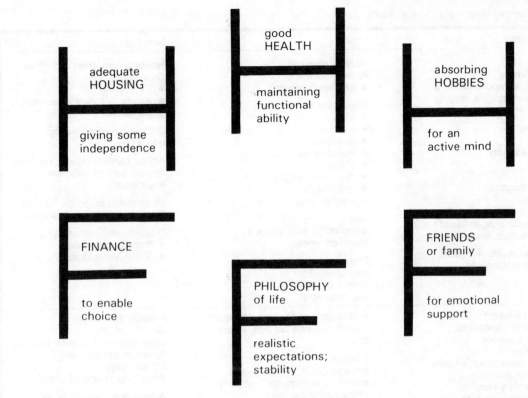

Fig. 7.5 Some factors affecting retirement.

- blood pressure problems and
- the effects of some drugs.

Hazards include things like slip mats, trailing flexes, and inadequately lit stairs (Mitchell, 1984). Frances McCabe (1985) studied some 110 housebound old people said to be at risk of falling, and concluded that careful forethought was necessary for the prevention of falls. She found many seemingly useful ideas were not acceptable to the old people in her study, and she pointed out that any interventions must be in line with old people's 'felt needs', the way they perceived the problem. She described how a simple test of balance and discussions about their recent falls, history and the drugs they take, can help draw old people's attention to ways they may avoid falls. RoSPA (1981) have a very good self-assessment safety checklist for old people, which could stimulate a wide range of thought and discussion.

Nora Saddington (1983) made suggestions as to how professionals can help with inexpensive aids to prevent a person falling and, as a consequence, becoming extremely cold. She also described how to recognise and deal appropriately with hypothermia. Warmth has been shown to be a basic problem in this country in winter. Within two days of a cold spell, deaths from coronary disease and, soon after, deaths from other diseases increase significantly. It seems that governments have failed to make these facts known for fear of pressures on resources being created by public demand to overcome these problems (Taylor, 1982).

Financial support

Advice on financial help with heating, together with advice on matters like insulation, payment schemes for gas and electricity and what to do in case of disconnection, is provided by Age Concern (1985). This organisation has produced some very useful and readable booklets for old people, par-

Box 7.5 Family health needs — the elderly

Environmental	Health	Social
Housing *Neighbourhood* shopping, transport, health & recreational facilities, helping agencies and friends *Household* Heating: type, accessibility Safety Falls: • steps: supports, • lighting • floor covering: frayed/slippery • high cupboards: awkward storing • bath: surface, supports Burns and scalds: fireguard, cooking arrangements	**Health, physical** Known disease? • involves handicap? *Check* e.g. • sight • hearing • dentition • incontinence • balance • degree of mobility • foot defects • weight Diet: what, when, who cooks it Meals on wheels Drugs taken: side-effects? correct dosage? non-prescribed	**Hobbies and other activities** Sedentary: • TV, reading • access to library, newspapers, magazines Creative: sewing, writing, handicrafts Active: garden, repairs, rambling, cycling, paid or voluntary employment Membership of groups: church, OAP clubs, WI, luncheon club Disability limits activities? • home help service? • Social Services aids?
Financial support *Benefits* and allowances Retirement pension War pension Disability allowances: mobility, attendance, invalid care Supplementary pension extra entitlements: help with heating costs, dental and other care Local authority rent rebates, grants for insulation Occupational pensions	**Philosophy of life, mental health** *Attitude* towards old age, illness, death *Emotional* disturbance: depression, grief, confusion, withdrawal, instability, intellectual impairment	**Friends and family** *Social contacts* Lives alone/with spouse or family Extent of contact with confidant(e)s What help at time of crisis Animal: e.g. cat/budgie as companion and 'dependant' Possible cause of voluntary isolation: • incontinence • fear of falling

ticularly *Your Rights* (Age Concern, 1983), which explains about local authority rent rebates, supplementary pensions and the various allowances available. Health visitors would probably find it very helpful to have this booklet available in their bag. The address for Age Concern's publications list will be found at the end of the reference section. The Department of Transport (1982) has printed a guide to the transport benefits which are available to disabled people, which some older people may find useful.

HEALTH FACTORS
Physical aspects

The aim in preventive care for the elderly is to maintain the best possible level of functional ability rather than to cure disease. Urinary and mobility problems tend to be under-reported, endured and accepted, wrongly, as an inevitable part of the ageing process (Williamson, 1981). Also, the effects of drugs can be misunderstood. If neglected, these problems can severely limit a person's ability to cope and remain reasonably independent in the community.

The elderly can be specially sensitive to certain drugs and their side-effects (MacLennan, 1981; Bliss, 1981). Many have difficulties in being able to see and differentiate between tablets (Hurd & Blevins, 1984). These factors and evidence of old people's lack of understanding about drugs, together with a correlation between reduced compliance with instructions and increased complexity of dose schedules (Kiernan & Isaacs, 1981), show a need for special care to be taken. It is a nursing as well as a medical problem and old people will benefit where the primary health care team work together to find a scheme to monitor what drugs their elderly population are given and are taking. Literature such as the Family Doctor booklet on medicines (Lewis, 198(2)) may help some individuals understand the drugs they need (or need not) take.

The ability to be independent can be helped in many ways. There is an increasing amount of interest in exercise for old people to improve their physical condition (Copple, 1983; Clapham, 1980; Hooker, 1981, pp. 133–139; Lawrence, 1981; Fentem, 1981) and in helping people prevent and overcome foot problems (Collyer, 1981; Turnbull, 1981; Foulston, 1981) in order to maintain their mobility. However, whatever their basic skills in this field, if old people suffer from incontinence they will be liable to loneliness and isolation through fear of going out. Dr Trimmer (1982), Vivien Rooney (1984) and Sally Robbins (1984) describe how important it is to have a clear history of an old person's incontinence problems and how a clear picture can lead to some very beneficial progress. This topic was also discussed in Chapter 6 (p. 113).

Mental health

It is said that to be forewarned is to be forearmed. Some older people may find very helpful two booklets that describe how to cope with death, both from emotional and practical points of view (Parkes, 1981; DHSS, 1979). These booklets would probably be particularly useful in pre-retirement discussions or classes.

If the primary health care team can have early warning of problems for old people such as the onset of dementia (see p. 124), it means that support services can beneficially be provided in good time (Williamson, 1981). Gilleard (1984, p. 62) describes the gradual stages of decline, the carers' bewilderment and then adjustment with each stage of dementia. They need sympathetic and practical support. The community psychiatric nurse (CPN) may be able to help. Age Concern have some booklets, such as the one providing advice for carers on 'reality orientation' for their relative (Dowdell, 1982), which can provide useful and practical ideas. Another problem of mental health is depression. This is relatively common amongst the elderly. There are, of course, many causes, one of them being the medication that old people take. Josephs (1982) lists some of the drugs, including alcohol, which can tend to precipitate depression.

SOCIAL ASPECTS
Hobbies and other activities

The sort of activities people choose or are able to undertake in old age will, of course, depend on many of the factors already touched on — finances, accommodation, physical health and mental attitudes. They are likely to reflect the earlier chances in, or style of, life and the interests developed prior to retirement. We have already considered, in the section on screening the elderly, the importance of looking out for incipient functional disabilities, in order to maintain old people's activities at the best possible level.

Friends and family

Loneliness can be a problem. It has been suggested by Dorothy Walster (1982) that owning a pet can help and can bring significant therapeutic benefits, mentally, physically and socially. She says the caring professionals and other visitors call and leave, whereas the pet provides 24-hour companionship.

Full-time companionship, however, can have its problems. When an old person has become dependent and moves in with a member of their family, it can sometimes cause significant tensions and, from time to time, can involve 'granny abuse'. Eastman and Sutton (1982) quote Green's observations that there is a correlation between high dependency and abuse where:

- increasing disability sours an originally loving relationship
- the care-giver accepted the old person reluctantly when s/he was unable to continue to live alone
- the family is, anyway, under stress.

Box 7.6 Signs of strain and, perhaps, violence (derived from Eastman 1984)

A number of factors *occurring together* in a household caring for a dependent old person should trigger the health visitor into considering further investigation and *increased support* for the family. Significant factors are, for example:
Where the old person:
- is dependent upon the key care-giver
- is known to be shouted at by the care-giver
- has frustrating behaviour, e.g. incontinence or shouting at night
- has a history of falls with vague explanations
- is sleepless
- has facial bruising

When the care-giver:
- has been obliged to change her life-style significantly
- is responsible for another family member
- has a history of mental ill-health
- frequently visits GP for 'nerves'
- is drinking heavily
- suffers from sleeplessness

Where there is evidence of:
- role reversal between adult child-parent
- family isolation and lack of emotional support
- inadequate accommodation
- financial problems
- marital conflict or divorce
- unemployment in the family

Eastman (1982, 1984) suggested that factors that should alert professionals to the possibility of abuse are a cluster of any of those characteristics listed in Box 7.6. If a number of these features apply to a household, then he feels the situation warrants further investigation. He says the most important thing is for there to be available emotional support and someone prepared to listen.

There is evidence of the great problems these carers face with little or no help from the services (Equal Opportunities Commission, 1980; Wright, 1983; Walker, 1983), often on account of ignorance of what is available to help them. Heather McKenzie (1984), of the National Council for Carers and their Elderly Dependants, has described how her organisation has now been emulated by others in sending out information packs to their members. They now also provide a granny-sitting service in various parts of the country. Dinah Tedman (1982) offers advice on supportive 'care for the carers' and emphasises the need for professionals to listen, to offer suggestions and emotional support and to keep any promises they make.

A health visitor, Geraldine Drummond (1984) and someone from Age Concern, worked together to set up a relatives' support group. The phases and stages through which the group went are described. It was found to be very helpful and went on to become an independent self-help group. This sort of proactive work will, hopefully, be widely emulated.

In this section, we have looked at some of the factors listed in the health needs format in Box 7.5, some of which have already been mentioned in the earlier sections. The chapter concludes with two examples of visits to elderly people.

EXAMPLES OF WORK WITH THE ELDERLY

Of the two examples given, one shows how a person may be encouraged to take timely action over problems: secondary prevention aimed at maximising functional ability and maintaining independence. In the second, the health visitor was not involved until problems had reached crisis proportions. Preventive care, mainly tertiary at this late stage, was fortunately successful in this case.

EXAMPLE ONE: MRS PERKINS

Miss Helen Voisey (HV) has planned and is now undertaking an assessment scheme aimed at contacting all the elderly people listed in a suburban group practice. She started by contacting all the over-80s and is now gradually meeting all the over-75s. The aim is to make 70 the routine age of contact within a year or two.

Mrs Bella Perkins, a 77-year old, was identified through reference to the age-sex register. An introductory, explanatory letter suggested a day when the health visitor would call.

Having introduced herself and checked that the visit was in fact convenient, HV found herself warmly welcomed and invited in. After some slight initial apprehension, Mrs Perkins showed a great deal of interest in the assessment scheme. She was shown her record card. She was very cooperative and chatty as they gradually worked through the prescribed format. Much of the relevant information on Mrs Perkins' circumstances will be found listed in Box 7.7.

Mrs Perkins walked with evident discomfort. Her health though was generally good. However, she had not been to the optician for 12 years and her dentures were painful, ill-fitting and 15 years old. She said her friends had had to 'pay a fortune' for their replacement spectacles and dentures. She did not 'have that sort of money'. There was a tendency for Mrs Perkins to be somewhat fatalistic about her problems, especially about her painful feet and loss of mobility, and to assume it was to be expected in old age.

Mrs Perkins was asked if she considered her finances too private a matter for discussion. She did not. There ensued a lively conversation about the advantages of being on supplementary benefit — especially with regard to free optical and dental care. Mrs Perkins decided to make appointments for treatment.

Waiting list places for chiropody were some 3 or 4 months long. As Mrs Perkins was then liable to remain relatively housebound for a while, visitors from Age Concern and the local school OAP Aid Scheme were suggested to supplement her social contacts. The

Box 7.7   Example one: Mrs Perkins

Environmental	Health	Social
Housing Home: owner occupied·	**Physical health** Reports poorer vision Ref. optician	**Activities** Reads and sews less than previously
Shops and other facilities: 1/2 mile	Painful dentures no longer wearing lower one for eating Ref. dentist	Limited mobility • feet
Garden unkempt, referred to local school OAP Aid Scheme		
Safety: Carpet wall to wall Reports hand rails • stairway • bathroom Fireguard available	Feet: thickened nails, painful corns and callouses Ref. chiropody	Copes with housework
		Shopping mainly delivered to door
	(Might need voluntary car service)	OAP Luncheon Club monthly
	No regular medication	
	Enjoys cooking: concentrating on softer foods	
Financial status National Insurance retirement pension: currently being collected by friend	**Mental health** Scored well on tests	**Friendship networks** Lives alone
	Seems well adjusted to death of husband and to daughter's move away	Small group of friends of own age gradually dwindling
Says would be entitled to supplementary benefit — too small to bother: 30 p per week: advantages explained	No regular medication	Next of kin: daughter in Scotland, three grandchildren
Rate rebate applied for: advised by neighbour		Welcomed idea of visitors
		OAP Aid Scheme may provide regular contact with young
		Age Concern visitor

schoolchildren would be keen to help in practical ways, for example by gardening and shopping.

On parting it was agreed that HV or the geriatric assistant would call monthly for a while, hoping to see Mrs Perkins soon with better glasses and dentures (and improved nutrition). The date of the next visit was arranged. It was suggested that, if possible, Mrs Perkins should wear open-toed sandals instead of slippers and her laced or barred shoes to hold the foot back and avoid further friction.

The health visitor left feeling there was a good chance that Mrs Perkins would follow up most of the ideas that had emerged during the assessment and that her independence and health would be maintained on account of it. This proved later on to be so.

EXAMPLE TWO: MRS DEAN

Mr Harold Vosper (HV) is attached to a group practice where there was not, at the time, a scheme for initiating contact with their elderly.

Mrs Dean, a 76-year old with osteo-arthritis, was referred to HV by one of the doctors. Mrs Farley, an only daughter with whom she lived, had come to the surgery saying that her mother would 'have to go into a home'. The doctor had listened as she talked about her problem. He visited Mrs Dean at home. The basic problem was the demands that caring for the mother and her constant presence in their small house was making on the Farleys. It had been brought to a head by a recent row between the couple. They had not yet reached a decision on what they hoped to do and seemed to have very little knowledge about what services might be available.

A visit by Harry Vosper was arranged. Some of the family's circumstances are outlined in Box 7.8. Mrs Dean described pain in her wrists, hips, knees and neck and chose to take no drugs for it. She tended to remain inactive. HV encouraged her to talk about her circumstances and feelings. She was resentful about her

Box 7.8 Example two: Mrs Dean

	Environmental	Health	Social
M	**Housing** Bedroom in daughter's home since death of husband 5 years ago, Warm, well kept Bathroom adjacent Safety factors: no loose mats or unguarded fire; rails in bathroom	**Physical health** Osteo-arthritis: reported significant deterioration in recent years Uses walking sticks Bedbathing service not wanted Refuses medication Possible deafness: ref. GP	**Activities** Sedentary: reads, radio and TV Said to spend most of day in bed or in chair by window Difficulty in walking to toilet Occasionally carried downstairs in a wheelchair
D	Owner-occupied 2 bed home, thro' lounge Near shops and other facilities Transport: no car, bus — 1/2 mile	Some backpain since frequent lifting of mother: liaison with Soc Services about aids	Gave up work 2 yrs ago to be with M Activities home based No holidays away Pops out to shops
S	Circumstances as above	Reportedly good	Clerk DIY redecoration
M	**Financial status** Retirement pension collected by son in law Attendance and invalid care allowances not applied for — leaflets NI.205, NI.212 and SB1 given	**Emotional health** Described as difficult, uncooperative and demanding Alert mind Deeply resentful of 'being treated like a child' and loss of useful role	**Friendship networks** Main contact by banging walking stick to summon daughter Few local friends, moved from 10 miles away No 'grannie sitter' Day centre and holiday schemes suggested
D	Significant drop in income now no longer contributing to family budget	Frequent arguments with mother — uses avoidance tactics to minimise tension Strong feeling of responsibility for mother	Neighbours call in Fears relationship with husband deteriorating Now considering minding service
S	Full-time employment	Said to be resentful of wife's absorption in her mother	No longer socialising with same friends as wife

Key: M = Mother; D = Daughter; S = Son in law

situation but gradually showed, more and more, her sympathy for her daughter's predicament. Mrs Dean was very anxious not to be cut off from her family. The nearest 'home' was many miles away and far from a bus stop. She responded positively to the ideas of a day centre place and volunteer visitors.

Before he returned downstairs, HV called Mrs Farley so that he could witness their management difficulties in getting Mrs Dean to the toilet. He demonstrated lifting techniques. The manoeuvres gave HV an opportunity to follow up a hunch he had had during his earlier conversation. He had suspected some deafness and found that Mrs Dean did not respond to low voice sounds when her head was turned. Both ladies were somewhat surprised at the idea of deafness and happy that the GP should follow it up.

Mrs Farley listened earnestly to what services and benefits might be available for the family. She was anxious to discuss some of the suggestions with her husband and her mother. It was important to her to have her mother nearby. She was beginning to feel it was much more possible to keep her mother with her, but did not yet want to commit herself. She remarked on how helpful it had been to talk about her problems. There was a discussion about the extent to which Mrs Dean's 'uncooperativeness' might be due to misunderstandings on account of hearing loss. Mrs Farley reminisced and recalled that they had not had these problems in the early years. Aids were discussed. A hoist, a zimmer frame and a commode were suggested. HV undertook to make tentative enquiries about this and other equipment that might be helpful, such as the loan of a stair lift.

The next few visits were made as the family requested — weekly for a month, and were mainly of a supportive nature. Mr and Mrs Farley decided that, with the aids and hospital day care, and later day centre support, with volunteer visitors, grannie sitters, holiday schemes and National Insurance allowances, they would be able to manage. The discussions at the primary health care team meetings on this and other cases has led to the decision to try to contact old people in the practice before their situation reaches crisis proportions. An assessment scheme is now being prepared.

USEFUL ADDRESSES

Age Concern England,
Publications Department,
Bernard Sunley House,
60 Pitcairn Road, Mitcham,
Surrey CR4 3LL
Tel 081 640 5431

HVA Special Interest Group for Older People
c/o Jill Carter,
Executive Committee Secretary,
Health Visitors' Association,
50 Southwark Street,
London SE1 1UN
Tel 071 378 7255

The Pre-Retirement Association
19 Undine Street, Tooting,
London SW17 8PP
Tel 081 767 3225/6; 081 767 3854

RoSPA, Cannon House,
The Priory Queensway,
Birmingham B4 6BS
Tel 021 233 2461

Workers Educational Association,
Temple House,
9 Upper Berkeley Street,
London W1H 8BY
Tel 071 402 5608

REFERENCES

Abrams M 1985 Falls in the home. New Age Winter: 22
Age Concern 1983 Your rights, 11th ed. Age Concern, Mitcham, Surrey
Age Concern 1985 Fact Sheet on Help with Heating. Age Concern, Mitcham, Surrey
Antrobus M 1981 Self-care in sickness and in health. Nursing Times Community Outlook 77, 42: 342–350, 357
Barber J M 1981 Screening and assessment: a challenge to GPs. Geriatric Medicine 11, 4: 39–45
Bliss M R 1981 Prescribing for the elderly. British Medical Journal 283: 203–206
Brown P 1982 The other side of growing older. Macmillan Press Ltd, London

Burkitt A 1977 Life begins at forty. Hutchinson Benham, London
Butler A 1982 Alarms that reassure. Health and Social Services Journal XCII: 734–736
Clapham J 1980 Keeping fit in retirement. Health Visitor 53: 532
Collyer M I 1981 Maintaining the elderly patient's mobility. Geriatric Medicine 11, 12: 27–30
Cook B, Phillips S 1988 Loss and bereavement. Austen Cornish, London
Copple P 1983 The concept of exercise. Nursing Times 79, 32: 66–69
Dartington T 1980 Family care of old people. Souvenir Press (E & A) Ltd, London

Davies L 1981 Three score years — and then? A study of nutrition and wellbeing of elderly people at home. William Heinemann Medical Books Ltd, London

Davies L, Holdsworth M D, Purves R 1982 Who needs meals on wheels? Community Care 407: 12–13

Day L 1981 Health visiting the elderly in the 1980s — do we care enough? Health Visitor 54: 538–539

Day L, Mogridge J 1981 Health visitor who stayed. Health and Social Services Journal XCI: 1114–1115

Department of Transport 1982 Door to door. A guide to transport for disabled people. Department of Transport, London

DHSS 1978 A happier old age. A discussion document on elderly people in our society. HMSO, London, p 33

DHSS 1979 What to do after a death. D49/Aug 79 Department of Health and Social Security, London

DHSS 1981 Growing older. Cmnd 8173 HMSO, London

Dodsworth A J 1976 Screening the elderly. Nursing Times 72: 909–910

Douglas-Jones A 1980 Screening for a healthy future. Geriatric Medicine 10, 5: 67–68

Dowdell T 1982 Forgetfulness in elderly persons. Advice for carers. Age Concern, London

Drennan V 1988 Working with groups of elderly people. In: Drennan V (ed) Health visitors and groups: politics and practice. Heinemann Nursing, Oxford

Drummond G 1984 Laughter is better than medicine — a support group for caring relatives. Health Visitor 57: 201–202

Dyne G (ed) 1981 Bereavement visiting. King Edward's Hospital Fund for London

Eastman M 1982 'Granny battering' a hidden problem. Community Care 413: 12–13

Eastman M 1984 Old age abuse. Midwife Health Visitor and Community Nurse 20: 162–165

Eastman M, Sutton M 1982 Granny battering. Geriatric Medicine 12, 11: 11–15

Equal Opportunities Commission 1980 The experience of caring for elderly and handicapped dependants: survey report. Equal Opportunities Commission, London

Fentem P 1981 Do you ever prescribe exercise? Geriatric Medicine 11, 8: 53–56

Foulston J 1981 Make the best use of your chiropodist! Geriatric Medicine 11, 7: 44–49

Geriatric Medicine 1981 Alarm call systems: an aid in emergencies. Geriatric Medicine 11, 3: 45–47

Gilleard C J 1984 Living with dementia. Croom Helm, London

Godber C 1980 Complications of bereavement. Geriatric Medicine 10, 5: 81

Gray J A M, McKenzie H 1980 Take care of your elderly relative. George Allen & Unwin, London

Grindel P 1981 Help for the bereaved. Health Visitor 54: 330–333

Halladay H 1981 A geriatric team within the health visiting service. Nursing Times 77, 38: 1039–1040

Harwin B 1975 Psychogeriatric screening. In: Hart C R (ed) Screening in general practice. Churchill Livingstone, Edinburgh

Hodgkinson P E 1980 Treating abnormal grief in the bereaved. Nursing Times 76: 126–128

Hooker S 1981 Caring for elderly people, 2nd ed. Routledge and Kegan Paul, London.

Hurd P D, Blevins J 1984 Aging and the color of pills (letter). New England Journal of Medicine 310: 202

Isaacs B 1981 Why do the elderly fall? Geriatric Medicine 11, 3: 17–13

Josephs C 1982 Depression. Geriatric Medicine 12, 12: 24–25

Kerr I F W 1975 Women in the middle years. In: Hart C R (ed) Screening in general practice. Churchill Livingstone, Edinburgh

Kiernan P J, Isaacs J B 1981 Use of drugs by the elderly. Journal of the Royal Society of Medicine 74: 196–200

Lawrence N 1981 Age and exercise. Geriatric Medicine 11, 1: 78–79

Lewis R J R 198(2) Is your medicine really necessary? British Medical Association, London

Luker K A 1981a Health visiting and the elderly. Nursing Times Occasional Paper No 35 77, 51: 137–140

Luker K A 1981b Elderly women's opinions about the benefits of health visitor visits. Nursing Times Occasional Paper No 9 77, 12: 33–35

Luker K A 1982 Evaluating health visiting practice. Royal College of Nursing, London

McCabe F 1985 Mind you don't fall. Nursing Mirror 160, 26: 52–56

McKenzie H 1984 Viewpoint. New Age, Autumn: 24

MacLennan W J 1981 Drug side-effects and the elderly patient. Geriatric Medicine 11, 9: 52–58

Milne J 1982 Care-less. The Guardian April 21st: 17

Mitchell R G 1984 Falls in the elderly. Nursing Times 80, 2: 51–53

Neil M 1982 It's nice to know that someone cares. Nursing Times Community Outlook 78, 37: 243–246

Nuttall D 1980 Bereavement. Health Visitor 53: 84–86

Parkes C M 1972 Bereavement: studies of grief in adult life. Tavistock Publications, London

Parkes C M 1981 Facing death. National Extension College, Cambridge

Parkes C M, Weiss R S 1983 Recovery from bereavement. Basic Books, New York

Parnell J 1982a Continuity and communication — 1. Nursing Times Occasional Paper No 9 78, 13: 33–36

Parnell J 1982b Continuity and communication — 2. Nursing Times Occasional Paper No 10 78, 14: 37–40

Pike L A 1975 Men in the middle years. In: Hart C R (ed) Screening in general practice. Churchill Livingstone, Edinburgh

Player D A, Irving G, Robinson R A 1971 Psychiatric, psychological and social findings in a pilot community health survey. Health Bulletin XXIX: 104–107

Powell C, Crombie A 1974 The Kilsyth Questionnaire: a method of screening elderly people at home. Age and Ageing 3: 23–28

Robbins S 1984 Incontinence in the elderly mentally infirm. Nursing Times Supplement 80, 14: 25–27

Robertson C A 1984a Health visitors and preventive care. Nursing Times 80, 34: 29–31

Robertson C A 1984b Screening for health. Nursing Times 80, 35: 44–45

Rooney V 1984 Incontinence in the elderly in the community. Nursing Times Supplement 80, 14: 13–14

RoSPA 1981 Safety in retirement HS/108/1981. The Royal Society for the Prevention of Accidents, Birmingham

Rowlings C 1981 Social work with elderly people. George Allen and Unwin, London, p 63

Saddington N 1983 Winter of discontent? Nursing Times 79, 43: 10–11

Shukla R B 1981 The role of the primary care team in the care of the elderly. The Practitioner 225: 791–797

Skeet M 1982 The third age. Darton, Longman and Todd, London

Stanton A 1979 A first experience of planning in a group practice. Health Visitor 52: 310–319

Stott D 1982 Running a pre-retirement course. Health Visitor 55: 360

Taylor G 1982 Cold comfort. Nursing Times 78: 181

Tedman D 1982 Carers need care. Nursing Times Community Outlook 78, 10: 71–76

Tinker A 1984 Health and housing. Nursing Times 80, 18: 57–59

Trimmer E 1982 About incontinence. Midwife, Health Visitor and Community Nurse 18: 386

Townsend P 1963 The family life of old people. Penguin, London, Ch. 11

Turnbull E M 1981 The practical problems of footwear, hosiery, and aids. Geriatric Medicine 11, 12: 33–36

Walker A 1983 Care for elderly people: a conflict between women and the state. In: Finch J, Groves D (eds) A Labour of Love. Women, Work and Caring. Routledge and Kegan Paul, London

Wallis M 1982 An extended talking service. Nursing Mirror 155, 10: 24–28

Walster D 1982 Why not prescribe a pet? Geriatric Medicine 12, 4: 13–19

Wilcock G K 1982 A review of dementia. Midwife Health Visitor and Community Nurse 18: 378–384

Wild D, Nayak U S L, Isaacs B 1981 How dangerous are falls in old people at home? British Medical Journal 282: 266–268

Williams I 1974 A follow up of geriatric patients after medico-social assessment. Journal of the Royal College of General Practitioners 24: 341–346

Williams I 1979 The care of the elderly in the community. Croom Helm, London

Williamson J 1981 Screening, surveillance and casefinding. In: Arie T (ed) Health Care of the Elderly. Croom Helm, Beckenham, Kent

Williamson J, Lowther C P, Gray S 1966 The use of health visitors in preventive geriatrics. Gerontologia Clinica 8: 362–369

Wilson F G 1970 Social isolation and bereavement. The Lancet II: 1356–1357

Wright F 1983 Single cares: employment, housework and caring. In: Finch J, Groves D (eds) A Labour of Love. Women, Work and Caring. Routledge and Kegan Paul, London

Yorkstone P 1981 Bereavement. British Medical Journal 282: 1224–1225

FURTHER READING

Age Concern 1985 Age well ideas pack. Health Education Council, London — Age well: a campaign to promote health activities for and with older people.

Age Concern 1988 Age well ideas pack. Health Education Council, London — Age well: a campaign to promote health activities for and with older people.

Barber H 1988 Self screening by the elderly using a new personal health record. Health Visitor 61, 3: 73–74

Bowling A 1985 Tracking down the elderly at risk. Health and Social Service Journal XCV, 4937: 254–255

British Geriatrics Society and Health Visitors' Association 1986 Health visiting for the health of the aged. A joint policy statement. British Geriatric Society/Health Visitors' Association, London

Burridge R 1988 The role of the health visitor with the elderly. Health Visitor 61, 1: 20–21

Chamove A S, Young M G 1989 Surveillance evaluation for the elderly. Health Visitor 62, 10: 301–302

Drennan V 1985 Working in a different way. A research project examining community work methods and health visiting. Community Nursing Service Paddington and North Kensington Health Authority, London

Drennan V 1986 A feasibility study into the screening of elderly people in an inner city area. In: While A (ed) Research in preventive community nursing care. John Wiley, Chichester

Drennan V 1988 Working in a different way. Senior Nurse 6, 1: 11–13

Drennan V 1988 Celebrating age. Nursing Times Community Outlook 84, 23: 4–6

Enderby V 1989 Ageing well in Thetford. Health Visitor 62, 2: 61

Gooch S 1988 Writing on the wall? Nursing Times 84, 9: 22 — Advocating greater health visitor involvement in care of the elderly.

Gruetzner H 1988 Alzheimer's. A caregiver's guide and source book. John Wiley and Sons, Chichester

Harrison S, Martin E, Rous S, Wilson S 1985 Assessing the needs of the elderly using unsolicited visits by health visitors. Journal of the Royal Society of Medicine 78, 7: 557–561

Itzin C 1987 Screening elderly people. Nursing Times 83, 48: 47–50

Kalache A, Warnes T, Hunter D 1988 Promoting health among elderly people. A statement from a working group. King's Fund, London

McClymont M, Thomas S, Denham M J 1986 Health visiting and the elderly. Churchill Livingstone, Edinburgh

Machell S, Mackenzie K, Phillips W 1988 Ageing well in Riverside. Health Visitor 61, 1: 21–22

Mondal B, Ganguli A, Cooke E 1987 Keeping out of the cold. Nursing Times 83, 38: 54–55 — Assessing vulnerability to hypothermia.

Omambala T 1987 An advisory health clinic for the elderly. Health Visitor 60, 10: 323–324

Organisation for Economic Cooperation and Development 1986 Road transport research. Guidelines for improving the safety of elderly road users. Report prepared by an OECD scientific expert group in cooperation with WHO. HMSO, London

Phillips S 1988 Health visitors and the priority of the elderly. Health Visitor 61, 11: 341–342

Phillips S 1988 Growing old gracefully. Nursing Times Community Outlook 84, 23: 15–18

Scrutton S 1989 Counselling older people. A creative response to ageing. Edward Arnold, London

Steel K 1989 Taking care to the over-80s: case-finding in one practice. Geriatric Medicine 19, 1: 43–49

Stevenson O 1989 Age and vulnerability. A guide to better care. Edward Arnold, London

Sutcliffe D 1989 In at the deep end. Nursing Times 85, 24: 28–31 — Advocating training schemes for carers.

Tester S, Meredith B 1987 Informed? A study of information and support for elderly people in the inner city. Policy Studies Institute, London

Vetter N, Jones D, Victor C 1986 Health visiting with the elderly in general practice. In: While A (ed) Research in preventive community nursing care. John Wiley, Chichester

Wakelin S 1988 Views on health visiting the elderly. Health Visitor 61, 1: 23

Wickham C 1989 Falls in the elderly. Nursing Times 85, 40: 50–51

Williams P 1987 Family feeling. Nursing Times Community Outlook 84, 2: 9–10

The health visitor cycle is the framework used to highlight important aspects of record making. Examples of records schemes are given, using case histories from earlier chapters. Evaluation is considered from three viewpoints: the clients', the health visitors' and by looking at quantifiability. A discussion about confidentiality concludes the chapter.

8

Records and evaluation

STATING WHAT HAS HAPPENED

Records are necessary for communication and investigation. The basic essentials that should be recorded to provide for these requirements are suggested as follows: firstly, key matters that have been reported by the family members or observed by the health visitor; secondly an indication of the service given by the health visitor; and thirdly an evaluation, through what the family has reported and changes the health visitor has noticed. Arrangements undertaken between visits, or at the next visit, can also be noted.

Evaluation can take many forms (Luker, 1985). Here it has been classified into three ways it might be experienced by a practising health visitor: firstly, trying to gain an understanding of the family's perspective and the way they value the work; secondly through self- and peer group assessment; and thirdly, by looking at ways in which aspects of the work can be quantified.

Record making and monitoring the work have implications for confidentiality. Particular care with regard to people's personal information and family dynamics is recommended and also that the clients should be enabled, if they wish, to be aware of what is written in their health visiting records.

RECORDS

BASIC REQUIREMENTS
Communication and investigation

Some of the many reasons why records are needed are listed on this page, Box 8.1. They are needed as a means of communication with self and, potentially, with others. Firstly, they help health visitors recall what has happened at previous visits and, on account of this, aid both planning and the actual provision of the service. They make an excellent aide-mémoire when reports and referrals are needed in communications with other health and welfare workers, and can act as a source of inspiration when health visitors want to publish descriptions of the sort of work they do by providing (anonymously, of course) specific types of real life examples.

Secondly, good records help to demonstrate to (the very few) other people who have a right to see

Box 8.1 Reasons for keeping records

A. **Accurate communication**	1. As aide-mémoire:
	  a. basis on which to plan work
	  b. and aid implementation
	2. To inform others:
	  a. client
	  b. successors/stand-in
	  c. co-professionals: referrals and reports
	3. Publish, to tell:
	  a. professions — health and welfare
	  b. public

B. **Investigation**	1. Evaluation of own work: individual cases, group sessions, clinics, aspects of caseload
	2. Data for research: own/other
	3. Accountability:
	  a. in law — memory aid, if immediate recording
	  b. to health authority NM; DHA/DOH
	  c. to public — Ombudsman

the notes, the key issues emerging from a visit. For example, they can help show clients how the health visitor has interpreted each encounter and help to improve their understanding of the purpose of health visiting. As another example, they can show a health visitor's successor, or anybody temporarily standing in, what has happened to date.

Records are invaluable when the work is being investigated in any way. This applies when health visitors are looking at and evaluating their own work as well as when others are undertaking the research. These matters are considered in the next section of this chapter. There are also other situations in which health visitors need good notes in order to be able to describe the work that was undertaken. Records can be used as a memory aid in a law court, providing they were written up contemporaneously.

Records are also needed because health visitors are accountable to their employing authority to provide some evidence of their work. Health visitors also provide various descriptions of trends, facts and figures for their nurse manager, their Health District and/or for the Department of Health. Furthermore, if ever the Health Services Commissioner were requested to investigate a case, or a health visitor's conduct were called into question in any way, full, clear and contemporaneous notes would be an obvious advantage (Whincup, 1981).

What should be included?

It is not always easy to know how much to write in the records. Health visitors know of the need for full notes. However, it is obvious that it would be impossible, for example, to record on paper everything that one would be able to see and hear in a video recording of a twenty or thirty minute visit, and even less possible to show a full picture of the environment in which the family lives. It is a question of trying to select out that which is felt to be important and to portray the key issues.

The problem of inadequate recording is well known. It has been a common fault amongst health visitors and is partly associated with the structure of their work, the fact that they see so

Notes

1 February 1988

Children seen, speech satisfactory. Playing with bricks.

Fig. 8.1a Hazel Vickery's visit to the Trent family.

Notes	Action
	req'd (√)
1 February 1988	done (X)

TRENT FAMILY - Transfer in

PARENTS
Decorating new home: short visit. Father has constructed wide safety gates to
provide large, safe play area. Mother given HV visiting care and list of clinics
and mothers' groups. Mother enjoyed previous HV's mothers' groups: seeks similar
"educational" group.
NB - contact "Help for Health" re educational groups in area.   X

CHILDREN - Mary, 3; Ann, 2.
Playing together with bricks. Mary building towers and bridges; asking many
"what, where, who" questions. Ann's two-year assessment at next visit.   √
Toddler negativism discussed.

REVISIT - Monday 15 February, am.   √

Dictated 1 February, am.   Signed/date H.A.Vickery.....4-2-88..

Fig. 8.1b Visit to the Trents: alternative case notes.

many people in a day and do not always have the clerical support they need (Robertson, 1982). June Clark (1985) says health visitors tend to write only what they have observed and not what they have done. An example of poor notes, written up very sparsely, is given in Figure 8.1a. It is a record of the visit making contact with the Trent family from Chapter 2. It will be seen that a picture of the key issues within that visit is demonstrated much better by the record of that same visit shown in Figure 8.1b.

The question is, what, in general terms, are these key issues that should be noted down? There are innumerable family health needs, potentially of importance in health visiting, that might be worth a mention, as can be seen from a quick glance at the various chapters of this book. There is no simple formula for choosing, and each individual health visitor has to use his or her professional judgement as to which actual/potential need/problem and what action taken are important enough to warrant a mention.

THE HEALTH VISITOR CYCLE

It may help a little, however, to look at writing records from another point of view. By returning to the health visitor cycle we can consider which of its thought processes and stages might be the most informative and the most logical to record. It will be recalled that the health visitor cycle, introduced briefly in Chapter 1 and developed in Chapter 2, is a development of the nursing process which concentrates on the data on which decisions are made: (a) background knowledge, (b) information available prior to the visit, (c) information available at the visit and (d) that available as a consequence of the visit.

This model has been extended a little to show, in Figure 8.2, the factors that most need to be recorded. The stages seen in the Figure in capital letters are suggested as those which provide the best vehicle and the simplest approach to drawing out the necessary key issues. Those in brackets are the parts of the cycle which do not seem to need, specifically, to be stated in the notes.

Key points: what has been 'Said, Seen and Done' (SSD)

1. The most important items to record after any visit are those matters which the family members have raised as issues, be they, for example, any worries they may have, reports

of developmental attainments or any particular requests.
2. Also important to mention are any significant observations by the health visitor, which might be, for example, that an old lady had difficulty in walking, a child's developmental attainments seen or the evident anxiety of a mother.
3. The next thing that needs to be made clear is what service has been provided: in effect, the action taken on immediate objectives (see Ch. 2, pp. 31–33), for example, 'A range of strategies for sleeping problems discussed: book lent' or 'Baby's hearing tested'.

If what has been said, seen and done is made clear, then the 'assessment' and 'plan' that lie behind the action decided upon should be able to be logically deduced, particularly by other health visitors. They are trained to have a similar background knowledge and would therefore be expected to go through similar thought processes. If the records are very clear and the factors involved are simple, then even a layman should be

Fig. 8.2 Records and the health visitor cycle.

able to work out the underlying assessment and plan. It is proposed, therefore, that it should not really be necessary to make these factors explicit in the vast majority of cases.

4. Evaluation, in terms of how the family members see the outcome of any strategies and ideas that were tried, and any significant observations by the health visitor on what has been achieved, are important to record. However, much of this information will not be available until the next meeting. It can then be recorded as 'what has been said' and as 'what has been seen' within the normal recording of that (following) encounter.

This information is needed, anyway, for assessment and planning that meeting and, although labelled under a separate heading in the model shown in Figure 8.2, does not necessarily need to be separated in the notes. What is important is that a note should be made of the results of the activities emanating from the previous contact.

5. Conclusions as to what activities, if any, the health visitor should undertake between visits, notions that evolve out of evaluation and deliberations during a visit, should also be included: for example, 'Promised to contact bereavement service' or 'Liaison with midwife'. Any arrangements about the next appointment should, of course, be noted.

Ordinary, everyday short- and long-term objectives, discussed in Chapter 2, should not really need to be recorded. Once again, they are part of the shared basic knowledge of practising health visitors and, as the subject matter of this book shows, are far too numerous to list out in normal health visitor records. Objectives which have turned out to be particularly important at any visit should be able to be logically deduced from the rest of the records of what has been said, seen and done, as above. However, this information could be supplemented by, for example, a note of particular thoughts about or promises for further care made by the health visitor with regard to future visits. This style of recording is demonstrated below using the Manners family case history as an example (see pp. 150–151).

Exactly what is written in any given case depends, of course, on each individual visit, and varies according to the issues the family members have raised and their responses to health visitor led ideas. It is not always easy to find the right balance. The level of content of the records should convey enough information to another member of the health visiting profession, to enable him/her to take over in the absence of the current health visitor. It should also be understandable and logical for the client. The aim is for succinct notes containing key 'factual' indicators: opinions could be more confusing than informative.

To summarise, it has been suggested here that the basic and key points that should be mentioned in records of a home visit are: what has been said, seen and done and, where necessary, what is intended. The ideas have been mapped out on the health visitor cycle depicted in Figure 8.2 and the reasons for the selection of these particular factors have been outlined.

SOAP DERIVATIONS

There is, of course, no absolute or set way in which records should be presented, and some very interesting experiments have been undertaken in this field (Marsden, 1985; Clark, 1985; Rogers, 1982; Hendy, 1983). Some people feel it is important to draw out and make a specific point of an assessment and a plan in the records, sometimes advocating the use of written objectives set out as a needs or problems list.

Many of the ideas for this approach evolved from the basic SOAP or SOAPE model used as a guide for recording (Hendy, 1983; Clark, 1983; 1985; Luker, 1985). In these models, the letters S, O, A, P and E signify, more or less, as follows:

- S: subjective data (client history)
- O: observed (by the health visitor) data
- A: assessment (health visitor's conclusions)
- P: plan/goal for each need or problem
- E: evaluation.

The equivalents of 'S' and 'O' in the health visitor cycle will be found on the right in Figure 8.2, as what is *said by client* and what is *seen by*

H.V. Under either model, as Kate Robinson (1983, 1985) has made quite clear, the health visitor's data is no less subjective than the client's. The equivalents in the health visitor cycle of 'A', 'P' and 'E' are, of course, '(assessment)', '(plan)' and 'evaluation' on the left side and at the bottom of the model. In the SOAP(E) approach to recording, each of these stages is supposedly made explicit and recorded. A list of problems and needs are listed, frequently on a separate sheet.

One disadvantage of a needs list is that it might prevent abandonment of impressions (and prejudices) of a previous visit. Also, a full written list of objectives brings with it the implication that something needs to be done about each of these particular issues. It could, then, tend to act as a muzzle to further thought, rather than as a vehicle for creative ideas, a tool to help respond to what seem to be the most important and relevant *current* needs from the family's point of view.

On the other hand, a needs or problems list could encourage follow-up of earlier worries. It might also help to give clients a better idea of the purpose of health visiting. This latter benefit assumes, of course, that the contents of the records are, in fact, shared with or shown to the clients, a matter returned to below.

Open records

An open and frank approach to health visiting is made much easier when contents of records can be made known to the families being visited. June Clark (1985) used her notes in conjunction with her clients. It can be done in many ways. The records might, for example as in Figure 8.3, physically be shown to the people being visited, or alternatively, written on site with the health visitor speaking aloud whilst writing. Everyone develops their own style in these things. This open approach, however, is very demanding and might be time consuming. Not all health visitors, nor the families they visit, feel confident enough to be able to take part in this style of communication.

One important factor in whether or not the records are shared will be the health visitor's style and approach to recording. For example, recording certain aspects of the health visitor's

Fig. 8.3 Open records: for education and trust.

assessment could act as a distinct disincentive to open records. Asking health visitors to set down their view of the situation and their impressions may encourage them to write down a personal view of, for example, family dynamics, which might tend to be derogatory or patronising. This they would obviously prefer not to share with their clients. Either way, they should not be writing about these aspects of family life.

A statement of what has been heard, seen and done, on the other hand, is based on matters which should provide the client with no surprises and, if properly written, no insult. As a basic principle, nothing in the notes should cause offence, with or without open records. A clear description of what has happened, as advocated above, should provide evidence enough of anything that really worries the health visitor: recording the facts on which any concern is based.

The moral question, of course, arises: if it worries the health visitor should it not, anyway, be shared with the client? If a family are not aware of the predicament they may be in, such as, for example, being suspected as child abusers, how can they do anything about it? Another side of the issue is that if records have been shared with a family who have run into this sort of trouble, it is much better for both the health visitor and the family later on. It becomes easier to approach the parents for permission to share some of their confidential information with co-professionals at a case conference, and/or to show the parents the health visitor's report to be submitted about their case (UKCC, 1984). The advantages of making this sort of sensitive issue part of 'what has been said' in the records, is obvious.

Sharing the contents of notes with clients as shown in Figure 8.3, is helpful, both educationally and for trust. When a client can see the matters which a health visitor selects as important enough to record, it probably demonstrates better than anything else the areas of interest within health visiting, and its purpose. Centile charts for a child's development and weight, a questionnaire for postnatal depression and so on, can all add to the understanding and, as mentioned in earlier chapters, lead to useful questioning and discussion. Trust is likely to be enhanced. By seeing the actual range of concern of health visitors and what they write, people will more readily comprehend that the intention is for support and not education and not for social policing.

Parent-held records

Sharing child health records is facilitated by a booklet specially designed by the Society of Area Nurses, Child Health (Owen, 1980). This booklet and another developed in Oxford were distributed to over 300 mothers attending clinics in Oxford (Green & Macfarlane, 1985). There was a high level of both parental and professional approval of both booklets from those who responded at the end of the survey, and helpful suggestions were made for improvements.

Further research has been undertaken on giving parents custody of the normal type of child health clinic records (Green & Macfarlane, 1985; Saffin, 1985). This has been welcomed by most parents. Improvements to the records to help with educational aspects of the notes are under way. In her study Pauline Pearson (1985) found that a propor-

tion of the doctors and health visitors involved with parents holding the small booklet failed to fill it in. This, as Kate Saffin pointed out, is not a problem when parents hold the primary document. The new national child health record aimed at greater parental involvement, was launched in 1990 (Crabbe, 1990; Jackson, 1990).

Whether they were parent-held or not, notes designed for a schedule of complex and regular child health medicals may have discouraged parents from contacting the doctor when they first suspected a problem. Dr Nicoll (1983, 1984) said the implications of the old MCW46 forms, universal and frequent examinations for all children, led to an overcrowded and rather cursory service at the clinics. Attendance levels decreased as the likelihood of a problem occurring increased. Client-centred health visiting in a flexible system was found to be a much better way in which to identify difficulties. We should be warned not to be hedged in by records systems, and always to be questioning whether we are actually achieving our objectives rather than merely filling them in!

The importance of not allowing our work practices to be driven by records systems becomes absolutely critical in the light of the Körner requirements for information and increasing computerisation of records. The Körner-in-practice emphasis on surveillance and almost total lack of space given to educative and supportive work, be it home, clinic or group-work based (Smith, 1987), means a very limited picture of our work is being fed upwards to the Department of Health decision-makers (Barker, 1987). Computerised records also provide a very narrow perspective (Holland, 1984; Little, 1988; MacInnes, 1989).

The hazards are, for example, that we *feel* expected to undertake very low priority surveillance work merely to complete the forms. Also, the strong emphasis on surveillance in the recording system will give the impression that (child) surveillance is all we do. Even worse, some health visitors might be persuaded to change the emphasis in their service and begin to provide mindless surveillance with little time available for education and support. We shall return to this theme later in the chapter.

```
Notes                                                         Action
                                                             req'd  (√)
5 August 1988                                                done   (X)


NANCY MANNERS - antenatal: 28 weeks
Nancy says is 'keeping off baccy an' booze' and has been using hospital dining
room for main meals.  Cooking facilities in bedsitter.  Will claim benefits;
on housing list: expects flat - one year.  Hopes to use hospital creche.
Seeking information on breastfeeding whilst at work: discussion and Messenger
and Garner books recommended.  Not attending A/N classes.
Nancy's mother (lives Mychester) said to have been 'moderately firm; listened
to reason':  Nancy hopes to be same sort of mother.  Personnel department and
nursing friends 'supportive' but says her mother's attitude was the key to her
decision that she could cope as a single parent.
I promised to tell about organisations - Gingerbread and National Council.         √
                                                                                   √
APPT - Tuesday 6 September, am.

Dictated 5 August, am.             Signed/date  H. S. Van der Haastreht 8.8.88


6 September 1988

NANCY MANNERS - ANTENATAL: 32 weeks
Nancy says studying hard to help when she returns to training and more busy
with baby.  Eating well, especially salads.
Had discovered full time creche charges everywhere far too expensive for her:
bitterly disappointed.  Says her mother will care for baby (half by coming
to Overhampton and half in Mychester) on the days Nancy works, just until she
qualifies.  Nancy plans to stop work then until child care becomes possible.
She talked at length: fully aware of current difficulties re free nursery
places.
Messenger breastfeeding book found helpful; discovered several books at library.
Now more confident about breastfeeding.
One-parent family organisations discussed.  Gingerbread address, meeting place and
time provided.  Immunisation programme discussed.  Hesitant about whooping cough:
literature given.  Says does not intend to attend A/N classes - anticipates
prejudice; midwife very informative.

APPT - Tuesday 3 October, am.                                                       √

Dictated 3 September, am.          Signed/date  H. S. Van der Haastreht. 6.9.88.
```

Fig. 8.4a The 'said, seen and done' records scheme: an example — visit notes for the Manners family.

RECORDS IN ACTION

We conclude this section by looking at examples of ways in which health visitor recording can be undertaken, and indicate some of the non-computerised experiments and schemes recently in progress.

SSD RECORDS

An example

First is what we shall call the 'Said, Seen and Done' (SSD) approach to recording, the one ad-vocated earlier in this chapter. The illustrations in Figures 8.4a and 8.4b show how the antenatal visiting and birth visit to Nancy Manners, examples from Chapters 3 and 4, might have been recorded under this scheme. The visit notes alone are shown. The face card is not reproduced in this example.

Explanation of the example

We can now demonstrate the rationale of this simple system by looking at the SSD records in Figure 8.4 in the context of the features of the health visitor cycle in Figure 8.2:

```
Notes                                                          Action
                                                               req'd    (✓)
                                                               done     (X)
3 October 1988

NANCY MANNERS - antenatal: 36 weeks
Garner book found reassuring.  Has visited Gingerbread 3 times: establishing
friendships.  Immunisation discussed.  Nancy thinks her baby will 'have the lot'.
List of clinics given.
Developmental assessment discussed.  Local scheme shown.  HMSO Sheridan
booklet lent.
                                                                         ✓

Dictated 3 October, am.        Signed/dated ...H.S. Van der Haastrecht. 4.10.88
```

```
11 November 1988

Birth visit with midwife for 'handover'.  Nancy has her mother, Mrs Manners,
staying to help.  Caesarian delivery and 'bonding' discussed.  Nancy feared
inadequate bonding.  Rayner booklet used:  lent till next visit.          ✓✓
Mrs Manners intends to buy HMSO Sheridan for monitoring baby ' for fun'.
Developmental assessment discussed.  Local scheme shown. Local clinic
described.  Nancy talked of friendship networks; intends to join Gingerbread
babysitting circle.

PAULINE - 2 weeks
Breastfeeding 3 to 4 hourly: midwife's support appreciated.  Pauline wakeful
in evening: not seen as a problem.  Hearing tested with hand clap: startled.
Eyes clear; umbilicus dry.  Passing urine; stools loose.  Baby looks well;
colour good, fontanelles normal.  Making eye contact.  Weight 3 kg.         ✓
Visit  next week requested: especially re breastfeeding.

APPT - Tuesday 15 November, am.                                            ✓

Dictated 11 November, am.       Signed/ dated ...H.S. Van der Haastrecht 14.10.88
```

Fig. 8.4b Visit notes for the Manners family, overleaf.

1. and 2. What said by client and seen by HV

In these records, what the *mother said*, for example, about her diet, benefits, housing and crèche plans and arrangements are noted, as is *health visitor observation*, for example, that the cooking facilities were available and the baby's condition.

3. What done: service provided

The assessment and plan could be derived from reading what had been said and observed and from what *service* had been *given*: in this case, for example, the need for and plan to give information on breastfeeding, the attempt to assess attitudes towards 'mothering' and the need for and plan to give information on potential friendship networks.

4. Evaluation: what said and seen

The *evaluation* can be found in what the *mother reported* at the following visit, for example, having found The *Breastfeeding Book* (Messenger, 1982) very helpful, and what the *health visitor observed* in her manner, i.e. being now more confident about breastfeeding and about being able to continue for a while after starting back at work. In the October visit it was reported that the referral to the Gingerbread Group seemed to be providing a useful friendship and self-help network. This was reinforced in the visit of 12th November, the birth visit, as Nancy stated she intended to join their babysitting circle.

5. Action planned between visits

There was, in this example, no action planned

between visits. However, there *might* have been a plan to contact the secretary of the Gingerbread Group after the visit of 3rd September, to arrange for a member of the group to visit Nancy and take her to the meeting and introduce her round. This action was not undertaken here, either because Nancy did not feel it was necessary or, perhaps, as the health visitor did not feel it was worth suggesting.

Objectives

A note of a particular short-term objective which Hannah Van der Haastrecht wanted to remember is seen, for example, in the records of the 5th August visit, in the reference to the promise 'to tell about organisations — Gingerbread and National Council'. Another can be found at the end of the notes on the birth visit (12th November) regarding Nancy's seeing breastfeeding as an important factor to be covered at the next meeting, scheduled for the following week. Ticks in the action column draw attention to the items/objectives needing to be followed up. These are subsequently crossed through to show they have been attended to.

Other everyday health visiting objectives, for example concern over nutrition and the intention to explain about immunisation programmes, have not been given a special mention as objectives for further visits. However, the presence of such objectives can be derived from the fact that these matters were included in the conversations and hence in the notes of subsequent visits.

Open records

If this health visitor had shared the content of the records with her client, then Nancy would have been able to see what points the health visitor saw as key issues during the conversation. She would also have been able to further her own understanding and give the health visitor an opportunity to explain about her work and intentions, by asking about the content of the records. For example she could have asked, if it had not already been explained during the conversation, why the remarks

about her relationship with her mother were included.

Had our fictitious health visitor felt, as many health visitors seem to, that matters of family dynamics are too sensitive and too private to be recorded, then the conversations associated with the attempt to assess attitudes on 'mothering' and potential for depression or stress, might have been left out. The health visitor's understanding of the family interactions from such conversation would then simply be stored in her memory.

Prerequisites

It can be seen that no specially printed record cards are needed for the 'said, seen and done' scheme of recording. The prerequisites are for enough space to record full notes, and preferably with a dictaphone and an audio-typist clerical support system to help neaten and speed up the record-making (O'Connor & Willis, 1985).

SOAP(E) RECORDS

DIY formats

Problem-oriented recording as proposed by Karen Luker (1985, pp. 149–153), does not need specially designed new record cards either. She explains how this approach to record making was pioneered by a doctor in the late 1960s for medical records and gives an example of how it can be modified for and used in health visiting.

Experimenting with a more complex system is also possible without specially printed record cards. June Clark (1985) has described how she ruled up A4 paper and photostatted it in order to have the ability to classify her records as she wished. She designed assessment/plan sheets for the family and the child and for the neonatal visit, and a problem/needs list for when several problems emerged and needed to be clarified and sorted out. A contact record card was used for short-term plans and records of telephone conversations and contact with other agencies. She felt her structured approach helped her find problems she had previously missed. The limiting effects that can be associated with the checklist approach, incorporated to some extent in Dr Clark's scheme, were discussed in Chapter 2 (p. 30).

Tailor-made formats

Specially designed cards were described by health visitors from Portsmouth and South East Hampshire (Rogers, 1982; Wilson & Cowan, 1982; Hedley et al, 1982). Record cards Mark I and II (Rogers, 1982) are now superseded by Mark III. Interest in their work was so great that they marketed a work pack on their method of recording.

Developments by Portsmouth's neighbours in Southampton and South West Hampshire have been described by Marjorie Marsden (1985). They have devised a family history card and a child record card. In this latter, on one side they have set out four columns in which they state:

1. a pre-visit reason for making contact and observations
2. objectives
3. action taken and short- and/or long-term objectives
4. whether or not objectives have been achieved

An example

Experiments with schemes derived from the problem-oriented approach to recording have emerged elsewhere. Richmond, Twickenham and Roehampton Health Authority health visitors have produced an interesting one. On their records, the series of visits to the Manners family, our example from Chapters 3 and 4, might be recorded as shown in Figures 8.5a to 8.5d.

In this scheme, there would also be other cards. For example, there would be one for a confidential household profile which describes the family circumstances. There would be another recording information about the type of birth and the reasons for it and other matters, such as the general appearance and condition of the baby when newly born. This card also has space for screening tests undertaken, prophylaxis and childhood illnesses.

This records system is versatile and has space to show, in the way that the writer chooses, what:

- the client said
- the health visitor saw
- was done
- was intended to be done
- has been achieved.

Detailed notes about any encounter between the family and the health visitor can easily be contained in records systems such as these. However, actually getting the notes written up is another matter. In many authorities, health visitors still have no clerical support and no access to the services of an audio-typist able to transcribe tape-recorded messages from a small pocket-sized dictaphone.

Writing full, clear and neat records by hand and, conversely, deciphering tightly packed hand-written notes to try to find the key issues, can be very time consuming. When multiplied by the hundreds of people seen in their homes and at clinics each year, it is potentially quite an encroachment on possible home visiting time. However beautiful and accommodating any records scheme may be, there may well be a tendency towards skimping on records, both in reading them and writing them, in order to protect time to visit. In the end it comes down to choosing whichever system the health visitors and their employers feel is most appropriate for their area and for their circumstances.

To summarise, when choosing a scheme for recording, be it SSD, SOAP or some derivative of them, there are some key questions to be asked such as: is it *simple to use* and does it help enable:

- health visitors to note down and take into consideration the families' aims and wishes?
- families to understand the purpose and make good use of health visiting?
- key observations and the service given by health visitors to be clearly noted?
- results of the work to be shown, not only as the health visitor sees it, but also as the family report the situation?

In effect, does the chosen system of record making facilitate good communication and enable appropriate investigation?

NAME MANNERS

ADDRESS Room 2, 14 Mountgrove Road, Overhampton

ASSESSMENT AT FIRST VISIT – DATE 5· 8· 85

A visit was made to Nancy – a student nurse, who is 28 weeks pregnant and is at present living in a 'bedsit' with cooking facilities. She is hoping to resume her nursing training postnatally. Nancy has given much thought, both to her practical arrangements for the expected baby and her capabilities and attitudes towards being a single parent. She has a very supportive mother who has encouraged her to look after her own baby. Her landlady, her nursing colleagues and the Personnel Department have also been supportive. Nancy appears to have a very positive attitude and is keen to find information that will help her be a good mother.

DATE	LONG TERM AIM	EVALUATION	SIGNATURE
5· 8· 85	① To enable and encourage Nancy to accept and enjoy the responsibility of being a mother. To support her through the difficulties of being a single parent so that the bonding between her and her baby will be established, thus enabling her child to develop emotionally and physically within a secure environment.		
	② To detect as early as possible any signs of ill-health, or abnormalities through regular visiting, developmental checks and health education.		
	③ Promotion of health through health education, immunisation and regular visiting		H.S. van der Haastrecht 5th Aug. '85

Fig. 8.5a Problem-oriented records: an example. 1. Health visitor care plan.

DATE AND TIME	CODE	NEED AND OBSERVATION	PLAN/ACTION	REVIEW	SIGNATURE
5 · 8 · 85	H	Nancy is now 28 weeks pregnant and is hoping to continue working. Concerned regarding her future accommodation and is hoping to be rehoused by the council in one year. She will claim social security benefits when baby is born and hopes to use hospital crèche.	① Check place on housing list.		
			② Advice on diet.		
			③ Invitation to A/N classes.		
		Nancy says she is "keeping off bready and stodge" and is eating hospital meals.	④ Information given on health education literature for pregnant mothers and support groups ie. Gingerbread and National Council.	3 · 9 · 85	HS vander Haadrecht 5 · 8 · 85
3 · 9 · 85	H	32/40 Nancy more confident and eager to talk. Is studying hard to alleviate pressure when she returns to nursing, postnatally. : eating well, especially salads. Is bitterly disappointed that crèche charges are too expensive and that there is a shortage of free nursery places. Has decided to stop work after qualifying until suitable care can be arranged.	① Encourage attitude towards breastfeeding.		
			② Encourage interest in reading material regarding immunisation programmes.		
		Has decided against A/N classes as she anticipates prejudice. Midwife and mother very supportive.	③ To discuss with mother the arrangements for looking after the baby until Nancy has completed her training.	1 · 10 · 85	HS vander Haadrecht 3 · 9 · 85

FAMILY NAME MANNERS

CODE: H = HOME VISIT C = CLINIC
T = TELEPHONE S = SURGERY
O = OTHERS

Fig. 8.5b Problem-oriented records: an example. 2. Health visiting record — family.

DATE/TIME	CODE	NEED AND OBSERVATION	PLAN/ACTION	REVIEW	SIGNATURE
1·10·85	H	36/40 Nancy has found Garrer book reassuring and has made three visits to Gingerbread meetings: establishing friendships.	① Immunisation and developmental checks for baby discussed.		
			② Information given re clinics in area.		H. S. Vander Haarstrecht 1·10·85
			③ Local assessment schemes described and discussed.		
2·11·85	H	P/N visit with midwife. Maternal grandmother Mrs Manners staying to help Nancy with baby Pauline. Midwife very supportive. Long discussion re- Caesarian delivery and bonding as Nancy anxious re "inadequate bonding".	① Developmental assessment and clinic described.		
			② Appointment for developmental check.		
			③ Ongoing encouragement re bonding with baby Pauline.		
			④ Rayner booklet lent.		
			⑤ Encouragement and support over breastfeeding.		H.S. Vander Haarstrecht 12·11·85
			⑥ Encouraged to join Gingerbread babysitting circle.	19.11.85	

Fig. 8.5c Problem-oriented records: an example. 3. Health visiting record — family, overleaf.

HEALTH VISITOR CARE PLAN — GIRL

CODE: H - Home Visit   C - Clinic   O - Other
         T - Telephone   S - Surgery

NAME **MANNERS** Pauline   ADDRESS 14 Mountgrove Road.

DATE/TIME	CODE	NEED AND OBSERVATION	PLAN/ACTION	REVIEW	SIGNATURE
2.11.85	H	2/52 'Handover' visit with midwife. Breastfeeding 3–4 hourly. Wakeful in evening – not seen as a problem. Maternal grandmother helping and intends to buy H.M.SO Sheridan for monitoring for 'fun'.	① Hearing tested : hand clap ✓ ② Eyes clear ③ Vision : eye contact ; responds to facial expression. ④ Umbilicus dry ⑤ Buttocks ✓ ⑥ Passing urine ; stools loose ⑦ Baby's colour good ⑧ Fontanelles ✓ ⑨ Weight 3 kg	19.11.85	H.S. vander Haasbrecht 12.11.85

Fig. 8.5d   Problem oriented records: an example. 4. Health visitor care plan — girl.

EVALUATION

Three approaches

Overlapping meaning in commonly-used terminology such as evaluation, assessment and measurement, masks some of the differing concepts involved. 'Value', 'assessment' and 'quantification' are terms used in this section to try to draw out three approaches to evaluation in which health visitors can become involved in their day-to-day work. Figure 8.6 shows a cartoonised and very simplistic version of these three viewpoints: the clients', the health visitors' and that involved in wider management and planning.

The best judge of the *value* of a service is, for the most part, the person who actually receives it.

We know the *value* of the service, to us

I try to *assess* to what extent the service helps them

Quantification tells me something — but what?

Fig. 8.6 Three approaches to evaluation of health visiting.

The people who give the service can only make a guess at its value to their clients and try to find out from them to what extent it is helpful. The providers can, of course, think about what they have planned to offer and about their overall aims. They can then try to *assess* the degree to which their goals and tactics seem to have been effective and, more importantly, decide whether the chosen goals and tactics were, in the event, the most appropriate. It may be felt that these two viewpoints are too subjective, but, as Karen Luker (1985) shows, all evaluation carries some measure of subjectivity.

The third approach to evaluation, *quantification*, involves numerical measurement of certain aspects of the service provided, such as the number of babies or old people discovered to have defective hearing, the number of health visitors employed or homes visited. These measures can vary significantly in the extent to which they are able to show what has been achieved in the work.

Both of the first two approaches, investigating the value of the service and critical self-assessment by health visitors, mostly involve a broad-based descriptive or narrative approach. They have the advantage of being able to encompass consideration of all aspects of the current service, potential aspects and a range of possible alternatives. Quantification, on the other hand, in measuring a range of specific items, covers a narrower field and is, of course, restricted to current practice or practice at the time it was carried out. However, such measurement can, when founded on soundly-based criteria, be an extremely useful tool. A well thought out combination of the three ways of evaluating the work is likely, in practice, to give the most helpful view.

FAMILIES' EVALUATION

The value of the service to the families receiving it is a key issue and seems the most important to research. The way the service is seen as, for example, instructive, supportive and courteously provided or not, directly influences whether it is received either as relevant and acceptable or is rejected and amounts only to misdirected and wasted effort by the health visitor.

We have referred in earlier chapters, particularly in Chapter 2, to some important studies of client opinion undertaken by health visitors. It will be recalled, for example, that about 70 mothers with their first babies were interviewed by Jean Orr (1980). As a consequence of her investigations, she was able to give some very useful advice to health visitors on important features of the provision of the service. The study involving in-depth interviewing by Jane Robinson (1982), who was seeking reasons for non-use of the service, was also very instructive. Although undertaken with very few families, it was able to show how people can feel about the different styles within health visiting and to draw attention to some of the factors that seem to affect take-up of the service.

In Chapter 7, we looked at Karen Luker's (1982) scheme for finding out old ladies' opinion of the service. This sort of format, outlined on page 126, Box 7.2, could be used by other health visitors to find out what people think of their work. It could be used for getting people's opinions about clinic or group work as well as about home visiting.

An investigation does not necessarily have to be on a large scale to be useful. Pauline Pearson (1984) tape recorded her conversations with the parents of sixteen babies. She asked open-ended questions and discovered a wide range of needs and views. She found quite divergent opinions about a similar style of health visiting. One mother, for example, was grateful that the health visitor did not say 'you should do this and you should do that', whereas another mother was yearning for 'an honest bit of advice': two very different responses to a non-directive approach. This sort of research does not provide simple guidance on exactly what to do or how to do it. It is, however, well worthwhile. It can give some useful leads, is thought provoking and is, as we said above, the best way to get to know the *value* of health visiting to the families receiving it.

There is, of course, a value in health visiting of which the family may be unaware or, perhaps, discounts. For example, immunisation against whooping cough on a large scale helps protect the most vulnerable in society, the extremely young babies, from the consequences of the disease —

providing a value to society as well as to the individual. Here we have been concerned directly with the view-point of the families on how they see the value of the service as it affects them.

In the later chapters, particularly in chapter 12, we look at the importance of client opinion of service provision at an earlier, planning stage of our work, as well as in the later evaluation.

ASSESSMENT BY HEALTH VISITORS

Health visitors, like the families they visit, are, of course, constantly assessing and coming to conclusions about each encounter they have. Here it is suggested that in addition to this everyday evaluation of each case, health visitors should make a conscious decision to step back from their work every so often and look at some individual cases and at their caseload overall, in order to think in a broader way about what has been achieved to date.

Peer group discussion can provide a very good environment for assessment of the work. It can encourage a wide-ranging view of possible alternative strategies for care. Brain-storming sessions in these groups could give health visitors courage to follow up and act on latent ideas for improvements in their service. Ann Stanton (1984) has described how 'peer group auditing' was set up in Edinburgh. She said that they had, unknowingly, following Shirley Goodwin's (1983a) ground rules for success in starting and running such a group. It seems the group was very successful. The auditing was described as having become addictive and plans were being made for looking at and assessing even more aspects of practice.

Another side of peer group assessment can be seen in the time spent with the nurse manager talking about cases that are of concern or present some dilemma, or in discussing the relative merits of new ideas for promoting the health of the local community. In these deliberations and assessments, nurse managers and their health visitors will have many factors to consider.

The fundamental question will be, of course, whether the aspect of health visiting under scrutiny is making or is likely to make a contribution to fulfilment of the aims and objectives of the work.

If stated in terms of the prevention and family health needs models of this book, then the questions will ask whether the service being provided, or proposed, is likely to help

- *prevent the occurrence* of problems or conditions
- *prevent the development* of problems or conditions
- *prevent deterioration* in established problems or conditions

with regard to *environmental, physical, mental/emotional and social* aspects of people's health and welfare.

The well-known questions raised by the Children's Committee (1980) are very important, too. It was felt that they helped to indicate the extent to which the professional is practising in partnership with clients. The points raised were whether:

- parents were seen as central to the life of their child and treated in accordance with this
- parents were encouraged to help each other and were enabled to do so
- the service was sensitive to the families' cultural and social norms
- the service was easily understood by the parents.

Other important basic factors are whether the service being provided or proposed:

- allows for creativity and encourages innovation
- takes a proactive rather than a reactive approach
- is formulated and devised in relation to local small area OPCS evidence of social deprivation and other evidence of health need.

Records and evaluation

Health visitors wanting a peer support group or their nursing manager to help them assess certain aspects of their care, may find their records provide an important aide-mémoire about the details of individual family members' progress and problems (presented, of course, anonymously).

However, using records the other way round, that is attempting to assess how health visitors are performing their work *solely* on an inspection of their records, has distinct limitations. We looked at another aspect of this issue earlier in the records section of this chapter.

Although well-recorded and full notes can give an observer such as a nurse manager a professional picture of what health visitors have been doing on their visits, the records cannot necessarily show how appropriate these activities were in relation to other possible alternatives. One cannot tell the whole story (see p. 144) either on what did happen or what could have happened. Only the health visitors know what choice there was as they saw it, and as the family appeared to see it, at the time. Only they can make informed speculations as to what topics could, perhaps, have been discussed or expanded and what possible alternative approaches there might have been. However, nurse managers who have been community trained understand the possible innuendoes and complexities within a visit and can empathise when these matters are discussed.

Normal health visitor records necessarily show only an outline or provide an index of what happened at any encounter. Robert Dingwall (1977, p. 113) observed that

the major part of what a field health visitor knows about her clients is in her head.

For this reason, assessment by outsiders benefits from being founded, for the most part, upon discussions with the health visitor involved. Also, the records cannot portray the appropriateness or otherwise of a health visitor's style and approach. This, too, is probably best ascertained, where no client view can be gained, through conversation in a counselling sort of environment and, perhaps, using some of the eight criteria said to be associated with interviewing skills and listed by Karen Luker (1985, p. 137), for example 'willing to listen and empathises' and 'shows human warmth'. Another possible basis for discussion could be provided by health visitors tape recording their own visit (Robinson, 1986).

Report writing provides another way of setting out the issues which need to be discussed in an assessment of the service. Much can be learned from the approach to evaluation taken in community health development (see Ch. 12) and it is likely that more and more health visitors will use such reports to help managers understand about the finer points of health visiting. Further aspects of the ways managers and health visitors can help each other assess the work is considered in the latter part of chapter 14.

In this section we have looked at peer group analysis which where it is supportive, constructive and creative, can be extremely helpful in enabling health visitors to share and evaluate their problems and concerns. It can provide a very important back-up for individual health visitors' own attempts to stand back and *assess* their work.

QUANTIFICATION

There are an enormous number of measurable entities that are available to analyse and provide some guidance. Both health visitors and their managers need to understand the implications of what is being quantified and how it is being measured. Also of importance is what evidence is being particularly singled out and used to guide the allocation of resources and the choice of projects to be undertaken.

What quantified?

When some aspect of health visiting is being measured, it is important to know, for example, what are the particular entities that have been selected for measurement, whether these entities are being assessed against pre-set and validated criteria on a pre-selected group, whether there is also a control group or the research could be replicated, and if it is a prospective study.

The Child Development Project (1984) provides an excellent example of this sort of well thought-out and 'scientific' approach. The research involved assessment over a three year period of parental environment and children's development and how this correlated with a particular style of health visiting. The style is one in which the parent is encouraged to take the initiative with the health visitor acting as a resource, as opposed to the rather more old fashioned style which sees the parent as the recipient of 'expert' health visiting advice.

In this research, an enormous amount of information has been coded and computerised for analysis. A variety of aspects is being studied. For example, a child development profile is being built up on each child by using parental reports, the researcher's observations and researcher assessments of the child's ability to complete a wide range of tasks. A child activity level questionnaire, a child's progress form and a maternal self-esteem questionnaire are being used. A nutritional questionnaire, concerned with what the children are being fed and the environment in which they are fed, has been used in some districts. It will be some time before the study is fully complete and all the results become available. However, early feedback was optimistic and success has been confirmed in a comprehensive review of the project's first phase (Barker & Anderson, 1988) (see Ch. 3, p. 38 and Ch. 5, p. 81).

The most important aspect of this research is that it shows that, given the expertise and the resources, it *is* possible to monitor and evaluate practices in health visiting in terms of indicators, for example, of good and bad health, the quality of the home's developmental environment and the child's progress.

The information traditionally collected has not been so useful. Knowledge of the number of homes visited or classifications of clients seen, for example, may be useful for maintaining the status quo regarding the staffing-level management of the work. However, it does not give any indication of what has been achieved and in what way the service could provide more effective care. The Körner Committee (Steering Group on Health Services Information, 1984) information system for services to the community will help to give a better picture of a variety of aspects of health visiting — some, such as immunisation, more successfully than others. Unfortunately, it looks as if educational and supportive aspects of the work will largely go unrecorded. The Commit-

tee expects greater use to be made of OPCS small area statistics and computerised age-sex population data as a guide to the need for the preventive service and how it should be allocated.

Hopefully, information about health surveillance and early detection of disease will identify people who have been missed by the normal provision of services, so that funds can be set aside for the more costly and time consuming follow-up of, for example, children of working mothers whose families can only be visited in the evening.

It has been suggested that there is a need for increased understanding of the benefits to the child, the health visitor and to management of centralised records for pre-school developmental screening to bring about improved reliability and validity of the central records. Under-recording has been shown to be associated with inefficient methods of data collection and lack of interest by staff who did not know the use to which such information could be put. This, it is suggested, would be as much of a problem with computerised as with handwritten data (Lambert et al, 1985). These factors will be important to remember as new systems are implemented.

The best solution for many reasons (see Ch. 14), is to involve health visitors themselves in the analysis and interpretation of the statistical output (Hull, 1989). In fact it is essential. Any information that is not meaningful to the staff providing it, is bound to be meaningless and therefore useless in any practical planning terms, to the recipient (Wilson, 1985; 1987).

The problem comes when this factor is not openly recognised by the managers or officials receiving the data. Many will be unaware of their ignorance. Field-level staff forced by the system to provide meaningless information, need repeatedly to send reports with it providing positively useful descriptions and data. Incredible amounts of health visitor time are spent in administrative tasks (Hull, 1989), particularly on Körner and other clerical work (Smith, 1987; Bishop & Thorogood, 1988; Brojaka, 1988; Little, 1988; Mills, 1988; Phillips, 1988; Smith, 1988; Howkins, 1989). In the short term, it must be worth spending a little more on writing reports (see Ch. 12 and Ch. 14) and/or in meetings, in order to press for implementation of a balanced and meaningful system which provides useful feedback for field-level planning.

The Körner Committee itself was aware of the problems and provided some ideas for improvements. It recognised that the enormous variety of activities involved in services to the community meant that a count of contacts could not be taken as a measure of the work done. They said that the proposed broad classifications give only a general indication of activity during the contact (para 7.9) and that a deeper description of what happens during that contact is necessary. Sadly, the categorisation of activities they suggest in Annex III is still at a distinctly general level from a health visiting point of view. It does, however, provide at least a chance to expand on the 'main purpose' categorisation of the extremely simplistic 'surveillance' or 'professional advice and support'.

It is good that the Committee made such a clear statement about the inability to measure health visiting by a count of contacts. Health visitors do sometimes tend to feel that they are being judged on the number of visits that they make. Robert Dingwall (1977, p. 114) explained how he thought this comes about. During his study he observed that management stressed emphatically that the quality of visits and not their quantity was what was important. However, he noticed guidelines were proposed for the number of visits at various phases of a child's life. This and management's preoccupation with classification of visits for the weekly returns, gave health visitors the *impression* that work was being monitored from a quantitative point view.

Records as quantifiable evidence

The sort of records kept in a study such as the Child Development Project or Karen Luker's (1982) research into the health needs of 120 old ladies, have to be very detailed, well planned and in accord with certain validated criteria. Health visitor records are not, for the most part, of this sort of calibre and such detail could probably only be justified in specifically planned experimental research or those few specific projects which it has been agreed health visitors should participate in. Normal health visitor records, however full and

well presented, are not generally able on their own, to provide reliable, quantifiable evidence and are really only useful at the self- and peer-assessment level of evaluation described above.

Local statistics

Infant mortality figures in Sheffield and Gosport, Portsmouth, have improved remarkably (see Ch. 5, p. 93). Health visitors there are undertaking special surveillance schemes aimed at lowering the rate of sudden and unexpected infant deaths. June Clark (1983) questioned whether it can be proven that it was the health visitor intervention that caused this to happen because the actual health visitor–client activities undertaken were not described. Only if described could they be tried out again, and only if repeated, and with similar results, could proof be assumed. However, since she wrote, Carpenter et al (1983) have given a detailed account in *The Lancet* defending their case that the factor that made the difference was, in fact, the health visitor contact. Also, the Portsmouth study (Powell, 1985) has become very well known and so it should be fairly easy to try it out again and thereby verify the matter or not so far as this is possible.

In Chapter 2 (pp. 19–20) we looked at the sort of local statistics that are available to help demonstrate where health visiting effort should be concentrated. Doreen Irving (1985) shows how scoring systems can be used. It seems the British Medical Association has decided to adopt an eight point scoring system to help identify areas eligible for special help in improving the services. It is described as a crude but 'good enough' device for identifying need. Doreen Irving says free copies of the figures for electoral wards in any specific district can be supplied by Peter Rice and that John Yates is producing analyses of district figures for health authorities.

Evaluation of health visiting outcome must go hand in hand with investigations of levels of health and ill health in the community. This is necessary to show, as far as is possible, not only the overall need for the work but also its overall effect, such as on infant mortality rates and increased public participation in health promoting activities.

It will be interesting to see to what extent John Dobby's (1984) research can contribute towards this. He experimented with certain classes of information which may be able to help health visitors estimate both the effectiveness of and the constraints on their work and help decide priorities for health visiting activities in their area.

What evidence is chosen?

There is, then, an increasing amount of evidence currently and potentially available which can give some guidance on various ways in which health visiting services might be organised or allocated. Probably the most important question regarding evaluation of health visiting is 'To what use is the evidence being put and, of all that is available, which aspects do managers choose to guide their decisions?'

Are health visitor managers encouraging, for example, up-to-date monitoring of local mortality and morbidity statistics? Are they taking into account the evidence from recent research into health visiting, such as that from the Child Development Project? Perhaps even more significantly, are they prepared, where necessary, to change the structure of the traditional staffing patterns and work schedules, as is necessary for this programme (Child Development Project, 1984)?

Health visitors are, in general terms, the health workers most closely aware of social needs and situations in the various corners of their District. To what extent do they share this knowledge? Do they and their managers use the OPCS and other statistics available locally to demonstrate to people allocating the resources where need seems to be greatest and why and where they recommend special efforts to be concentrated?

Nora Saddington (Nursing Times, 1984) was quoted as warning that the minimum data collection recommended by the Körner Committee would not be enough to make informed decisions about priorities in health visiting. It seems she gave two examples of how, in Birmingham, health visitors had used social information in addition to the data assembled by the health authority managers and, in this way, had identified the whereabouts of the people most in need of intensive health visiting.

Discovering and deciding on 'need' in a community is a complex matter. Jean Orr (1985) has described many of the issues and difficulties involved and has advocated that health visitors should compile, and keep up to date, a community health profile from which to plan and provide health visiting activities. We look at some of the practicalities of community and caseload health profiling in Chapter 15.

These quantitative matters, that is looking at and using 'facts' and figures, are an important aspect of evaluation, as is, in the day to day work of the practising health visitor, self- and peer-assessment and attempts to understand what value the families put on the work.

CONFIDENTIALITY

Confidentiality is an important issue both in recording and in the evaluation of our work. Trends towards records which are becoming increasingly geared for evaluation and, in some cases, pressures towards closer oversight of the records, bring the matter to the fore. In general terms, any information given to a nurse is given with the expectation that it will go no further. Matters of an impersonal and general nature are less likely to be categorised in this way, but clinical and personal matters are given to the nurse with the underlying assumption of confidentiality (Bailey, 1980).

There is a need for health visitors to be particularly sensitive to this issue and also to the vulnerability of their clientele in this respect. Working in the informal way that we do in people's homes, on occasions using questioning techniques or some other approach to help people express how they feel, confidential information is often entrusted to the health visitor within the natural course of conversation. Personal information, however casually it appears to have been given, whether in the secrecy of the person's home, in a quiet corner of the clinic or anywhere else, should never be treated casually. This is one of the areas where 'full recording' and describing every activity and key issue at a visit become difficult, not for lack of space or time, but on grounds of confidentiality.

Individual health visitors have to make their own ethical decisions on this matter. Should health visitors note down, for example, how someone is quarrelling with his/her spouse or, perhaps, how a woman has revealed that the true paternity of her child is not the father thought by everyone else to be so? The important question is: what risks to confidentiality or what benefits for the family are likely to result from recording personal details? Is the better alternative to record 'Personal problem discussed' — or to write nothing?

In a small way, this problem was touched on with regard to Nancy Manners' relationship with her mother (p. 152). Would Mrs Van der Haastrecht have made a note of a poor relationship, where, for example, the mother was said to have beaten her? This would have implications for Nancy's need for extra support and, perhaps, her own tendency later to treat her child in the same way, an issue returned to in Chapter 11. In some cases it is no simple matter to gauge just what should be committed to paper. Perhaps 'when in doubt, write nought' should provide the final guidance.

Robert Dingwall (1977, p. 93) in his study, noted that the health visitor's records did not reflect the degree to which conversation at visits was in fact concentrated upon the mother's welfare and feelings. It could be that this tendency reflected the health visitor's intuitive protection of client confidentiality over personal issues. If it is not written then it cannot be leaked, for example, either to a manager or later by some subsequent health visitor working with the family.

The protection of confidentiality may mean that, from a records point of view, the work will inevitably portray a medical model, for example showing a bias towards surveillance of developmental progress and interest in physical aspects of adult health. Supportive aspects of the work associated with a relationship-oriented model and with health visitors' social awareness, may remain largely invisible and secret by being unrecorded.

As Kate Robinson (1985) says, we do not yet have enough knowledge of what actually happens in health visiting to know what approaches and philosophies are actually involved. Moreover, it seems that normal health visitor records are not going to tell us the whole truth about the work, whatever records scheme is invented.

With the moves to make health visitor records (a) more explicit and/or (b) more subject to review, comes an increasing need for these issues to be discussed at length, both among health visitors and between health visitors and their managers. Currently, general agreement seems the norm, presumably because managers with a health visitor background can empathise over the problems involved.

There may be difficulties, however, when an employing authority requests information which involves a breach of confidentiality. Joan Bailey (1980) suggests that if facing such a dilemma the nurse should seek advice. This could be, for example, from a professional organisation, such as the RCN or HVA, and especially from the Professional Conduct Division of the UKCC who specialise in matters of confidentiality. Miss Bailey explains that in general it is felt that employers have no legal entitlement to confidential information and that it is therefore wrong for the nurse to provide it. This has been confirmed in the United Kingdom Central Council's (UKCC, 1987; Nursing Times, 1987; Willis, 1987) recent guidance on confidentiality.

The Health Visitor Association has drawn up a useful guide on confidentiality (Health Visitor, 1980). Advice is given, for example, on disclosure at case conferences, obtaining clients' permission before handing on information and how to approach requests to break confidences in a court of law. Peter Godber (1981) said that requests to disclose case notes in court should be contested, and quotes a Court of Appeal decision which protects health visitors from having to surrender them. However, he advised that they should take their notes with them into the courtroom, in order to remind themselves of the facts and give more accurate evidence.

Guidelines on confidentiality are also available from the Royal College of Nursing (1980). There will, however, always be grey areas where it is difficult to be sure what is for the best, and manager and peer group support and, perhaps, contact with the UKCC can clarify ideas and the issues involved.

Open records

Perhaps the best way to ensure having an appropriate and ethically acceptable balance of information, which is neither surprising nor offensive to the families involved and states reasonably clearly what happened at a visit, is to share the content of the records with them. The exercise of going through it together should help to crystallise out key matters. Furthermore, if clients are encouraged to say what they think should be included from what has been observed, achieved or requested, it represents another move towards true partnership and gives one more opportunity to discover the families' viewpoint.

Shirley Goodwin (1983b) warned that sooner or later there will be legislation enabling people to have right of access to their records. She urges health visitors to think very carefully about what they are writing and its purpose. The Data Protection Bill is now in force; the DHSS issued a circular which states the general principles associated with people's rights to see their records in local authority social services departments (Health Visitor, 1983). In 1990, a private member's bill on access to health records was supported by around 70 national organisations (Nursing Times, 1990). There are ever increasing pressures for open access.

Health visitors can naturally be concerned by the prospect of notes and records, originally expected to remain unseen by their clients, becoming open for them to inspect (Anonymous, 1983). However, if all records are written by health visitors bearing in mind to what extent they would blush to read them, not only in court but also to the families concerned, it may help them to find an appropriate balance between what is useful and what is invasive and/or offensive.

It has been suggested in this chapter that statements of facts about what has been said, seen and done at a visit are proper to record, and that it should generally be unnecessary to make a note, specifically, of the health visitor's assessment or opinion, particularly over family dynamics and personal details. Three aspects of evaluation — the way clients value the service, health visitors' attempts to assess what they have achieved and numerical measurement of aspects of the work — were considered, as was the use of statistical information in planning priorities. Records, evaluation and confidentiality are distinctly interlinked and are very important aspects of our work.

USEFUL ADDRESSES

Health Visitors Association (HVA)
36 Eccleston Square,
London SW1 1PF
Tel 071 834 9523

The Royal College of Nursing of the
United Kingdom (Rcn)
Henrietta Place,
Cavendish Square,
London W1M OAB
Tel 071 409 3333

United Kingdom Central Council for
Nursing, Midwifery and Health
Visiting (UKCC)
23 Portland Place
London W1N 3AF
Tel 071 637 7181

REFERENCES

Anonymous 1983 Patients' access to records (letter). Health Visitor 56: 319
Bailey J M 1980 The law and the community nurse. Cumbria Area Health Authority, Carlisle
Barker W 1987 Counting heads. Senior Nurse 6, 1: 8–10 — Essential reading.
Barker W and Anderson R 1988 The Child Development
Programme: an evaluation of process and outcomes. Early Child Development Unit, University of Bristol
Bishop M, Thorogood M 1988 (letter) On implementation of Körner. Health Visitor 61, 1: 4
Brojaka P 1988 (letter) Support for Körner. Health Visitor 61, 11: 330
Carpenter R G, Gardner A, Jepson M, Taylor E M, Salvin

A, Sunderland R, Emery J L, Pursall E, Roe J, Sheffield Health Visitors 1983 Prevention of unexpected infant death. The Lancet I: 723–727

Child Development Project 1984 Child development programme. Early Childhood Development Unit, Bristol. p 17–20

Children's Committee 1980 The needs of the under-fives in the family. The Children's Committee, London

Clark J 1983 Evaluating health visiting practice. Health Visitor 56: 205–208

Clark J 1985 Delivering the goods. Nursing Times Community Outlook 81, 2: 23–28

Crabbe G 1990 Record holders. Nursing Times 86, 13: 22–23

Dingwall R 1977 The social organisation of health visitor training. Croom Helm, London

Dobby J 1984 Research into health visiting effectiveness (letter). Health Visitor 57: 292–293

Godber P 1981 Confidentiality of case records. Health Visitor 54: 193

Goodwin S 1983a Caring for the carers. Part 2: Coping with stress. Health Visitor 56: 46–48

Goodwin S 1983b Open secrets. Nursing Mirror 156, 26: 22

Green A, Macfarlane A 1985 Parent-held child health record cards — a comparison of types. Health Visitor 58: 14–15

Health Visitor 1980 Guide for health visitors on confidentiality. Health Visitor 53: 30

Health Visitor 1983 Disclosing information to clients. Health Visitor 56: 355

Hedley C, Grieve L, Hood J, Leyshom Y 1982 Using the need/problem orientated method of record-keeping. Health Visitor 55: 211–215

Hendy A 1983 The nursing process and health visiting. Health Visitor 56: 197–200

Holland T 1984 Computers for child health records. Nursing Times 80, 24: 48–49

Howkins E J 1989 (letter) Bureaucrat or health visitor? Health Visitor 62, 5: 165

Hull W 1989 Measuring effectiveness in health visiting. Health Visitor 62, 4: 113–115

Irving D 1985 How to identify the needy. Health and Social Services Journal XCV: 18–19

Jackson C 1990 To have and to hold. Health Visitor 63, 7: 221–222

Lambert C, Miers M, Edwards J, Farrow S 1985 Centralised records — who benefits? A discussion of issues raised by research into pre school developmental screening. Health Visitor 58: 11–13

Little J 1988 (letter) 171005 and all that. Health Visitor 61, 11: 330

Luker K 1982 Evaluating health visiting practice. Royal College of Nursing, London

Luker K 1985 Evaluating health visiting practice. In: Luker K, Orr J (eds) Health visiting. Blackwell Scientific Publications, Oxford

MacInnes A D 1989 The extent of computerisation in health visiting records. A survey of Scottish Health Boards and English Health Authorities. Health Visitor 62, 5: 145–148

Marsden M 1985 Implementing the health visiting process. Health Visitor 58: 166–167

Messenger M 1982 The breastfeeding book. Century Publications Co Ltd, London

Mills C 1988 (letter) Time is money. Health Visitor 61, 11: 330

Nicholl A 1983 Community child health services — for better or for worse? Health Visitor 56: 241–243

Nicholl A 1984 The value of selective pre-school medicals in an inner city area. Public Health, London 98: 68–72

Nursing Times 1984 How more data can alter priorities. Nursing Times 80, 46: 7

Nursing Times 1987 UKCC warns of careless talk. Nursing Times 83, 13: 5

Nursing Times 1990 Access to records Bill before the House. Nursing Times 86, 9: 8

O'Connor P J, Willis M 1985 Clerical help for health visitors. Health Visitor 58: 261–262

Orr J 1980 Health visiting in focus. Royal College of Nursing, London

Orr J 1985 Health visiting and the community. In: Luker K, Orr J (eds) Health visiting. Blackwell Scientific Publications, Oxford

Owen C M 1980 Child health record booklet. Midwife Health Visitor and Community Nurse 16: 156–162

Pearson P 1984 Images of a health visitor. Nursing Mirror 159, 19: 21–23

Pearson P 1985 Parent-held records — what parents think. Health Visitor 58: 15–16

Phillips P M 1988 (letter) Community oppressive? Health Visitor 61, 9: 264

Powell J 1985 Keeping watch. Nursing Times Community Outlook 81, 2: 15–19

Robertson C A 1982 Becoming a health visitor — an obstacle course? Nursing Times 78, 36: 1508–1512

Robinson K 1983 Talking with clients. In: Clark J, Henderson J (eds) Community health. Churchill Livingstone, Edinburgh

Robinson K 1985 Knowledge and its relationship to health visiting. In: Luker K, Orr J (eds) Health visiting. Blackwell Scientific Publications, Oxford

Robinson K 1986 (personal communication)

Robinson J 1982 An evaluation of health visiting. Council for the Education and Training of Health Visitors, London

Rogers J 1982 Introducing the health visiting process. Health Visitor 55: 204–209

Royal College of Nursing 1980 Guidelines on confidentiality in nursing. Royal College of Nursing, London

Saffin K 1985 Card carriers. Nursing Times 81, 13: 24–26

Smith A 1988 (letter) Evaluate for change. Health Visitor 61, 11: 330

Smith J 1987 (letter) On the implementation of Körner. Health Visitor 60, 11: 358

Stanton A 1984 A question of help. Nursing Mirror Community Forum 158, 21: i–iii

Steering Group on Health Services Information (1984) Fifth Report to the Secretary of State. Chairman Mrs E Körner. Department of Health and Social Security, HMSO, London

UKCC 1984 Code of Professional Conduct for the Nurse Midwife and Health Visitor. 2nd edn. United Kingdom Central Council for Nursing, Midwifery and Health Visiting, London. paragraph 9

UKCC 1987 Confidentiality. An elaboration of Clause 9 of the second edition of the UKCC's code of professional conduct for the nurse, midwife and health visitor. United Kingdom Central Council for Nursing, Midwifery and Health Visiting, London

Whincup M 1981 The duties of a health visitor. Nursing Times 77: 567—568

Willis S 1987 Confidentiality: duty or danger? Health Visitor 60, 7: 213

Wilson C R M 1985 Quality assurance: getting started. Ontario Hospital Association, Toronto

Wilson C R M 1987 Hospital-wide quality assurance.

Models for implementation and development. W B Saunders, Toronto — Strongly recommended reading.

Wilson M, Cowan J 1982 Putting the health visiting process into practice. Health Visitor 55: 209–211

FURTHER READING

Records

Hardy L, Engel J 1987 The search for professionalism. Nursing Times 83, 15: 37–39

Kratz C R 1988 Setting the records straight. Nursing Times Community Outlook 84, 10: 4

Stroud R N 1988 (letter) Making models work. Nursing Times 84, 12: 14

Evaluation

Guldager E 1988 Do health visitors improve children's health? Nursing Times 84, 18: 58

Luker K A, Chalmers K I 1989 The referral process in health visiting. International Journal of Nursing Studies 26, 2: 173–185

Luker K A, Chalmers K I 1990 Gaining access to clients: the case of health visiting. Journal of Advanced Nursing 15, 1: 74–82

Royal College of Nursing 1989 Standards of care for health visiting. Royal College of Nursing, London

Winn E 1986 Making use of community health services information, King's Fund, London

Confidentiality

Melia K 1989 Computer ethics. Nursing Times 85, 29: 62–63

Newton T 1986 Protecting data. Senior Nurse 4, 3: 10–11

In Chapter 9, we look at health visiting and handicap, mainly through the perspective of the prevention model, describing in passing important ideas from the Warnock Committee Report. We conclude with two examples of health visiting families who have a handicapped child, one example using the prevention framework and the other the family health needs format.

9

Families with a handicapped child

THE PREVENTION MODEL AND SOME WARNOCK IDEAS

The role of the health visitor is considered in this chapter by using the prevention framework, that is:

- preventing the occurrence of handicap and of later problems if an impairment is already present. This mainly involves health education and anticipatory guidance
- preventing the development of problems by discovering handicap early, or discovering other aspects of handicap where impairments are already known to exist. These are important in order to enable timely care to be given
- rehabilitation and containment of the problem and support for the family. This is aimed at prevention of deterioration in the case of established handicap. It involves appropriate support through the emotional crisis and giving information on practical help.

Several ideas from a 1978 governmental report are very relevant to this work. Table 9.1 shows an outline of the prevention framework in this context and indicates where these ideas are particularly useful.

Warnock Report

Some important concepts for health visitors were contained in the Warnock Committee Report. The government published a brief guide (Warnock,

Table 9.1   Health visiting and handicap: prevention framework

Aims	Some activities	Warnock ideas
To prevent occurrence of handicap or later problems	*Health education:* Public: for greater understanding	Wider concept
	Parents: anticipatory guidance	
	Genetic counselling/ abortion	Partnership with parents
	Pre- and antenatal care	
	Immunisation: e.g. rubella, polio	
To prevent development through early diagnosis and care	*Surveillance, screening and referral:* Find hearing, vision, neurological problems; refer for assessment	Early discovery and education and partnership with parents
	Listen to parental fears: act on them	
	Monitor for multiple problems; assess functioning	
	Clear records, share reports with parents:	
To prevent deterioration through rehabilitation and containment	*Practical and emotional help:* Support in stress: bereavement; marital tensions; morale boosting	
	Practical advice and information	Named Person and partnership with parents
	Guidance on services and agencies	
	Tell about voluntary organisations	
	Catalyst for emergent groups	
	Liaison with other professionals	

1978) as well as the report itself, a sure sign that it was intended that the ideas in it should be read about and acted upon! Perhaps the four most im-

portant ideas for our work were those concerning, firstly, a wider concept of handicap, secondly, early discovery and education, thirdly, parents as partners and, lastly, the notion of a 'named person'.

1. The report proposed that special educational need, not medical impairment, should determine the kind of schooling a child was given. It pointed out that, taking a wider look at handicap, it could be seen that some 20% of children would need special help at some time in their school career.

It was envisaged that a range of educational provision should be available, including that enabling attendance at normal school backed by appropriate health services. It was hoped that a more positive approach to handicap would emerge.

2. and 3. Early discovery of handicap, early education and the health visitor's part in these were discussed. The Court Report (1976) surveillance recommendations were endorsed, as was the need for parents to be involved in their children's assessment.

The report stressed that there should be a partnership between parents and professionals and that parents need advice, information and practical help in their important role as the main educators of their children.

4. Research undertaken for the Report (Warnock Report, 1978) showed that a very high proportion of parents found it difficult to obtain the advice they needed. It was therefore proposed that a designated Named Person should provide the main point of contact for families where a handicapping condition has been discovered.

As it was found that health visitors were in general the most, sometimes the only, helpful professionals in the early years, they were recommended as the Named Person up to school age. It was suggested that multiprofessional assessment might show another worker in frequent contact with the family to be more appropriate as the Named Person. He/She would, therefore, be designated to this role. Also, arrangements were proposed which would enable parents to ask to be put in touch with another professional, should their designated Named Person prove to be unsatisfactory.

A guide and advocate needed

A designated Named Person is very much needed. Many studies have shown that families caring for handicapped relatives tend not to receive full advice on services and entitlements to which they have a right. Sam Ayer's (1984) three-year study of 132 mothers caring for their severely mentally handicapped children led him to conclude that the current policy of 'community care' meant, in reality, 'institutional care in the community'. Despite the rhetoric, supportive facilities were so poor for these families looking after their own children that 'community care' could not be referring to family care.

Many of the families in Dr Ayer's study did not know about basic services available to help reinforce their efforts to care for their children themselves. High proportions did not know, for example, about a nappy service, home adaptations and the home help service. He said few acute crises are generated by these families' chronic problems of long-term management. It seems social workers do not tend to see them as 'appropriate' or 'deserving' cases. Dr Ayer drew up a checklist, outlined in Box 9.1, which, he suggested, parents and those seeking the welfare of

Box 9.1 Community care for families: checklist (from Ayer, 1984)

> Services providing reinforcement to help parents to care for their own mentally handicapped children
>
> A full range of support from specialist services
> Home visits, at least two monthly, by specialist social worker and/or community mental handicap nurse
> Regular reports from these visits made available to parents
> Short-term relief, counselling, classes etc.
> Full information given to parents on statutory services
> Priority placement on housing list for these families
> Parents' workshops
> Full laundry service
> Special equipment available
> Day care in school holidays

these families could use to evaluate the provision of services locally.

Where there are enough specialist social workers and/or community mental handicap nurses to provide frequent, regular visiting, then the health visitor is unlikely to be nominated the Named Person. These services do not yet seem to be widely available, leaving the health visitor in the main, to speak for and support parents of both physically and mentally handicapped children.

INCREASING AWARENESS

There are two sides to preventing the occurrence of difficulties. One is aimed at preventing the handicap ever happening and the other aims at trying to prevent problems arising out of known disability. We look first at the former and lead on into the latter.

PREVENTING HANDICAP

Aspects of everyday health visiting to do with increasing people's awareness of health needs, play a part in helping prevent handicap, for example in newborn babies. Enabling people to understand the value of vaccination and immunisation, particularly the vaccination against rubella, and public knowledge about the value of, for example, pre-conceptual and antenatal care regarding nutrition, smoking and alcohol, all help to produce healthy, normal babies. Other vaccinations, such as those against measles or polio, help prevent handicap occurring in otherwise healthy people as a consequence of those diseases.

Genetic counselling

A health visitor might tell parents about services that can help prevent handicap. For example, genetic counselling can help prospective parents understand the degree of risk attached to giving birth to a baby with an inherited genetic disorder. People who have a baby with, for example, multiple handicap may, after assessment and diagnosis of the baby's condition, be able to receive guidance about risks regarding future pregnancies. Cousins marrying or parents over 35 years may seek information. It has been suggested that genetic disorders occur in about one in twenty babies born alive (Winter, 1984).

PREVENTING LATER PROBLEMS

Through counselling

A service has been described in which a specialist health visitor was employed to follow up genetic clinic consultation with home visits (Harris & Weetman, 1982). This was done, for example, where it was felt that extra explanations would help people to better understand the risks. It was also given where people were thought to have great anxiety, or where blame seemed to be attributed to a particular member of the family.

Counselling was also undertaken, where necessary, to help parents overcome the problems of bereavement associated with having passed on a damaging gene to their child: the depression, the feelings of guilt and hostility. Follow-up visits were also made for counselling women who have an abortion following amniocentesis. This aspect of the service helps prevent the occurrence of later chronic emotional problems, which could affect the family.

Increased public understanding

Parents can feel shunned by society. Occasionally there may be a chance for health visitors who give talks to women's groups and others to help increase public awareness. They may be able to help engender the wider concept of handicap which enables greater acceptance and equal chance for children with these special needs. In this way, potential problems which many parents suffer over the social stigma attached to having a handicapped child in the family, could to some extent be avoided. The attainment of good public understanding and a caring attitude is a huge task and health visitors may be able to play some small part in it.

Anticipatory guidance: in general . . . .

The health needs of handicapped children are the same as those of other children, except for the special requirements associated with their impairment. The families, therefore, may wish to discuss various aspects of, for example, nutrition, hygiene, safety, immunisation, dental care and illness recognition in the same way as families with normal children described in earlier chapters.

Stimulation and play with the baby or young child is one of the subjects that may be discussed between parents and their health visitor. This is classified in this chapter as part of a supportive programme aiming at containment and rehabilitation (see p. 181). However, attention has been drawn here to a special consideration within these stimulation programmes.

. . . . and on the attachment process

Studying Down's syndrome children with their mothers, Berger and Cunningham (1983) felt that care has to be taken to prevent a problem occurring over the attachment and bonding between baby and mother. This is not so easy for babies with a difficulty that involves sensory impairment, such as movement disability, mental handicap or blindness. These can present something of an obstacle to the socially important and enjoyable two-way interactions in which parent and baby smile, vocalise, touch and gaze at each other (see Ch. 4, p. 63). Furthermore, misinterpretations and interactive failures may lead to negative feelings and avoidance, on both sides, of further attempts towards emotional involvement.

Although slow to begin, Down's babies generally smile and maintain eye contact by about three months. In their small study, Berger and Cunningham found that after that age mothers of Down's babies played with and talked to their babies more often. However, they did not tend to leave time for their babies to respond, thereby reducing the potential for social interaction. In comparison, mothers with normal babies conducted more two-sided communications.

After experimenting with various interactive

approaches, it was found that parents imitating their baby's behaviour most increased the baby's responsiveness and improved parent–baby interaction. Berger and Cunningham concluded that it should be explained to parents that:

- although mostly a few weeks delayed, smiling, eye contact and cooing invariably appear
- Down's babies need more time to cope with and to respond to stimulation
- their baby's gaze and eye contact show readiness to interact
- imitating their baby is one possible way of improving their social interaction with their baby.

In this way it is hoped that parents' increased awareness can help prevent the occurrence of problems with their emotional relationship with their baby on which so much depends.

In this section, examples have been given of health visiting work aimed at preventing the occurrence of handicap and of later problems. A wide range of 'normal' health visiting is relevant. It may also be possible to help public understanding of the 'wider concept of handicap'. In helping parents cope with the special needs, perhaps for genetic counselling or regarding bonding and attachment, another Warnock concept is employed by working in 'partnership with parents' to enable the best possible results and prevent the occurrence of later problems.

ON THE LOOK-OUT

The second and third of the Warnock ideas mentioned at the beginning of this chapter feature very strongly in secondary prevention: working in 'partnership with parents' in order to try to achieve 'early discovery and early education' for any incipient potentially handicapping problem. Screening and surveillance procedures and modes of discovery, keeping in touch with the District Child Development Team and good clear re-

cords and reports, are all part of this aspect of the work.

DISCOVERY

Only a very small number of handicaps are discovered at birth. For example, only 7 of the 82 handicapped children selected for the Child Study Sample of four-year olds by Chazan et al (1980) were discovered then. These were cases of Down's syndrome and spina bifida. A further 3 children with handicaps were discovered in the following few weeks. In some cases an episode such as an epileptic fit, meningitis or heart failure dramatically heralded the problem.

In most cases, however, a child's handicap reveals itself more slowly. Often the disability is apparent a long time before it becomes a handicap. Chazan et al said parents or professionals notice some aspect of functioning or behaviour which is unusual or absent. When, over time, it does not resolve itself, they become concerned about the implications. Often some triggering event crystallises the parents' or the professional's apprehensions and they decide to seek further advice and assessment. Chazan et al (1980, p. 40) gave an example of a mother who expects her child to say a word by 15 months. As the months go by and no word is spoken she becomes increasingly uneasy until a precipitating factor, such as a neighbour's comment on the child's speechlessness, causes her anxiety level to reach such a peak that she turns to some professional for advice.

Centile charts perform a very useful role in providing the necessary precipitating factor. They are drawn with demarcation lines which show quite clearly at what point a referral for further assessment should be made. Screening and surveillance of babies and young children were looked at in Chapters 5 and 6. We have looked at the importance of following up at home families who find it difficult or prefer not to attend screening clinics in order to discover problems as early as possible. Again centile charts are highly desirable because one can tell at a glance to what extent they have been completed. An additional consideration, once a handicap has been discovered, is the possibility, in some cases the probability, for example of deafness in Down's syndrome, of multiple handicap. The presence of further defects has always to be borne in mind.

Quite a range of handicap, including a high proportion of severely handicapped or disturbed children, was included in the Chazan et al (1980, p. 8) study sample. They investigated who discovered the handicap. 35 of the 82 in this sample had been discovered by professionals and 29 by parents who had then sought advice. In 2 instances, the mothers had been unable to persuade professionals of their children's problem, being dismissed as 'over-fussy' or 'over-anxious'. This highlights yet again the need to listen carefully to parents' views and anxieties. Quite a proportion of the mothers in this study were not fully aware of their child's problem. Many of these were from deprived and difficult circumstances. The 'partnership with parents' does not seem to have been put fully into effect.

Another important study of the discovery of special needs children is that undertaken in Dundee by Drillien and Drummond (1983; Bax & Whitmore, 1989). It highlighted similar patterns to those in the study above.

An inverse proportion of facilities

A factor well known in health visiting was also highlighted (Chazan et al, 1980, pp. 25–26). The health visitors tended to have around the same sized caseload per head of population. However, some had as many as three times more children with problems than their colleagues working in another district. Added to this, the districts in which there were more problems had fewer facilities available, such as nurseries and playgroups. The researchers pointed out that this meant the health visitors were less able to share the care of these children with other workers and, inevitably, these families were receiving a lower standard of care.

It seems that in some cases, post-war housing policies had led to a very large number of children with problems being concentrated in a comparatively small area. This situation is reminiscent of Sue Phillips' (1986) problem. She was permitted, indeed encouraged, to spend time and effort acting as a 'catalyst', helping to create a much needed family centre which included day care and play facilities. This response to community need was successful, both in itself and from a health visiting point of view. Sue Phillips remarked, however, that in a health authority in which a daily quota of visits must be completed, there would not have been time for this sort of work. The community's needs would remain unmet.

ASSESSMENT OF FUNCTIONING

This screening and surveillance aspect of health visiting is much more than just discovering potential problems and handing them on for assessment, diagnosis and treatment. Discovery of handicap has significant implications for the family and the child. The question arises as to how to attain the best possible functioning for the child, how the handicap affects functioning and, from that, what special needs the family and child may have. Chazan et al's Screening Schedule Two, outlined

Table 9.2 Scheme for measuring functioning

Behaviour	Aspect
Sensory-motor	Locomotion
	Use of hands
	Vision
	Hearing
	Hand/eye coordination
Self-help	Feeding
	Toileting
	Dressing
	Competence around the house
Language	Expressive language
	Speech articulation
	Receptive language
	Listening to stories
Modes of activity	Level of activity
	Restlessness
	Constructiveness/destructiveness
Social, emotional and behavioural adjustment	Cooperation with adults
	Dependence
	Aggression
	Withdrawal
	Reactions to stress of deviant behaviour

From Chazan et al (1980, Appendix A)

in Table 9.2, can be a useful tool in thinking, with the parents, about the overall situation they currently face. The Schedule looks at five main behavioural areas, each aspect of which carries ratings on a five point scale ranging from normal functioning to severe handicap.

This sort of assessment, combined with problem oriented and detailed planning similar to that demonstrated by Barber and Kratz (1980), could provide a very useful basis from which to set the problems and planning in perspective. Barber and Kratz showed in a case study how the situation facing a family with a severely handicapped baby could be set out in the SOAP format. Immediate problems concerning the management and development of the baby, physical, emotional and social concerns regarding the mother, emotional problems for the father and problems the parents shared, were listed. Incipient environmental problems associated with long-term care, the baby's death and subsequent offspring, were covered separately. The functioning of the family and the child is inevitably a dynamic and changing process and therefore needs frequent review.

District child development team

The need for multiprofessional involvement and regular review was emphasised in the Court Report (1976). It recommended the setting up of more District Handicap Teams. Dr Christie (1986) has outlined the work of District child development teams, which in some areas provide the clinical and operational functions recommended for the District Handicap Team. These were:

- investigation and assessment
- to arrange for coordinated treatment
- to provide professional advice for parents and professionals involved in the care of the family
- a source of information on handicap and services available
- a training role.

Catriona Rouf (1983) argued that parents should be active participants of the care group, that they be told what is wrong with their baby and be involved in planning the care. She feels professional secrecy places an extra burden on the parents, leaving them feeling that they are without emotional or practical support.

Records and reports

Health visitors who do not attend the child development centre sessions may well need to write reports for the team. Sharing the information in the report or planning the contents of it with the parents, can make a contribution towards their involvement and their understanding of their baby. Parents now have a right to have a copy of any advice, information and evidence used in the Education Authority's Statement of Special Educational Needs (Health Visitors' Association, 1985). Health visitors' records, including those of assessment and referral, are likely, therefore, to be available to the parents as of right.

Inform education authorities

The implications of the Education Act, 1981, concerning the rights of parents over information about the special educational needs of their child, their rights to assessment when their child is under two years and the Health Authority's statutory obligation to inform the Education Authority when the child is over two, were described by Dr Macfarlane (1985). He explained the parents' rights to participate fully at all stages of the subsequent assessment procedure and about their right to appeal if they do not agree with the final statement by the Education Authority. We return to this issue on page 179.

In this section we have taken a wide look at aspects of screening and surveillance in the health visiting care of families with a young handicapped baby or child.

PRACTICAL AND EMOTIONAL SUPPORT

The Warnock concept of 'parents as partners' has been highlighted in the earlier two sections: it is just as important with regard to helping parents attain the best possible life for their child with these special needs and for the family as a whole, despite the handicap. The parents need to have someone to whom they can turn, a 'Named Person', to help them find and sort out information about available services and agencies which will enable containment and rehabilitation of the problems they face. They need that person, too, to act in liaison with these agencies, and also to care and give support with bereavement counselling, morale boosting and optimism in order to overcome emotional problems.

EMOTIONAL SUPPORT
Knowing how it feels

It is impossible for professional workers who have not, themselves, had a handicapped child to truly understand what it feels like. Some idea of the emotions involved can, however, be gleaned from books written by people who do know. There are, for example, two books about having given birth to a Down's syndrome baby. One tells of parents who decided they did not wish to take their baby home (Milne, 1982). The other described the circumstances and the parents' feelings surrounding the nine months their baby lived. The good times as well as the grief and the shock were described (Boston, 1981).

Personal experience provided a very sound basis from which Helen Featherstone (1980) was able to write about the anger, fear, loneliness, guilt and self-doubt which people can feel. She described too how these emotions and the burdens of physically coping can impose strains on the marriage. The emotions associated with visiting a severely handicapped son in hospital and the importance of the staff's attitude and approach were outlined in a short article by J E Dean (1982).

The bereavement process
Informing the parents

The experience of being told about their child's impairment is one which lasts in the parents'

memory. It has been recommended that they should be told:

- the simple facts
- as soon as possible
- together
- in a quiet room
- by the consultant
- with a specialist health visitor in attendance.

The health visitor is then able to provide continuity, enabling further explanations and questions to be answered as necessary and providing the link with community services (Gath, 1985). Melvyn Hall (1987) offers further advice.

Know thyself

We have already looked in Chapter 7 at some aspects of bereavement counselling including the feelings of inadequacy that people can have when trying to help those who are grieving and the need for personal adjustment on attitudes towards death. Ann Fillmore (1981) has described how some professionals find it difficult to come to terms with their own grief and, consequently, are unable to advise their patients appropriately. Being inadequately aware of their own, and not facing up to their patients' natural reactions of sorrow, guilt, anger and need for acceptance of their own mortality, can lead them into using evasive tactics. This might result in, for example, a doctor refusing to allow parents to be informed about the terminality of their child's condition. This, in turn, can lead to emotional difficulties in the family which the health visitor will have to find some ingenious way of sorting out.

Giving support

Ann Gath (1985) and Yvonne Heavyside (1985) have discussed the stages of grief with regard to families with a handicapped baby. Yvonne Heavyside quoted a model of the various phases of the bereavement process, which maps out the way these phases manifest themselves and the way that the parents need, and can be given, help as each stage is reached. She also pointed out that it is important for nurses to:

- touch and handle the baby
- say something nice about the baby
- boost parents' morale regarding their ability to handle their baby
- respect parents' wishes if they do not wish to discuss their feelings
- answer questions simply
- admit it if they do not know any answer and find out who does
- encourage hopefulness and optimism
- encourage assertiveness in the parents.

Most parents are likely to have to insist on their rights at some point on behalf of their child. The way that parents are able to cope, as with other critical life experiences such as the birth of a first child or adjusting to unemployment, is influenced by their emotional background and personality. Some people are more vulnerable than others. What has been shown, however, is that the optimism associated with early intervention programmes in which parents are involved, working with a trained home visitor to stimulate their baby, is emotionally beneficial. These programmes have a morale boosting effect (Gath, 1985) and can do much to alleviate depression, common amongst these mothers (Burden, 1980).

Studies of marriage breakdown related to having a handicapped child seem to indicate that it may be the early emotional trauma rather than the 'wear and tear' of looking after a difficult child that causes the marital tensions and later breakdown (Gath, 1985). It is also possible that parents of Down's syndrome babies fare better, on average, than parents of other sorts of severely educationally subnormal children (Gath, 1985) and tend to make a good emotional adjustment (Murdoch & Ogston, 1984). The research is inconclusive at the moment, but is providing some indicators.

Morale boosting and reassurance using video

In North Devon, five videos were produced for parents of handicapped children at the various stages of their child's development and their emotional adjustment (Walker, 1984). The videos are concerned with:

- reassuring parents that help is at hand
- the child's right to lead as normal a life as possible
- the effects of stress on marriage and the siblings
- special needs in the child's development and education
- what will happen when the parents are too old to cope.

Support literature is left with the parents which reinforces the reassuring information in the video. The videos had first to be tested and then were to be made available to other health authorities at a nominal cost. The problems raised in these programmes are all touching on areas about which parents may have many questions and which they may wish to discuss with their health visitor. Having someone who is prepared to listen and let them think through their worries and feelings can help dispel anxieties, help them work through the grieving process and prevent pathological consequences.

Emotional support cannot really be separated from practical support which, in itself, offers optimism through involvement, explanations and concrete assistance. For the parents to feel cared for, any help offered needs to be given in response to what the parents themselves see as important.

PRACTICAL INFORMATION AND ASSISTANCE

Finding out

Parents become the experts on their handicapped child, but not without help. If the health visitor does not have a good knowledge of the condition and of the services and aids that pertain to the particular family needs encountered, then it is important to take steps to find out about them. The proportion of handicaps within any given caseload is very small. In addition to this, even within a given diagnosis, the nature of each individual child's circumstances can be very different. Generalist health visitors, therefore, cannot be expected to be fully informed on any particular handicapping condition that they might meet, nor, of course, the many variations within it.

The need then, is to find people and agencies who can give guidance. Perhaps the first people to turn to should be the:

- specialist health visitor, if there is one
- consultant paediatrician or other specialist in charge of the case, for up-to-date and accurate information
- medical librarian, for appropriate literature
- health visiting nurse manager, for moral support!

Agencies that may be able to give some help are organisations such as the National Children's Bureau, the Voluntary Council for Handicapped Children and library services such as 'Help for Health' (see Ch. 2, p. 20). Robert Gann (1986) gives some good leads in his book about resources available for self-care. He has a section which gives information about the wide range of health care directories and journals which publish information on the statutory and voluntary services available. He provides a brief synopsis of the contents of each directory and source mentioned.

There are another two books that show families with special needs and their health visitors how to find help. One is the Mental Health Foundation's wide-ranging directory of around 10 000 self-help and community support agencies throughout the British Isles (Webb, 1985). These organisations are classified and listed according to the sort of problems that people may have. By using the key coding at the foot of each page a great deal of information can be learned about local groups and agencies. The other book is the Disability Rights Handbook (The Disability Alliance, 1991), which is revised every year to produce up-to-date, comprehensive guidance on the rights, benefits and services available to disabled people. The further reading list at the end of this chapter contains more recent examples of useful directories.

It is worth searching round, too, for books writ-

ten for parental guidance. There are, for example, the constructive and positively written books that help parents of Down's syndrome children. There is one that helps parents have a better understanding of the implications of their child's condition for themselves and their child (Cunningham, 1982), and others that help them give their child a helping hand (Cunningham & Sloper, 1978; Brinkworth & Collins, 1973).

There are also books available for parents who have children with other sorts of handicap. For example, there are two based on a behavioural approach: one group oriented, concentrating on communication with the child (Newson & Hipgrave, 1982), and the other providing more of a step-by-step guide to everyday problems (Carr, 1980).

In Griffiths and Russell's (1985) book, there are explanations of broad classifications of problems such as

- disorders of motor development
- visual handicap
- communication disorders
- special learning difficulties
- mental handicap
- multiple handicap

as well as explanations of assessment and 'parents as partners', which parents might find informative.

Taking another perspective, Diana Millard's (1984) book gives brief explanations of conditions such as

- cleft palate
- dislocation of the hips
- talipes
- cerebral palsy
- limb deficiency
- muscular dystrophy
- epilepsy
- diabetes
- cystic fibrosis

and describes practical ideas for coping with the everyday life of a handicapped child. In this book, recommended reading lists are provided for the child, for the parents and for the professional helper. Most of the books for parents have lists of useful addresses, providing, too, of course, useful guidance for professionals as well as the parents.

One book written for professionals working with developmentally handicapped children makes an excellent reference book for health visitors. Zelle and Coyner (1983) have provided a wealth of information on assessment and intervention for these children's first two years of life. Dipping into the appropriate sections may enable a better background understanding of the philosophy and the aims and purpose of the work.

Rights to information

Parents now have a statutory right to know about voluntary organisations that are able to give them advice and assistance (Macfarlane, 1985). The Named Person will need to make sure this information is given. A widely available introductory booklet is the Voluntary Council for Handicapped Children's (Russell, 1976). This lists some of the organisations that can help, and gives a brief overview of services available. Many Community Health Councils now produce a booklet which describes local facilities and organisations such as the one produced by Southampton and South West Hampshire Community Health Council (1979). Health visitors may also find it useful to have available the latest DSS pamphlets that explain the rights to attendance allowances from the age of 2 (Henwood, 1990) and mobility allowances on reaching the age of 5 years (Lakhani, 1990a; 1990b).

Rights regarding assessment and education under the 1981 Education Act are explained in booklets written for the Advisory Centre for Education (Newell, 1983; Newell & Potts, 1984). They provide parents with a guide to various aspects of the Act, give tips, for example, on how to request assessment and appeal against decisions, suggest how letters might be written and, generally, help parents to be assertive and attain the services that they feel are most appropriate for their child. The equally important teamwork aspects of successfully getting a handicapped child into mainstream schooling have been described by Norma Pollard (1990).

Informal support

Groups

One in every three self-help groups is started with close cooperation with professionals (Robinson, 1978). Health visitors can quite often assume a catalytic role. Also, there is a need for some background support: this is hardly surprising as there are several inherent difficulties. Judy Wilson (1982) pointed out that they are generally organised and run by people who have problems in common with the members. This can present problems to the group because a leader with obligations to care for an ill child may, for example, suddenly have to cancel an evening with the group.

In many cases, members have not been 'joiners' before and may suffer, somewhat, from lack of experience in running a group. Added to this, the group is used as a stepping stone back to normal life, so that people are liable to leave when their situation has improved rather than stay on as lifelong members. Judy Wilson's research led her to feel that support for groups being set up is very important.

Research in general shows that around half of the parents with disabled children belong to a group. Cooke & Lawton (1984), however, found that considerably fewer than half of the 400 families with 10-year-old handicapped children they studied belonged to such a group. They pointed out that this finding matches a tendency found in another study of decline in membership after the child reaches six years of age. Parents who were members seem to have found them helpful. This was, however, mostly for the emotional support and practical advice they could give. Very few had received financial or practical help.

Friends and family

It is interesting to note that informal support from friends, neighbours and family was found *not* to help on a day-to-day basis, but might help at a time of crisis. Babysitting was a problem for parents with severely handicapped children. It seems relatives and friends can be 'non-plussed' by the complexity of the problems involved, making parents unwilling to leave them. In effect, the informal support was found to be no greater for the families with severely than for those with mildly disabled children.

Cooke and Lawton found, too, that it was the mothers who bore the main burden of responsibility. Fathers were found to give help, where it was given, with child care and minding rather than with housework. There was a tendency for them to help even less where the child was severely handicapped. Baldwin and Glendinning (1983) also found women bore the brunt. The care of the handicapped children lessened their chances of returning to work which would have provided social and psychological benefits away from 'the daily grind'. Also these mothers were less able to subsidise the family income and help compensate for the increased costs associated with the care of a severely handicapped child.

Fellow feeling

Some people find that it is very reassuring to meet another family with a child with special needs similar to theirs. It can lessen the feeling of isolation and make it possible to find someone who is able to listen with empathy, without necessarily having to join and attend a group.

Health visitors are sometimes able to put people with unusual and obscure complaints in touch with each other through an information column in the Health Visitor journal. Dunning et al (1986) are concerned that the variation in disorders and in the way they affect people, might lead to a mismatch between people and cause distress. They suggest that health visitors contact their Regional Genetic Counselling Centre to enquire about families with similar problems who would be willing to be put in touch with their family. Whether or not people do, in fact, need to be protected from meeting a variation of their problem, the genetic counselling service does provide a useful link.

Providing services and advice

The Named Person, or the person acting as such, should ensure that parents are offered all services to which they are entitled and any relevant advice.

The aim is to help them increase the functioning of their child and the family as a whole to the best possible extent, in order to live as normal a life for them all as can be attained. This means, for example, helping parents find out about mobility aids and entitlements (Tarling, 1985; Nursing, 1985; Stevens, 1985), offering them respite care — before a crisis occurs, and, perhaps, working out with them their child's current functional needs so that appropriate services and advice can be offered. Sadly, many families have been found to have been inadequately advised and provided for (Ayer, 1984; Chazan et al, 1980, p. 101; Disabled Living Foundation, 1979, pp. 43–55). Bathing, dressing, mobility and feeding are but a few of the problems that may be encountered and require habilitation.

Assignment of responsibility

A study by Gillian Parker (1984a) of the provision of incontinence services for handicapped children showed that the adequacy of the provision of services varied with the organisational structure of the community health services. In the districts in which the health visitor, or the health visitor and subsequently the school nurse, had sole responsibility for the service, the service was properly provided. Where responsibility was divided between various people, it was much poorer.

Another factor was whether the service was offered spontaneously by the nurse or health visitor, as people hesitate to ask. Lack of knowledge of the service was the main reason for non-take up of the service. Gillian Parker (1984b) also found that advice tended to be inadequate on what steps parents could take towards improved continence for their child. Many did not realise, until their child started school, that an improvement could have been possible before. She thought that the Portage type of programmes would alert health visitors to just what could be achieved.

Pre-school training

Health visitors seem to enjoy being involved in Portage and other pre-school training programmes aimed at improving the child's abilities (Mansell,

1981; Cunningham et al, 1982; Cameron, 1982). Also, the programmes seem to engender positive feelings in the mothers taking part (Sloper et al, 1983). Sloper et al were a little apprehensive lest the mothers become dependent upon the visiting therapist and afraid to do what they feel is intuitively right. Another fact that emerged was that in some cases parents seemed to feel that the more effort they put into the programme, the more their child would improve. The fallacy of this was mentioned earlier in the chapter, in discussion about the need to aim for good interactional processes (see pp. 172–173). Sloper et al felt that perhaps more emphasis should have been put on explaining the interaction of maturational, environmental and inherent factors on the potential for development, and on teaching the underlying philosophy. This approach would aim at helping the parents understand, not only what to do, but more importantly why they are doing it. An overview of the sort of work undertaken in Portage schemes and the way it is planned, has been provided by Cameron et al (1984) whilst replying to what they felt were 14 criticisms of the system.

LIAISON

There may be many people involved in the care of a family with a handicapped child, particularly in the first year or so. There may be, for example, many visits to clinics, hospital and various agencies. The travelling can be costly and the experiences mentally exhausting. There is a great deal to be gained from liaison between the various people involved in this care, in order to successfully establish a coordinated service aimed at minimising, as far as possible, the confusion and trauma for parents.

It is best if the health visitor meets and knows, by name, the main people involved with the family. It might be possible to get to know several, for example, at a meeting of the District child development team. There may be, for example, a community physiotherapist (Sutcliffe, 1980), a social worker or community mental handicap nurse (Simon, 1981; Williams, 1980) alongside whom the health visitor might be working. Perhaps the most important professional to contact, preferably in the

first instance in person, is the local specialist most involved with the family. This cooperation can

Box 9.2 Generalist or specialist? Arguments in favour of both

	Generalist health visitor	Specialist health visitor
EARLY DAYS	Useful in the early days, when there is non-acceptance of handicap, by parents. HV visits everyone, therefore acceptable: not stigmatising	Prolonged and repeated visits in initial period: parents need intensive help then, to prevent later problems.
	Can monitor children not yet officially diagnosed, only suspected	Assuming service adequately funded, more free to provide service
	Involved very soon after birth, where diagnosis immediate: probably met antenatally; already known where condition discovered later	Particularly useful in inner city work, where crises more common and normal HV overstretched
LIAISON	Better liaison with primary health care team, for example over parental need for counselling, information and support	May be better able to coordinate, cooperate with and alert other services on a broader front, for example physiotherapy, psychotherapy, special aids, adaptations and voluntary organisations
	In contact with 'normal' families living locally, who may offer moral support and invite to 'normal' mothers and baby group, etc	May be able to work more closely with District Child Development Centre Team
EXPERTISE	Avoids 'expertosis' as HV and parent learn together — parent in control, with HV helping to find out sources of information and appropriate help	Learns from previous experience and special training: can build up special skills and knowledge
	Can maintain contact with other professionals involved — an advantage if HV able to attend relevant Child Development Centre sessions, with parents there, decision-making	Can share knowledge with and train other HVs

Especially useful where problems complex |

Box 9.3 A family with a handicapped baby: health needs of parents

Environmental	Mental/emotional	Social aspects
Adequate housing e.g. for safety and mobility	**Emotional** *support* Parents *told together* about handicap and follow-up at home (by GP?) and given chance to hear again what forgotten from initial interview	*Overcome potential isolation:* Meet other person(s) with similar problem e.g. local self-help group or National organisations or through special introduction
Financial support: (extra costs of handicapped child and one parent less able to work)		
Knowledge of *benefits and entitlements* — when attendance and mobility allowances become due and extra sources such as Rowntree Family Fund	Feel people prepared to *listen, and care;* encouragement to express anger, grief, resentment, guilt (these feelings likely to result in marital tensions)	*Time as normal family:* Home help service Babysitting (volunteer) Ability to have normal holidays — respite care
Encouragement to claim these entitlements	*Regular visits:* professional awareness of crisis periods e.g. when anticipated attainments are not achieved	*Overcome feeling of social stigma* Acceptance by relatives and friends
Knowledge of aids and equipment e.g. clothing, bedding, laundry, fares, adaptations	*Chance to talk* about worries about future	*Develop own interests* Especially the mother, perhaps opportunity to return to work
Physical		Encouragement to be *forceful* In order to gain entitlements and supportive services
Overcome tiredness — extra time and effort taken by care of baby, hospital appointments, etc. — home help?	**Knowledge** of condition and equipment, also training available, medical needs, including likelihood of surgery, etc.	
Knowledge about hoists and mobility and other aids, to help with *physical management*	Help with sorting out confusion of advice	
Genetic counselling re further children, if relevant	*Preparatory knowledge* about dressing, feeding, sleeping, toilet training etc.	
	Confidence to follow own initiative on care of baby/child	

provide two-way benefits: on one side, up-to-date and accurate information about diagnosis and treatment; and on the other, feedback for the specialist (assuming the family's permission is given) on how the family members are coping and what problems they are meeting.

Specialist or generalist?

Having researched the subject, the Disabled Living Foundation (1979, p. 63) found it could not prove the case either for or against specialist health visitors. However, it felt that overloaded generalist health visitors coping with a caseload of, perhaps, 7000 people would not have time to give adequate attention to families with a severely handicapped child. If they did give that time, then other work would have to be skimped.

Some of the arguments in favour, on the one hand of a generalist health visitor and on the other, of a specialist, are shown in Box 9.2. These families with a handicapped child face many problems. Some of them are outlined in a family health needs model in Boxes 9.3 and 9.4. Whoever looks after them, they need time and attention. Melinda Firth (1982) has made suggestions as to how generalist health visitors might be able to give an improved service to these families, for example, through training, information and reduced caseloads. Generally, health visitors with a specialist post tend to favour that approach (Disabled Living Foundation, 1979; Twinn, 1981). Cunning-

Box 9.4 A family with a handicapped baby or child: some health needs of the children

Physical	Mental/emotional	Social aspects

Handicapped baby/child
Play and fun:
 	
   Programme of exercises and/or activities appropriate to developmental attainments — stimulating but not overwhelming
 	
   Access to toys e.g. from Toy Library
 	
Regular developmental assessment and hearing, vision, communication, and measurements of head, length/height, and weight
 	
Special care according to need: e.g. Down's — skin, chest, extra vitamin supplement
 	
Safety relevant to developmental attainment level
	Loving home: to be accepted and without overprotection
	
	Attachment — allowed enough time to respond and take part in two-way interaction: time to respond to stimuli
	
	Overcome effects of separation e.g. hospitalisation and respite care
	
	   Play and fun and sleep, general behaviour, etc. — approach as appropriate
	
	Siblings
	Attention of parents (and professionals)
	
	   Discussion with parents regarding family tensions (due to anger, frustration and grief associated with adjustment to handicap)
		Normal absences from parents
		   Acceptable babysitter
		   Play and fun and satisfactory relationship with siblings, other children, grandparents, other relatives
		
		   Arrangements to be made for later access to playground or nursery class, if required
		
		Notification to Education Authority
		
		Approach: 'potential ability' not disability; special needs not 'handicap'
		
		Access to normal family life with parents — outings, holidays
		
		   Respite from extra household duties (especially caring older sister)
		
		May feel social stigma re handicap:
		   needs acceptance by friends and ability to bring them home

ham et al (1982) said that where a highly motivated generalist health visitor continued to call when a specialist health visitor was visiting to help with training, this combination gave the most satisfactory service.

Whichever way, be it specialist, generalist or both, if the area carries a high level of problems and a low level of staffing, then the service is going to be spread too thinly to be effective. In this situation, health visitors need to keep their managers informed and up to date, not only on what they are able to achieve, but also on what they cannot.

This chapter has considered the work of the health visitor regarding families who have a handicapped child. Using the prevention model as a framework, we looked firstly at health education aimed at preventing the occurrence of handicap and, when it has occurred, at preventing the occurrence of later problems. Secondly, there was screening and surveillance aimed at early diagnosis and care to prevent the development of incipient problems. The third aspect was practical and emo-

tional help aimed at rehabilitation and containment of the problems in the case of known disability or difficulty. The relevance of some of the concepts of the Warnock Report were included. Two examples follow, the first uses the family health needs framework from Boxes 9.3 and 9.4 and the second, the prevention format.

EXAMPLES OF WORK WITH FAMILIES WITH HANDICAPPED CHILDREN

The first example uses the family health needs framework (see Box 9.5) in outlining a health visitor's thinking on the way to visit a family recently informed of their child's diagnosis. The second, outlined using the 'prevention' approach (see Box 9.6), is about some aspects of work with a family with a Down's syndrome child.

EXAMPLE ONE: THE FIRTH FAMILY

On her way to visit the Firth family, Heather Vaughan (HV) thought about some of the special needs that the family now had. Their 4-year-old daughter, Anne, who now attended playgroup, was in full health. However, their 2-year-old son, Paul, had just been confirmed as a case of early cystic fibrosis.

Fortunately, the District used centile charts for weight, height and head measurements, and so the gradual move towards the 3rd centile (in spite of a good appetite) was easy to monitor. Frequent pungent smelling stools and then some chest infections caused HV to refer the matter to the GP before the measurements dropped below the 3rd centile. It would be necessary to continue the monitoring of Paul's growth. This was now likely to be mainly undertaken during, what would probably be, frequent visits to the hospital.

Paul would now be on a special fat-restricted, high calorie and protein diet with enzyme and vitamin supplements, physiotherapy and, possibly, antibiotics. His parents had a great deal of learning and work ahead of them. The health visitor intended to tell Mrs Firth about the Cystic Fibrosis Research Trust if she did not already know of it. The secretary of the local branch had been very helpful when HV had phoned. She had described the sort of information and emotional support the Trust was able to give. Ms Vaughan intended to tell the Firths what had been said and how they could contact the Trust if they should wish to.

In due course, HV would check that the Firths were aware of the benefits and allowances to which they might be entitled, and she would encourage them to take them up. However, just at the moment it was the need to listen, should Mrs Firth wish to talk about how she felt, that was likely to take greatest priority at the visit. At the most recent meeting of the primary health care team, talking about emotional adjustment Dr Green had said that the parents had been told the diagnosis by the consultant. Dr Green had known the date of the appointment and had visited the mother at home the next day in order to answer her queries and to show his concern.

The health visitor had a copy of 'Help starts here' in her pocket, but she would gauge the extent to which Mrs Firth was accepting the handicap before she produced it. It might be better to give it at the following visit. She knew

Box 9.5 Example one; the Firth family

Environmental	Mental/emotional	Social aspects
Parents Financial support: knowledge of benefits and entitlements	Emotional support: parents told: follow up by Dr Green and regular visits by HV	Overcome potential isolation: meet other people with similar problem, perhaps through Cystic Fibrosis Research Trust
Encouragement to claim the entitlements (high costs + mother less able to work)	Encouragement to express anger, grief, resentment and guilt (feelings likely to result in marital tensions) and to talk about worries about future	Overcome feeling of social stigma re coughing and smelly stools
Physical		Acceptance by relatives and friends: support group may help with ideas
Genetic counselling re further children, if relevant, and for emotional support		
Children: Paul Continued assessment, especially of measurements of height and weight, to monitor rate of disease	Loving home: to be accepted and as others, without overprotection	Arrangements for nursery, if required
Special care re physiotherapy, diet and supplements, ?chemotherapy	Overcome effects of separation through hospitalisation	Approach: 'potential ability', not disability
		Notification to Education Authority
	Anne Attention of parents, to minimise jealousy over extra attention to brother	Access to normal family life with parents — outings and holidays
		Meet other families with CF through Cystic Fibrosis Research Trust

Dr Green had not mentioned genetic counselling. That service would probably be able to provide good emotional support. This was another point HV would mention either at this meeting or the next one, perhaps the following week.

There would be the matter of notifying the Education Authority and, perhaps, arranging for a special nursery place, depending on the extent of any special needs. In order to be helpful to the mother, it would be important for HV to know just how much Paul's handicap was likely to affect his functioning and how, over time, he was, in fact, progressing. She had already made an appointment to see the consultant and expected to be in touch by telephone from time to time.

The health visitor could not help hoping that the couple would contact the Trust. She felt it was likely to be the best source of guidance, for example over jealousy by Anne and other problems associated with the great amount of attention that Paul would be getting. From the telephone conversation HV thought, too, that their approach would be optimistic and positive. She arrived on the doorstep a little apprehensive, partly in case some of the anger inevitably associated with bereavement processes would be directed at herself, and partly in case she misread some of Mrs Firth's feelings and wishes at this very difficult time.

EXAMPLE TWO: THE EDWARDS FAMILY

Honor Vincent (HV) had enjoyed seeing Amanda Edwards playing amongst the children at the playgroup she had just been visiting. It seemed she was presenting the staff with no particular problems. A Down's syndrome child, she was progressing well and clearly benefited from the stimulus provided by the other children.

After the early stages of grief over the handicap her mother had gone 'all out' for acceptance by the community. Mrs Edwards had been very keen to arrange a panel discussion session at the local Women's Institute on handicap and had asked HV and the GP to join her. It had been quite a success. They had talked in depth about the early days, the inevitable bereavement, grief for the loss of the expected normal child, and Hilda Edwards had been embarrassingly glowing about the professional support at that time. The Cunningham books had been found particularly reassuring and encouraging. Mrs Edwards had described how she had tried to encourage her

Box 9.6 Example two: the Edwards family

Aims	Some activities
To prevent occurrence of handicap or later problems	*Health education:* Public: joint discussion at local Women's Institute — Mrs Edwards, HV and GP Parents: anticipatory guidance as for all children, but especially on stimulation and on two-way communication for bonding Information about genetic counselling service; amniocentesis and abortion discussion
To prevent development through early diagnosis and care	*Surveillance, screening and referral:* Monitored for multiple problems; listened to parental fears and acted upon them; assessed especially for vision and hearing — teaching parents how (GP: heart, respiratory and endocrine disease) Assessed developmental progress and functioning Records and reports shared with parent — information for education authority
To prevent deterioration through rehabilitation and containment	*Practical and emotional help:* Support: active listening in bereavement phases, morale boosting, too Practical advice and information, e.g. financial entitlements and nappy service Information about voluntary organisation able to give advice and support: Down's Children's Association — accompanied mother to clinic Help due to special training in Portage scheme Contact with District Child Development team

daughter to do things, but only at her own rate, and to concentrate on two-way communication between them as they played.

The Women's Institute session was rather symbolic, in a way, of the fact that the HV, GP and mother had worked together as a team. For example, explaining about genetic counselling had been shared between HV and the GP. The mother had taken an active part with HV in monitoring for possible defects, in particular, hearing, vision and developmental assessment.

Dr Smith had regularly checked for heart and endocrine disorder and, fortunately, there had been none. Hilda Edwards had been worried about hearing, and the yearly visits to the audiometry clinic had paid off: significant deafness had been discovered at this most recent visit and arrangements were under way for a grommet operation in the near future.

When they had been assessing Amanda's progress, HV had always shown Hilda Edwards the records as she wrote them up. She also showed the mother reports, such as the ones for the Education Department, so that she would be informed on exactly what was being said and could contribute her opinion. There was no doubt that she had become the expert on her own child and that the help from the Down's Children's Association had played a significant part in that. Also, the emotional support from the local branch had been invaluable. A mother with an older Down's syndrome child had accompanied Hilda Edwards to the clinic to see her through the embarrassment she had felt in those early days, and a very good friendship had developed. They now frequently baby-sat for each other.

Amanda had been somewhat slow in becoming continent, so the Edwards had decided to take up the nappy service. However, toilet training was now being so successful they had just cancelled the supplies.

When she had visited the family soon after the birth of the baby, HV had felt remarkably ignorant and useless from a practical point of view, with nothing but a textbook knowledge of Down's syndrome. Fortunately, she had been able to attend a Portage scheme course and it had been fun working with the mother on it. They had both attended the District Handicap Team clinic sessions when Amanda was assessed. Liaison and teamwork had worked very well, both at this level and, of course, with the primary health care team.

Mrs Vincent wondered, as she walked back to her car, whether arrangements would be made, as the Edwards wished, for Amanda to attend their local school. She hoped so. Anyway, they knew how to appeal against any decision they felt unjust.

USEFUL ADDRESS

National Children's Bureau
8 Wakeley Street
London ECIV 7QE
Tel 071 278 9441

REFERENCES

Ayer S 1984 Handicapped children in the community. Nursing Times 80, 37: 66–69

Baldwin S, Glendinning C 1983 Employment, women and their disabled children. In: Finch J, Groves D (eds) A Labour of Love: Women, Work and Caring. Routledge & Kegan Paul, London

Barber J H, Kratz C R 1980 Towards Team Care. Churchill Livingstone, Edinburgh: p 93–99

Bax M, Whitmore K 1989 (letter) Identifying disabilities. Health Visitor 62, 4: 106

Berger J, Cunningham C 1983 Early interactions between infants with Down's syndrome and their parents. Health Visitor 56: 58–60

Boston S 1981 Will, My Son. The life and death of a mongol child. Pluto Press, London

Brinkworth R, Collins J E 1973 Improving babies with Down's syndrome and introducing them to school. National Society for Mentally Handicapped Children, Belfast

Burden R L 1980 Measuring the effects of stress on the mothers of handicapped infants: must depression always follow? Child: care, health and development 6: 111–125

Cameron R J (ed) 1982 Working Together. Portage in the UK. NFER-Nelson, Windsor

Cameron R, Chambers G, Martin S 1984 What is wrong with Portage? Health Visitor 57: 142–144

Carr J 1980 Helping your handicapped child. A step-by-step guide to everyday problems. Penguin, London

Chazan M, Laing A F, Bailey S M, Jones G 1980 Some of our children. The early education of children with special needs. Open Books, London

Christie P N 1986 Management of the handicapped child. Midwife Health Visitor and Community Nurse 22: 67–69

Cooke K, Lawton D 1984 Informal support for the carers of disabled children. Child: care, health and development 10: 67–79

Court Report 1976 Report of the Committee on Child

Health Services, Fit for the future. Cmnd 6684. HMSO, London

Cunningham C 1982 Down's syndrome. An introduction for parents. Souvenir Press, London

Cunningham C C, Aumonier M E, Sloper P 1982 Health visitor support for families with Down's syndrome infants. Child: care, health and development 8: 1–19

Cunningham C, Sloper P 1978 Helping your handicapped baby. Souvenir Press, London

Dean J E 1982 Communication between professionals and parents of handicapped children. Nursing Times 78: 1371

The Disability Alliance 1991 Disability rights handbook, 16th edn. A guide to rights, benefits and services for all people with disabilities and their families. The Disability Alliance, London

Disabled Living Foundation 1979 The specialised health visitor for the handicapped baby, young child and school child. A report. Disabled Living Foundation, London

Drillien C L, Drummond M 1983 Developmental screening and the child with special needs. A population study of 5000 children. Clinics in developmental medicine No 86. Heinemann, London

Dunning J A, Mueller R F, Smithells R W 1986 Information wanted (letter). Health Visitor 59: 29

Featherstone H 1980 A difference in the family. Life with a disabled child. Harper and Row, London

Fillmore A 1981 The dying child and professional withdrawal. Health Visitor 54: 328–330

Firth M 1982 How good is professional support following a diagnosis of mental handicap? Health Visitor 55: 215–220

Gann R 1986 Health information handbook: resources for self care. Gower Press, Aldershot

Gath A 1985 Parental reactions to loss and disappointment: the diagnosis of Down's syndrome. Developmental Medicine & Child Neurology 27: 392–400

Griffiths M, Russell P 1985 Working together with handicapped children. Souvenir Press, London

Hall M 1987 But what do we tell the parents? Health Visitor 60, 4: 110–112

Harris R, Weetman M 1982 Genetic counselling and the work of a medical genetics centre. Health Visitor 55: 343–345

Health Visitors Association 1985 The health visitor's role in child health surveillance. A policy statement. Health Visitors Association, London

Heavyside Y 1985 Handicapped babies and their families. Midwife Health Visitor & Community Nurse 21: 388–392

Henwood J 1990 Attendance allowance. Health Visitor 63, 1: 28

Lakhani B 1990a Mobility allowance. Health Visitor 63, 2: 62

Lakhani B 1990b Mobility allowance in practice. Health Visitor 63, 3: 98

Macfarlane J A 1985 The Education Act 1981. British Medical Journal 290: 1848–1849

Mansell C A 1981 Portage — not just another course. Nursing Times 77: 1807–1808

Millard D M 1984 Daily living with a handicapped child. Croom Helm, London, p 12–15; 39–47; 55–60

Milne P 1982 John David. The child that changed their lives. A novel. Virago Press Ltd, London

Murdoch J C, Ogston S A 1984 Down's syndrome children and parental psychological upset. Journal of the Royal College of General Practitioners 34: 87–90

Newell P 1983 ACE special education handbook — the new law on children with special needs. Advisory Centre for Education, London

Newell P, Potts P 1984 Under-5s with special needs. Pre-school children: the new law and integration. Advisory Centre for Education, London

Newson E, Hipgrave T 1982 Getting through to your handicapped child. A handbook for parents, foster-parents, teachers and anyone caring for handicapped children. Cambridge University Press, Cambridge

Nursing 1985 Civil and government benefits for the disabled. Nursing 2, 33: 966–967

Parker G 1984a Incontinence services for the disabled child. Part 1: the provision of aids and equipment. Health Visitor 57: 44–45

Parker G 1984b Incontinence services for the disabled child. Part 2: the provision of information and advice. Health Visitor 57: 86–88

Phillips S 1986 A centre for change. Nursing Times Community Outlook 82, 7: 15–17

Pollard N 1990 Laura starts school. Nursing Times Community Outlook 86, 28: 24–26

Robinson D 1978 Self-help in relation to health care. Midwife Health Visitor and Community Nurse 14: 265–267

Rouf C 1983 Parents care too. Health and Social Services Journal XCIII: 415

Russell P 1976 Help starts here. For parents of children with special needs. National Children's Bureau for the Voluntary Council for Handicapped Children, London

Simon G B 1981 Local services for mentally handicapped people: the community team, the community unit and the role and function of the community nurse, social worker and some other members of the CMHT. British Institute of Mental Handicap, Kidderminster

Sloper P, Cunningham C C, Arnlijotsdottir M 1983 Parental reactions to early intervention with their Down's syndrome infants. Child: care, health and development 9: 357–376

Southampton and South West Hampshire Community Health Council 1979 Information booklet for parents with mentally handicapped children. Southampton and South West Hampshire Community Health Council, Southampton

Stevens T 1985 Aids centres and the Disabled Living Foundation. Nursing 2, 33: 968–971

Sutcliffe B J 1980 Physiotherapy in the community. Midwife Health Visitor and Community Nurse 16: 166–170

Tarling C 1985 Assessing the mobility needs of the dependent person. Nursing 2, 32: 947–950

Twinn S 1981 The specialist heath visitor for handicapped children: luxury or necessity? Health Visitor 54: 478–479

Walker E 1984 Sharing the video. Health and Social Services Journal XCIV: 350–351

Warnock M 1978 Meeting special educational needs: a brief guide to the report of the Committee of Enquiry into education of handicapped children and young people. HMSO, London

Warnock Report 1978 Report of the Committee of Enquiry into the education of handicapped children and young people. Cmnd 7212. HMSO, London, p 76–78

Webb P 1985 Someone to talk to directory 1985. A directory of self help and community support agencies in the UK and Republic of Ireland. Mental Health Foundation, London

Williams R 1980 A community service for mentally handicapped children. Nursing Times 76: 2011–2012

Wilson J 1982 Stepping stone to normal life. Health and Social Services Journal XCII: 1253

Winter R M 1984 Who needs genetic counselling? Update 28: 1159–1163

Zelle R S, Coyner A B 1983 Developmentally disabled infants and toddlers: assessment and intervention. F A Davis Company, Philadelphia

FURTHER READING

Finding help

Duin N, Jacka F 1987 Health help 87/88. Bedford Square Press/NCVO, London

FitzHerbert L, Bellofatto H (eds) 1987 A guide to grants for individuals in need. The Directory of Social Change, London — This should be read bearing in mind the main points in Ian Kerr's (1987) article below.

Jones I H 1988 Helping hands. A guide for nurses, other professional health workers and carers, on statutory and voluntary services available for people needing further help in the community. Macmillan Education, London

Kerr I 1987 Trusts, myth and magic. New Society Voluntary Action 80, 1273: ii — A note of caution

regarding the difficulties experienced by the providing agencies listed in the directories.

Knight S, Gann R 1988 The self-help guide. A directory of self-help organisations in the United Kingdom. Chapman and Hall Medical, London — Contains advice on obtaining self-help health literature and further information in addition to directory.

Macdonald F 1990 The health directory 1990. Bedford Square Press, London — Around 1000 self-help bodies listed with a brief outline of what each does.

National Council for Voluntary Organisations 1986 The voluntary agencies directory, 1987. Bedford Square Press/NCVO, London

In this chapter we look at some of the special problems encountered by families who have, during the past few decades, come to live in Britain. These problems might include health factors associated with environmental and social difficulties, a language barrier and cultural differences. In order to be able to help effectively, health visitors need to get to know about and to understand these families' particular viewpoint.

10

Recent immigrants and ethnic minority families

KNOWLEDGE AND UNDERSTANDING

First we consider the importance of health visitor knowledge and understanding of the particular customs and beliefs of the families they visit. We then use the family health needs format to look at some problems that may be encountered by families who have immigrated fairly recently and at the problem of sickle cell anaemia. In this model, seen in Box 10.1, matters are categorised into environmental factors such as accommodation and income, physical health and mental factors and, lastly, social factors such as the extended family and self-help groups.

The same but more so

Health visiting families who have come from abroad is, in essence, no different from that described in the rest of this book. The aims of the work and the range of matters discussed are just the same. The difference lies in the increased potential for communication difficulties and for health visitor ignorance of cultural factors. For example, a fundamental aim in health visiting is to tailor the preventive health care to suit the particular individual or family. This is obviously more difficult if the health visitor does not know about the family's cultural background and/or religion, or, for example, what it feels like to be a black person in a predominantly white population. It is never easy to know exactly what is in the mind of

Box 10.1 Family health needs framework showing health related factors described in this chapter

Environmental factors	Physical health	Mental/emotional health	Social aspects of health
Common problems • poor housing in inner city areas • low status, low paid occupation • work long hours, often at night • imported traditional food expensive *Very different* from home environment: • weather • traffic • socialisation patterns • city instead of rural • traditional clothing • food • colour prejudice	*Health education* 1. For feeding and other practices to improve perinatal morbidity and mortality rates 2. Nutrition, vitamins and exposure to sunlight to prevent rickets in children and osteomalacia in women 3. Lead in imported medicaments and cosmetics: danger re surma — updated health visitor tests for lead *Screening and support* re ethnic minority group related disease e.g. sickle cell disease — need screening for family members and counselling, as well as care services	*Knowledge* Language problems — a barrier to use of health and welfare services Health visitor could: Use • phonetic translation • Henley hints • flash cards Learn • Asian language Checklist • suitability of local health services Work with • linkworker (if available) • opinion leaders *Mental health* Potential for misunderstanding in cross-cultural interpretation of behaviour Strains of adjustment e.g. anxiety, guilt and shame on being obliged to break religious laws (e.g. by examination by male Dr)	*Religious practices* Health visitors need to: • understand these in outline • expect variation • respect views Recording religion (and ethnic origin) • sensitive issue • can help health care priority and resource allocation decisions *Support from:* • family • friends • childminding *Self-help groups:* • for support • as pressure group • source of information on needs of ethnic minorities

a client, but it is significantly more difficult where life experiences and language form a barrier.

The potential for stereotyping provides another example. This is always a possible trap, but perhaps, is more likely if the health visitor knows only a limited amount about the relevant religion and customs and makes assumptions about the family's beliefs and behaviour (Hunkins, 1983). These problems of communication and understanding, where they exist, are of course felt by client and worker alike.

The provision of practical care can also be more difficult. For example, it is not easy to help women overcome social isolation where there are few other women in the locality of the same or similar cultural background. The obstacles associated with being able to offer acceptable and relevant health education where the family has relatively uncommon cultural beliefs and little

has been written on the matter, provide another example.

To some extent, cross-cultural problems affect anyone who moves to a new environment, for example, from city to rural life or from 'the North' to 'the South' in Britain. However, the degree of adjustment and the challenges are significantly greater when moving between countries, particularly where the way of life is so different.

Guidance for health visitors

In these past few years, there have been series of articles which have given health workers an outline of the cultural beliefs and customs and some of the specific health problems of the main minority groups now in Britain (Schofield, 1981a, 1981b, 1981c; Henley & Clayton, 1982a, 1982b, 1982c, 1982d, 1982e, 1982f; Mayor, 1984a, 1984b; Black,

1986, 1985a, 1985b, 1985c, 1985d, 1985e, 1985f, 1985g). A number of health visitors have followed up their researches by visiting the country of origin of the people for whom they care (Pearson, 1982a, 1982b, 1982c; Rudge, 1983; Rhodes, 1985a, 1985b).

Organisations such as the Commission for Racial Equality, the King's Fund Centre and the Health Education Council are able to provide reading lists of books, articles, reports and pamphlets. Their addresses will be found at the end of the chapter.

Learning about life-style and religious beliefs is one thing. Getting to know about people's feelings is another. Brent Community Health Council (1981) provided a perspective of black people's relationship with the health service which many health workers might not have considered. Racism, stereotyping, and being used as cheap labour were among the matters described, and the booklet shows clearly how people can feel. Melba Wilson (1983) pointed out that there is not a 'black community' as some people imply, and that black people are as diverse as any other. Being seen as 'a problem' or being given an identity merely as 'immigrant' can be very hurtful. There are now many indigenous black people. They are bringing to society a new dynamic influence and this needs recognition.

Racial awareness courses should be part of the educational programme (Clark, 1985; Stevenson, 1985). These can help health visitors review their own assumptions about 'normal behaviour' and take a more empathetic and understanding approach in the study of other cultures. Health visitor students who are themselves members of minority groups could help with these learning processes (Stevenson, 1985) and if conversant with the language and culture, they might have an important role to play (Inter Departmental Consultative Group, 1984, pp. 8, 15; Clark, 1985). The handbook by Mares et al (1985) explores many of these key issues, as well as being a very useful resource and reference manual.

Health visiting nurse managers need to know to what extent their staff have the knowledge relevant to the people they visit. Twenty health visitors working in a multi-cultural inner-city area were questioned about their knowledge of Asian cultures in a small study by While and Godfrey (1984). In the main, the health visitors demonstrated a significant lack of knowledge and had not had post-registration training in this field. This ties in with June Clark's experience of the scarcity of appropriate courses.

It sounds as if 'do-it-yourself' is the solution until courses become available. Health visitors could ask religious leaders (Karseras & Hopkins, 1987, pp. 14–15) and the leaders and workers from local ethnic minority self-help groups to come and speak to them and, perhaps, lead discussions. There is so much to discover. However, if there is the will to learn about people's beliefs and customs, then a way can be found: and it is important that these customs should be understood in the context of the way they have been adapted, both to suit society as it is encountered and to contend with racism (Henley, 1986).

FAMILY HEALTH NEEDS

ENVIRONMENTAL FACTORS

Many immigrants to Britain find themselves obliged to settle in the very poor parts of cities and towns and to take badly paid jobs — two factors that increase the likelihood of poor health. Previous generations living in these areas also suffered from similar ill-health. For example, in the past there was a tendency for many children in central Glasgow to get rickets, just as there is now in their Asian counterparts (Dunnigan et al, 1985). Elizabeth Watson (1984) found poor housing and environmental factors increasingly significant over time regarding the health of disadvantaged mothers and infants.

In Batley where Hazel Rhodes (1985a, 1985b) worked, she found that unemployment was twice as high amongst the Asian community as amongst the indigenous community. Asian men tended to have the more poorly paid, lower status jobs, but worked very long hours and night shifts to increase their income. Although on similar incomes, 90% of the Asians owned their own homes, whereas less than 45% of the indigenous people did so. Overcrowding was commonplace for the Asian families. Three-quarters of their population had more than one person per room, compared with just over one tenth of the indigenous population, perhaps reflecting the Asians' need to band together and buy to overcome the difficulties of finding rented accommodation. These families are coping remarkably well in very difficult circumstances.

Several families had come from one area of the Gujerat and had settled into a relatively homogeneous community which had Asian shops readily available. This 'cornershop environment' meant the families were able to help each other. It also meant that for the women there was little contact with British culture and customs and that they could manage quite well without speaking English. There was also very little incentive for the men to learn any more than they needed to communicate at work.

These people came from a well-organised village and from relatively wealthy, prominent and property-owning families. Family members have a mutual obligation to help care for each other. They are unused to welfare provision by the government. A great deal of the women's and children's time there is spent in the fresh air, which enables socialisation between the women and safe play and exploration for the children. Life in their Yorkshire mill town is very different.

Many other people from abroad experience a similar change in their circumstances. For example, they have a lowered status, the climate is not so good and traffic can be very dangerous. 'Natural' ways of meeting and chatting with neighbours are not available, and it is not safe to let the children run free to play and explore their environment in the way that the parents themselves were brought up. They meet colour prejudice and/or racism.

Clothing which is an important part of the cultural heritage of some families is not always suitable, for example silks worn in winter. Traditional food, especially if imported, can be very expensive. The climate, the inner-city environment and the social structure of the British system are not supportive of the traditional patterns of behaviour of people, not only from India and Pakistan, but also from, for example, Vietnam, the West Indies, Africa and many parts of the Mediterranean. Not all are lucky enough to join a sub-community based on their own culture. Some people can be very isolated at the same time as they are trying to adjust to the new environment.

Health visitors are in a unique position because they call on families routinely, without the families having to request it. In this way, information can be given about the voluntary and statutory services available to help people cope with their difficulties. Advice and suggestions to promote good health and prevent ill-health form an integral part of this service.

PHYSICAL HEALTH

Examples are given here of the way that help can be provided, such as health education using an interpreter which seems to have helped to reduce the perinatal mortality rate. Two other examples are facilitating screening and providing counselling for families with a specific condition such as sickle cell disease, and giving advice on the acquisition of vitamin D in campaigns to eradicate rickets. Responding to specific difficulties, such as the possibility of lead in surma (an imported eye cosmetic popular in some cultures), helping to identify whether lead is present in it and warning of the potential for harm, provides the last example.

Health education with interpreters

Health visiting services have been shown to be effective and to help improve perinatal mortality rates for Bengali families in an inner London area. Elizabeth Watson (1984) studied the health of 100 women and small babies there and their use of the services by the time the baby was eight weeks old. 28 of the families were Bengali, 49 were from the indigenous population and the rest were a heterogenous group from ethnic minorities which she classified as 'English speaking immigrants'. With one exception, this latter group spoke English well and were able to communicate easily with the health service workers.

The children across all the groups were reported to have high levels of morbidity and admission to hospital in the early weeks of life. All the mothers used the services. The perinatal mortality rate had previously been higher for Bengalis than for the indigenous population. With preventive health service efforts, it had dropped to the same rate. However, subsequent interviews, when the babies were aged 8 months and 14 months, revealed an increasingly adverse influence of social conditions on the health of disadvantaged mothers and babies. The Bengalis in the study were distinctly appreciative of the health visitors' care, particularly over artificial feeding practices and the use of an interpreter. They had all learned to use the sterilisation units correctly.

It was suggested that it would be better to stress the value of breastfeeding than to concentrate on artificial feeding techniques (Watson, 1984). However, before becoming too zealous on this issue, it would be wise to ask the mothers more about their reasons for their choice. Lack of privacy in these young mothers' overcrowded homes and the lack of traditionally available family support may be important factors in their decisions on how to feed their baby (Mayor, 1984b).

Some of the specific health problems of children of parents from Asia (Black, 1985d), from the Mediterranean and around the Aegean Sea (1985e), from the West Indies and Africa (1985f) and from Vietnam or of Chinese descent (1985g) have been outlined by John Black. He drew attention to congenital abnormalities associated with a particular ethnic group, such as sickle cell disease in families of African descent or beta thalassaemia amongst Asian and Mediterranean families. He said that, if properly treated, these diseases tend to cause less distress and disability than, for example, cystic fibrosis, the commonest of the genetically determined recessive conditions in Europeans (Black, 1985a).

Sickle cell anaemia

It is surprising that neonatal screening for phenylketonuria, present in 1 in 7000–10 000 live births in the white races, is thought important enough to be fully available, whereas screening for sickle cell anaemia, which affects at least 1 in 400 of the West Indian community (Black, 1985a), is still limited

in its availability. It is important that the presence of sickle cell disease, in whatever form, is known both to the families and the professionals who care for their health. This is necessary so that the appropriate interpretation in illness can be made and anticipatory action taken (May & Choiseul, 1988; Black, 1985f; Konotey-Ahulu, 1985; Prashar et al, 1985; Serjeant, 1985; Anionwu & Hall, 1983; Gray, 1982; Anionwu, 1982).

Both the Sickle Cell Society (Health Visitor, 1982) and the Organisation for Sickle Cell Anaemia Research (OSCAR), whose new addresses will be found at the end of the chapter, can provide information about the disease and counselling. Anne Gray points out that there is a great deal of professional ignorance about the disease. She says that 'at risk' antenatal patients should be screened as routine and that specially trained health visitors should visit the homes of affected women to provide counselling and to arrange for other members of the family to be screened if they wish it. Health visitors should check on what facilities are available for this in their locality.

Rickets

Rickets is sometimes a problem amongst Asian children. Important factors are:

- inadequate exposure to sunlight
- strict vegetarian diet
- household cows' milk used for infant feeding
- inadequate maternal intake of vitamin D during pregnancy (Black, 1985d).

In a pilot study some Muslim, Sikh and Hindu women who were pregnant were interviewed by Val Box (1983) to find out the effectiveness of dietary advice and/or of information about exposure to sunlight in the prevention of rickets. She had an experimental group and a control group. Women who were counselled on diet were able to remember only about half of the advice. At such an interview there is a limit on what can be remembered, and all that group forgot they had been told about exposure to sunlight. Surprisingly, blood samples showed that the control group, who were not given special advice on food, had increased their levels of vitamin D to a greater extent than the experimental group. It was speculated that this was due to greater exposure to sunlight.

With the exception of very strict vegans, Val Box concluded that, as an Asian diet provides about the same amount of vitamin D as that of the indigenous population, health visitor education should be concentrated on exposure to sunlight and vitamin D supplementation. Dr Black (1985d) warned about the potential problem of overdosing for children given standard vitamin drops as well as foods fortified with vitamin D.

A campaign to reduce rickets in Glasgow was monitored by Dunnigan et al (1985). Low dose supplements were found to be so successful that the campaign had been extended to women at risk of osteomalacia. In another study, vitamin D given to pregnant women was shown to correlate with their babies having improved length and weight as compared with the babies from the control group who had no supplement. This was especially so when the babies were 9 and 12 months old (Brooke et al, 1981). An annual dose, either by injection or by mouth, was found to provide very good serum levels of the vitamin (Stephens et al, 1981).

Lead in cosmetics

Lead is sometimes used in medicines and cosmetics in the Third World. There has been considerable concern about lead sulphide in surma, an eye cosmetic popular amongst Asians (Aslam & Healy, 1982). Although it is illegal to import it, in actuality it is posted in as a gift or brought back from a holiday. The original surma was much safer and was made from matter such as soot or vegetable dyes. It may be applied to babies' eyes several times a day from about two weeks onwards. Children may rub their eyes and then suck their fingers and consequently swallow lead.

The problem is to find a way of discovering the presence, or otherwise, of lead in surma. Currently there is no completely satisfactory, non-hazardous test for use by the mother in the home. Drs Healy and Aslam (1984) have suggested tests which need particular chemicals and could be undertaken in the home by a health visitor in less than five minutes. Where the presence of lead was indicated,

confirmation would be needed by qualified personnel. Aslam and Healy have found that samples of surma coming into the country in hand luggage from Mecca and Medina invariably contain lead. They advocate education about the dangers of surma as, whatever is tested, new supplies are likely to be arriving. Posters and pamphlets entitled 'Surma, the gift that can be dangerous' are available from the Department of Trade and Industry Consumer Safety Unit (address and a video with the same title from Black Box at end of chapter). Karseras and Hopkins (1987, pp. 83–84) describe the feelings people may have as a result of a professional request that their surma be tested. These days significant costs of the test may add to the problems!

This section has given some examples of ways health visitors may be involved in preventing illness and promoting good health for families who have immigrated. The example of sickle cell disease might more properly be classified under the previous chapter on preventive health care regarding handicap as nowadays it is of concern to significant numbers of people whose parents immigrated decades ago.

MENTAL/EMOTIONAL FACTORS

There are basic health needs (a) for knowledge about health promotion and prevention of ill-health and (b) for stability and security to enable and promote good mental health. Language difficulties can prevent understanding and full use of health services. Moving to a new country inevitably brings with it stresses and strains.

Knowledge

The language barrier

It is important that health visitors find a way to overcome language problems. The service is bound to be inadequate for families who face this difficulty. In effect, they are debarred from the basic choice of whether or not to use it. An increasing number of foreign language health education pamphlets, leaflets, tape-slides, films and videos are becoming available (Health Education Council, 1986; Chauhan, 1980; Maternity Alliance, see useful addresses), but these do not solve all the communication problems. The best solution would be the employment of health visitors from the same cultural background or at least who speak the relevant language, but both are currently a rare occurrence.

A booklet for health visitors and midwives which will translate, phonetically, key questions and statements in a common Asian language, is being produced by Redbridge Health Education Service. Training in its use is planned and it seems likely to make a very positive contribution. Karseras and Hopkins (1987, appendix 2) provide lists of phonetically translated phrases useful for developmental assessment. A health visitor in East Suffolk has developed a portable tape recorded monologue in English and Bengali, which covers basic issues and requires no more than simple 'yes'/'no' answers (Kember, 1988). Many other schemes are being tried out (Wandsworth Council for Community Relations, 1978). June Clark (1985) suggested that there would be great benefits if health visitors went to classes to learn their clients' language. Even partial understanding would help overcome many problems.

Where no language classes are available, there might be a community leader or a family prepared to give some lessons. If health visitors were told how to say it, they might be able to write down the words phonetically for some of their favourite foreign language health education leaflets. Gradually the families visited could teach the proper pronunciation and there could be distinct advantages in this exchange of learning. It might help to provide a less formal atmosphere and would be especially useful in families where the women have not been taught to read.

Where the dialogue has to be in English with people whose knowledge of the language is limited, it may be much improved by using Alix Henley's (1982) hints on how to make it easier to get across the meaning. It is a question of a careful choice of words and a well thought-out approach. A list of her suggestions was reproduced in Community Outlook (1981). Another way of improving communication and helping people to understand

could be the use of flash cards. Barbara Rudge (1983) saw these used in health education projects in India and felt they might also be helpful here.

Many useful ideas were put forward in two workshops organised by Training in Health and Race and the Centre for Ethnic Minorities Health Studies. The booklet that was subsequently published described how initiatives were being taken to improve the uptake of antenatal services. It included a checklist of basic points about the accessibility and relevance of maternity services for recent immigrants, especially those who cannot speak English (Appendix II). Health visitors should be aware of the extent to which their local services measure up and should plan to help their clientele overcome obstacles (Pearson, 1985).

Cross-cultural understanding and acceptance

In many places interpreters are available, but the service tends to have its limitations. For example, like the health visitor the interpreter may come from a significantly different class (normally higher) and cultural background: this results in re-inforcement of the 'deference barrier' associated with contact with officialdom. Also these communications tend to be hospital- rather than client-centred and the service is not always easily available (Mays & Levick, 1985).

An advocacy scheme was set up in Hackney in 1980. Five women were employed on a wide-ranging basis. For example, as well as interpreting they not only helped people learn about their rights and spoke on their behalf, but also helped health workers to understand the problems and perceptions of non-English speaking women. These workers were specially selected on account of their language skills, their warm and compassionate personalities, and the fact that they had children themselves and came from the local community. The success of the scheme was easily demonstrated in the increased antenatal attendance, improved haemoglobin levels and baby birth weight for non-English speaking mothers (Winkler & Yung, 1981; Watson, 1984; Cornwell & Gordon, 1984).

This idea of employing workers from the community has spread. A DHSS report recommended a major new initiative in maternity services to take account of the problems of communication and cultural differences that discouraged Asian mothers. The Asian Mother and Baby Campaign was subsequently launched and now some ninety 'linkworkers' have been employed on a nationwide basis in areas with a large Asian population. Training videos are available (Alibhai, 1984).

The workers act as a bridge between the Asian communities and the health service, and work in partnership with the health professionals to help full communication in both directions between client and health professional. The project is to be evaluated and will assess health statistics, the subjective views of the people involved and changes in professional practice (Alibhai, 1984; Hadley, 1986).

The ways that innovatory ideas are accepted or otherwise in a community are complex. Philip Rack (1982, pp. 191–192, 237–240) explained the mechanisms and pre-requisites for change. He demonstrated the value of opinion leaders, for example the influence of the senior Asian women (especially the mother-in-law), in matters of pregnancy, childbirth and childrearing and of the Hakim or Vaid in general health issues. Linkworkers should be able to help health professionals understand these factors from a local and very practical point of view.

Mental health

Stresses and strains

Probably the best description and explanation for health visitors of mental illness in the context of cultural variation is that provided by Philip Rack (1982). He describes the feelings that immigrants can have during the processes of adjustment and the expected behaviour in various cultural groups, and gives thought-provoking examples of misunderstanding and misdiagnosis.

Health visitors attend seminars and seek advice from a unit especially set up in Islington in order to give psychotherapy and counselling, by people familiar with a variety of cultural backgrounds and languages (Francis, 1984). The cultural shock as a result of the unpleasant experiences associated with moving to Britain can manifest itself in various states of mental illness (Black, 1985a).

Hazel Rhodes (1985b) was able to compare the differences in the pace and way of life of Asian women whom she knew in Batley with their relatives whom she met in Alipor. In India they had servants and were freer from stress. In addition to the stresses and strains associated with employment and accommodation, the differences of culture can be very hurtful. She explained how the health of women and children is seen in Alipor as a family matter. The honour and status of the family is called into question if family difficulties and problems are made public. Zohra Ali Zubair (1984) described the deep anxiety, guilt and shame that women can feel when they are seen (and internally examined) by a male doctor, that is a man other than their husband.

Health visitors need to do their best to understand the problems of adjustment and to overcome language difficulties, as far as they can, in order that an appropriate and compassionate service is given which enables recently immigrated people to maintain a good level of health.

SOCIAL ASPECTS OF HEALTH

Respect for religious beliefs, social isolation and loss of family support, the need for childminding and the importance of self-help groups are examples of social matters that are pertinent, of course, to all health visiting care groups, but are particularly so for people who have recently immigrated.

Religious beliefs

It is important for health visitors to be sensitive and aware of the religious customs and spiritual beliefs of the people they care for, so that they can take these factors into account in their discussions and suggestions. A well-researched outline of the customs of a wide range of religions has been drawn up by Chris Sampson (1982). Within any given religion there is, of course, a great deal of variation and, as Sampson points out, an intermingling of ideas between the different philosophies.

It is important to be mindful of the particular views of any given family. Individuals may vary significantly in their degree of orthodoxy, or they may choose to put a different interpretation on certain matters within their religion. For example, Mary Peel (1983) pointed out that some members of a Moslem community may believe that birth control is forbidden by their religion, whilst others point out that Moslem scholars 'have regarded all safe legitimate contraceptives to be permitted'.

As with all families, it is worth making a note on the records of a family's religion if this is known and important to them, so that their beliefs can be respected. Recording this is less likely to be seen as a potential source of prejudice and discrimination than making a note of ethnic origin. Many modern health visiting records have a space for both of these features and health visitors have to think very carefully about their use. For example, the 1981 Census did not include a question on race or ethnic origin as it was felt it would not be acceptable (Population Trends, 1982), though it will be included in the 1991 Census. A statement of racial origin put on health visiting records gives no indication of how long it is since the person or the family members immigrated and about the degree of adjustment — nor whether they were born and educated in Britain! Religion gives more directly useful information. However, it is probably best to ask the family members how they feel about their religion being noted on the records.

Health visitors and their clients are more likely to be happy that health visitor records should include sensitive matters such as religion and/or ethnic origin if it is quite evident that the purpose is to provide equality of opportunity and/or to monitor the active implementation of such a policy. If they can see that the information is used, and used in a completely non-name-linked statistical and analytical manner, to plan and create local health and support services appropriate to the particular needs of the client groups — and to quote recent examples — then that would be evidence enough.

Where it is just a matter of labelling and with no apparent benefit, they are less likely to concur.

Family factors

The degree of family support and community companionship available varies significantly for individual immigrants. In Batley, many of the older generation of the family were still in Alipor (Rhodes, 1985a), though families lived close together as an extended family. The family circle may be able to cope with child-minding whilst the mother is at work or attending a clinic. In the study in Tower Hamlets, Bengali women were found to take their babies with them, as did 60% of the 'English speaking immigrants'. 'Indigenous mothers' were far more likely to rely on their mothers or other relatives to look after their child when they went out (Watson, 1984).

The Bengali men tended to undertake a much wider range of help at home than the other men in that study, but were less likely to take time off work so that they could be available when the new baby and the mother came home. Catherine Watson (1984) showed how domestic responsibilities and being unable to go out alone at night can limit the chances for non-English speaking women to learn the language. It seems, however, that the project workers in Hackney were helping some of the women to enroll in classes. Individual circumstances and opportunities can vary greatly.

Child-minding

There is some concern about the provision of day care for under-fives, particularly those of Asian and Afro-Caribbean descent. It is pointed out that research projects indicate that mothers from immigrant backgrounds are far more likely to work full time than non-migrant mothers. They are also more likely to have problems in finding and keeping a place with a child-minder. It was suggested that health visitors could be in a good position to recruit child-minders from amongst the Asian and Afro-Caribbean communities (Inter Departmental Consultative Group, 1984, pp. 12–14, 20; Clark, 1985).

Ideas for new initiatives for day care and schemes which help overcome racial disadvantage as well as sources of funding for such projects have been described by the Inter Departmental Consultative Group (1984) for Provision for Under-Fives. Ealing Council, the GLC and DHSS have got together on a project which is run by the Family Welfare Association. There are many activities, for example: play sessions are available; health visitors are there to advise on child care; a social worker gives advice on welfare services; and counselling sessions and classes are held in English conversation (Community Care, 1985).

Self-help groups

There has been a 'mushrooming' of self-help groups amongst the ethnic minorities in recent years. Many of the groups are health related, especially with regard to antenatal, child and adolescent health care and improved care for diseases which are specific to certain ethnic minorities. Melba Wilson (1983) found that many groups were founded in response to inadequacies, particularly a lack of understanding, in the health services. She quoted a DHSS circular which suggested that district health authorities should consult with representative organisations from ethnic minorities in order to form appropriate policies and allocate resources for health care.

However, it seems that dialogue between the health service hierarchy and the voluntary community groups is still a long way off. Health visitors, working with linkworkers where appropriate or possible, may be able to help bridge that gap. They will, however, need their managers' support if the messages from the groups are going to influence the 'health service hierarchy' and achieve a more appropriate service. In this chapter we have looked at the implications for health visiting with regard to some of the issues associated, in one case rather tenuously, with immigration. After an introduction about the need for adequate health visitor education and understanding, a family health needs framework was used to separate out and consider some of the environmental, physical, mental and social matters affecting health.

EXAMPLES OF WORK WITH ETHNIC MINORITY FAMILIES

The first example describes an antenatal visit to a Hindu household by a health visitor and a linkworker. The second is about background support given to a self-help group seeking sickle cell screening services in their area. The examples are outlined in family health needs formats in Boxes 10.2 and 10.3.

EXAMPLE ONE: AN ANTENATAL VISIT TO THE PATEL FAMILY

Hermione Verrall (HV) and Mrs Sharma, a linkworker, were visiting the Patels because Lalita Kumari Patel, the 19-year-old wife of the third son in a Hindu household, was pregnant. The family lived in a deprived inner city area where there was a small Hindu community.

The family were delighted to find that Mrs Sharma had come with the health visitor. Their teamwork was building up a good reputation. They were introduced to Lalita Kumari's husband who was at that time unemployed. He took no part in the subsequent discussions and left the three women of the household to converse with their visitors. One was Lalita Kumari's mother-in-law who had come to live some years previously with her oldest son on the death of her husband. The wife of the oldest son was also present.

With Mrs Sharma's help, HV conversed with all three women, seeking, in particular, the opinion of the mother-in-law, as it was likely to be held in high regard within the household. The women had heard of the lead-testing service the health visitor carried with her, and they brought three cosmetics for her to test. Two passed the tests and one needed to be checked by the pharmacists and arrangements were made for this.

Diet was discussed. The Patels explained how they had found good substitute foods for those that were normally unobtainable in Britain. A local shop made some traditional foods available. The value of exposure to sunlight was described as well as how to get hold of vitamin D.

Mrs Sharma explained that having heard the good news about Lalita Kumari's pregnancy through a neighbour, she had brought the health

Box 10.2   Example one: an antenatal visit to the Patel family

Environmental factors	Physical health	Mental/emotional health	Social aspects of health
Common problems • poor housing in inner city areas • low status, low paid occupation • work long hours, often at night for first and second sons • third son unemployed: Claiming supplementary benefit: entitlements in pregnancy explained *Very different* from home environment: • weather • traffic • socialisation patterns • city instead of rural	*Health education* 1. Value of vitamins and exposure to sunlight in prevention of rickets in children and osteomalacia in women Normal diet taken Explained about free vitamins and milk 2. Lead in imported medicaments and cosmetics: Family sought HV tests for cosmetics One item referred to Pharmacy Dept (*Plans* to • discuss immunisations • explain infant surveillance scheme)	*Knowledge* Language difficulties but minimised through work with linkworker Use of pictorial scheme to provide reminder of explanation *Mental health* Strains of adjustment: women seem well adjusted. Husband reported as anxious about unemployment	*Religious practices and traditional customs* Linkworker able to explain individual preferences and views of family members *Support from:* • family • friends

visitor to help explain the value of early attendance at an antenatal clinic and to answer any questions they might have, for example about welfare benefits. First she explained that the health authority had decided to start a midwives' clinic for Muslim and Hindu women in early pregnancy. Antenatal classes were discussed and, as her husband did not wish to attend, Lalita Kumari asked if her sister- or mother-in-law might come too. This was agreed and they opted to come to the series of classes in the local health centre, specially arranged for non-English speaking families. Mrs Sharma promised to be there.

The conversation then moved on to the free services (including milk and vitamins) available, as the couple were at the time on supplementary benefits. Whilst HV was explaining she filled in a pictorial chart to provide them with a reminder, as none of the women had been taught to read.

Another visit was arranged for two months later, when HV promised to discuss immunisations and the local infant surveillance scheme if they wished it.

As they walked towards the car, Mrs Sharma and HV talked about the success of the midwives' early pregnancy clinic where the women were able to have their own family with them at the examination — conducted by a woman. In due course, the success of the clinic

and evidence of the number of women wishing to be examined by women for religious reasons, led to the appointment of a part-time female obstetrician.

EXAMPLE TWO: 'THE GROUP' AND SCREENING FOR SICKLE CELL ANAEMIA

As she happened to be passing by at the right time, Henrietta Varley (HV) decided to look in on 'The Group', a health education based self-help association of young mothers in an inner city area of London. This group had grown out of a series of antenatal/postnatal classes in which many of the young women (or their husbands) had been at school together. HV slipped quietly in and sat in a chair on the edge of the circle where some twenty mothers were in hot debate over what constituted 'normal discipline' in the context of 'child abuse'.

Adele Brown, a mother whom HV knew quite well, caught her eye and indicated she would like a word outside. Mrs Brown came quickly to the point and explained that her sister's only child had recently died with sickle cell anaemia. It had not been diagnosed in the early stages of the illness and inappropriate treatment had been given (Konotey-Ahulu, 1985). 'The Group' had taken the matter very much to heart and had decided to do something positive about it by pressing for sickle cell screening services in their district. Had HV any ideas?

The health visitor asked what approaches had been considered and was told that they had thought of a petition to the district general manager. Mrs Brown's brother-in-law had sent a letter of complaint to the health authority about the tardy diagnosis, due mainly to inadequate screening services. They thought that that might help, but felt intuitively that a sickle cell awareness campaign would need to be launched, in order to get enough interest for the necessary allocation of funds for the service.

It seems that the group had no information on just how many people it might affect in their own area and in the district. However, as there were a large number of families of West Indian origin, it was likely to be a significant number. HV suggested that they tried to find accurate figures as far as they could, perhaps by using local population figures from OPCS small area statistics (Population Trends, 1982). She also suggested that they contact the Sickle Cell Society and invite someone to come and offer them guidance.

Mrs Varley undertook to ask her nurse manager whether health visitor records might give reliable information about the number of babies of Afro-Caribbean descent born locally. She said she would write a proposal for the Community Unit general manager and would be able to follow it up when he came on his next 'ground roots' visit which was scheduled in two months' time. It occurred to HV that it would be a good idea to look at the current District Plan to see if a screening service was planned and what priority it had been assigned.

Having asked how Mrs Brown's sister was, HV heard that her health visitor had been very supportive through the illness and since the death. Family and friends were helping the couple to adjust. They had been very pleased that 'The Group' had decided to take up the issue. HV left the premises feeling very glad she had called in. It was another six months before the screening was given top priority and it was in full swing a year after that.

Box 10.3 Example two 'The group' and screening for sickle cell anaemia

Environmental factors	Physical health	Mental/emotional health	Social aspects of health
Common problems • poor housing in inner city areas • low status, low paid occupations • poor facilities *But*—some parts of community very cohesive	*Health education* Self-help group discusses many aspects of physical health *Screening and support* re ethnic minority group related disease — sickle cell disease — need for screening facilities for forewarning of presence or possibility of disease	*Knowledge* Self-help group discusses many aspects of mental and emotional health Seeking to find information: will contact Sickle Cell Society *Mental health* Care for couple through bereavement period	*Self-help group* Provides focus for socialisation and mutual support Can act as pressure group Source of information on needs of ethnic minorities *Support for Mrs Brown's relatives* • family • friends • group members • HV in early days

USEFUL ADDRESSES

Black Box
10 Giltway
Giltbrook, Nottingham
NG16 2GW

Commission for Racial Equality
Information Department
Elliot House
10–12 Allington Street
London SWIE 5EH
Tel 071 828 7022

Consumer Safety Unit
Department of Trade and Industry
Millbank Tower
Millbank
London SWIP 4QU

Health Education Council
78 New Oxford Street
London WCIA IAH
Tel 071 631 0930

Maternity Alliance
15 Britannia Street
London WC1X 9JP

Redbridge Health Education Service
IIford Chambers
11 Chapel Road
IIford, Essex
IGI 2QS
Tel 081 533 0813

King's Fund Centre
126 Albert Street
London NWI 7NF
Tel 071 267 6111

Sickle Cell Society
Green Lodge
Barretts Green Road
Park Royal
London NW10 7AP
Tel 081 961 7795/8346

Organisation for sickle cell anaemia
research (OSCAR)
22 Pellatt Grove
Wood Green
London N22
Tel 081 889 3300/4844

REFERENCES

Alibhai Y 1984 Forging a new partnership. Nursing Times 80, 37: 19–20

Anionwu E 1982 Sickle cell disease. Health Visitor 55: 336–341

Anionwu E, Hall J 1983 A handbook on sickle cell disease: a guide for families. Sickle Cell Society, London

Aslam M, Healy M 1982 Present and future trends in the health care of British-Asian children. Nursing Times 78, 32: 1353–1354

Black J 1986 The new paediatrics: child health in ethnic minorities. British Medical Journal, London (*This is a reprint of the seven articles below*)

Black J 1985a The difficulties of living in Britain. British Medical Journal 290: 615–617

Black J 1985b Contact with the health services. British Medical Journal 290: 689–690

Black J 1985c Asian families I: cultures. British Medical Journal 290: 762–764

Black J 1985d Asian families II: conditions that may be found in the children. British Medical Journal 290: 830–833

Black J 1985e Families from the Mediterranean and Aegean. British Medical Journal 290: 923–925

Black J 1985f Afro-Caribbean and African families. British Medical Journal 290: 984–988

Black J 1985g Chinese and Vietnamese families. British Medical Journal 290: 1063–1065

Box V 1983 Rickets: what should the health education message be? Health Visitor 56: 131–134

Brent Community Health Council 1981 Black people and the health service. Brent Community Health Council, London

Brooke O G, Butters F, Wood C 1981 Intrauterine vitamin D and postnatal growth in Asian infants. British Medical Journal 283: 1024

Chauhan V 1980 Community information (Asian languages) directory. Commission for Racial Equality and Citizens Advice Bureau, London

Clark J 1985 Understanding the under-fives. Nursing Times Community Outlook 81, 11: 8

Community Care 1985 Shanti Niketan opens its doors. Community Care 547: 7

Community Outlook 1981 Chat sheet. Nursing Times Community Outlook 77, 28: 239–241

Cornwell J, Gordon P (eds) 1984 An experiment in advocacy. The Hackney multi-ethnic women's health project. Report of a conference organised by the King's Fund in collaboration with City and Hackney Community Health Council. King's Fund Centre, London

Dunnigan M G, Glekin B M, Henderson J B, McIntosh W B, Sumner D, Sutherland G R 1985 Prevention of rickets in Asian children: assessment of the Glasgow campaign. British Medical Journal 291: 239–242

Francis W 1984 Out of the textbooks and into the consulting room. Community Care 535: 19–20

Gray A 1982 Sickle cell disease. Nursing Times 78, 31: 1324–1325

Hadley A 1986 Mothers' advocate. Nursing Times 82, 6: 16–17

Health Education Council 1986 Health education for ethnic minorities. Resource list prepared by the Health Education Council, 2nd ed. Health Education Council, London

Health Visitor 1982 The Sickle Cell Society. Health Visitor 55: 341

Healy M A, Aslam M 1984 Identification of lead in Asian cosmetics – a test for use by health visitors. Public Health, London 98: 361–366

Henley A 1982 Asian patients in hospital and at home. Oxford University Press, Oxford

Henley A 1986 Nursing care in a multiracial society. Senior Nurse 4, 2: 18–20

Henley A, Clayton J 1982a Cultural patterns. Health and Social Services Journal XCII: 833–834

Henley A, Clayton J 1982b What's in a name? Health and Social Services Journal XCII: 855–857

Henley A, Clayton J 1982c Catering for all tastes. Health and Social Services Journal XCII: 888–889

Henley A, Clayton J 1982d Religion of the Muslims. Health and Social Services Journal XCII: 918–919

Henley A, Clayton J 1982e Five signs of Sikhism. Health and Social Services Journal XCII: 943–945

Henley A, Clayton J 1982f Illness and the life cycle. Health and Social Services Journal XCII: 972–974

Hunkins S V 1983 West Indians' sexual attitudes (letter). Health Visitor 56: 7

Inter Departmental Consultative Group 1984 Services for under fives from ethnic minority communities. Report of a subgroup on provision of services for under fives from ethnic minority communities. Department of Health and Social Security, London

Karseras P, Hopkins E 1987 British Asians: health in the

community. John Wiley and Son, Chichester — Essential reading.

Kember M 1988 Improving communications with non-English speaking families. Health Visitor 61, 12: 372

Konotey-Ahulu F 1985 Ethnic minorities and sickle cell disease (letter). British Medical Journal 290: 1214

Mares P, Henley A, Baxter C 1985 Health care in multiracial Britain. Health Education Council and National Extension College, Cambridge

May A, Choiseul M 1988 Sickle cell anaemia and thalassaemia: symptoms, treatment and effects of lifestyle. Health Visitor 61, 7: 212–215

Mayor V 1984a The family, bereavement and dietary beliefs. Nursing Times 80, 23: 40–42

Mayor V 1984b Pregnancy, childbirth and child care. Nursing Times 80, 24: 57–58

Mays N, Levick P 1985 When maternal instinct isn't enough. Health and Social Services Journal XCV: 870–871

Pearson M 1985 Racial equality and good practice maternity care. A report of two workshops held in Bradford organised by Training in Health and Race and the Centre for Ethnic Minorities Health Studies. Health Education Council and National Extension College for Training in Health and Race, London

Pearson R 1982a Understanding the Vietnamese in Britain. Part I: background and family life. Health Visitor 55: 426–430

Pearson R 1982b Understanding the Vietnamese in Britain. Part II: marriage, death and religion. Health Visitor 55: 477–483

Pearson R 1982c Understanding the Vietnamese in Britain. Part III: health beliefs, birth and child care. Health Visitor 55: 533–540

Peel M 1983 Islam and family planning (letter). Health Visitor 56: 436

Population Trends 1982 Editorial. Sources of statistics on ethnic minorities. Population Trends 28, Summer: 1–8

Prashar U, Anionwu E, Brozovic M 1985 Sickle cell anaemia — who cares? A survey of screening and counselling facilities in England. The Runnymede Trust, London

Rack P 1982 Race, culture and mental disorder. Tavistock Publications, London

Rhodes H 1985a From Alipor to Batley. Nursing Times Community Outlook 81, 24: 39–44

Rhodes H 1985b From Batley to Alipor. Nursing Times Community Outlook 81, 28: 8–14

Rudge B 1983 Health education, Indian style. Health Visitor 56: 373–376

Sampson C 1982 The neglected ethic. Religious and cultural factors in the care of patients. McGraw-Hill, Maidenhead

Schofield J 1981a Behind the veil: the mental health of Asian women in Britain. 1. Life in Asia, Health Visitor 54: 138–141

Schofield J 1981b Behind the veil: the mental health of Asian women in Britain. 2. Migration and life in Britain. Health Visitor 54: 183–186

Schofield J 1981c Behind the veil: the mental health of Asian women in Britain. 3. Preventing stress — the role of the health visitor. Health Visitor 54: 248–251

Serjeant G R 1985 Sickle cell disease. Oxford University Press, Oxford

Stephens W P, Klimiuk P S, Berry J L, Mawer E B 1981 Annual high-dose vitamin D prophylaxis in Asian immigrants. Lancet II: 1199–1201

Stevenson O 1985 Education for community care. British Medical Journal 290: 1966–1968

Wandsworth Council for Community Relations 1978 Asians and the health service. A directory of measures implemented by Area Health Authorities to meet the needs of the Asian community. Commission for Racial Equality, London

Watson C 1984 The vital link. Nursing Times 80, 30: 18–19

Watson E 1984 Health of infants and use of health services by mothers of different ethnic groups in East London. Community Medicine 6: 127–135

While A E, Godfrey M 1984 Health visitor knowledge of Asian cultures. Health Visitor 57: 297–298

Wilson M 1983 Networking for health. Health and Social Services Journal XCIII: 565–567

Winkler F, Yung J 1981 Advising Asian mothers. Health and Social Services Journal XCI: 1244–1245

Zohra Ali Zubair 1984 Preface. In: Cornwell J, Gordon P (eds) 1984 An experiment in advocacy. The Hackney multi-ethnic women's health project. King's Fund Centre, London

FURTHER READING

Denning S 1986 Barriers to health. Results of a survey of the health care needs of Bengali people in Kings Cross. Kings Cross Centre Campaign, 62 Marchmont Street, London WC1 Tel: 071 278 5069

Donovan J 1986 'We don't buy sickness, it just comes.' Health, illness and health care in the lives of black people in London. Gower, Aldershot

Elfer P, Gatiss S 1990 Charting child health services. A survey of community child health services provided by health authorities in England, Scotland and Wales. National Children's Bureau, London, Section Two — Recommended reading.

Ellis J 1989 Breaking new ground. Community development with Asian communities. Bedford Square Press, London

Health Visitors' Association Working Party 1989 Entitled to be healthy. Health visiting and school nursing in a multiracial society. Health Visitors' Association, London

Huntsman R G 1987 Sickle-cell anaemia and thalassemia. A primer for health care professionals. Canadian Sickle Cell Society, P O Box 131156, Station A, St John's, Newfoundland, Canada A1B 4AA

Iskander R 1987 Developing a black consciousness. Nursing Times 83, 42: 66–69

Larbie J, Mares P, Baxter C 1987 The trainers' handbook for multiracial health care. National Extension College, Cambridge

Wilson A 1987 Finding a voice: Asian women in Britain. Virago, London

This chapter considers some of the ways health visitors can help to prevent the occurrence, development or deterioration of situations involving child abuse and looks at some of the difficulties for health visitors in this field of their work.

11

Child abuse

SMALL BUT IMPORTANT

The framework

Child abuse should be studied in the context of cross-cultural family and societal violence. Here it is possible to take only a limited look at the topic. We use the prevention model (see Table 11.1) as a framework for outlining some of the aims of health visitors with regard to child abuse and neglect, that is their attempts to:

- prevent the occurrence of such problems, for example by improving people's understanding of the basic needs and development of babies and children and of the factors associated with child abuse, in order to engender good bonding and good parent–child relationships and interaction.
- prevent the development of child abuse and neglect where strains and tensions are becoming too great, for example by trying to identify the most vulnerable people, and ensuring a 'life-line' (someone to talk to in a crisis) and that help such as a day nursery place is available, to help relieve the stress in the household.
- prevent deterioration of the situation in cases in which child abuse has or seems to have occurred: for example, by keeping in touch with the family if their child is taken into care and helping them cope with their child's behavioural problems on return to the family.

Table 11.1 Prevention model of health visiting aims regarding child abuse

Aim	Through	Examples
To prevent occurrence of child abusing situation	Teaching	Parenthood courses • in school • antenatally Child abuse discussions, e.g. incest
	Normal supportive services	Tell about groups and agencies
To prevent development of stress & tensions leading to child abuse	1. Identifying those vulnerable 2. Enabling extra support for them	In liaison with midwives Observations of health visitors Tell of self-help groups, eg. OPUS Health visitor special initiatives More frequent visiting
To prevent deterioration where child abuse seems to have occurred	Child-centred decisions with nurse management support	Use social and clinical evidence Full and contemporaneous records Multi-profession decision & action Evidence in court where necessary Continued support for parents if child removed

Keeping up to date

Child abuse has always been a feature of society (Radbill, 1980; Korbin, 1980; Borkowski et al, 1983). Attitudes towards it have changed over the past twenty years since interpretation of X-rays alerted doctors to patterns of physical violence towards children. More recently, concern has also focused on child neglect and emotional and sexual abuse.

A feeling that something could and should be done about child abuse has been developing rapidly. In recent years, there has been a great outpouring of literature intended to help guide health and welfare workers. Early literature was mainly devoted to alerting people to the problem and to encouraging them to take action. Suggestions on how to discover the people most prone to this problem have been proliferating. Now a number of research projects are being undertaken, leading to increasingly perspicacious commentary. For example, Nigel Parton (1985) has brought together a great deal of the available data and has drawn attention to the need for clearer definitions of child abuse and for a more wide-ranging and supportive solution to the problem.

Ideas will change as informed understanding of the subject improves. It is therefore important that health visitors have plenty of opportunities to keep up to date by going on courses, by reading and through mutual support groups and nurse manager help (see Ch. 2, pp. 20–21). However, it is becoming more difficult to attend courses now that resources are being cut back (Thorneley, 1986). For this reason, the nurse managers' role in facilitating and enabling the best possible practice becomes very important.

A small part of health visitors' work . . . .

Helping parents overcome the strains and tensions of child care is an integral part of most health visitors' everyday work. Child abuse pertains to a very small part of this and lies at one extreme of the range of need for care and support (see Fig. 11.1).

The government does not collect statistics on child abuse. Normally the numbers quoted, such as 7000 children physically abused by their parents in England and Wales in 1984, are derived from an extrapolation of figures from National Society for the Prevention of Cruelty to Children (NSPCC) teams who have access to statistics which cover less than 10% of the country. The figures quoted can therefore provide only an indicator (Laurance, 1985). The numbers of reported cases of child abuse and neglect have been increasing over recent years. However, it may well be due to a greater readiness to report the problem.

Where more firm figures are available, it can be seen that serious and acknowledged child abuse

Fig. 11.1 Continuum showing range of child care supportive work. Above the continuum shows the extent of health visiting involvement, below shows parents' feelings and skills.

and neglect represent only a very small proportion, if any, of most health visitors' work. For example, there are very few children involved in care proceedings, a matter of about 4 children per 10 000 each year (Dingwall, 1983). Also, only a small number of pre-school deaths caused by 'violence or accident' are due to child abuse. In Ontario, for example, they amounted to around 4 to 8% of the deaths (Greenland, 1986). In comparison, accidents in the street or in the home account for extremely high numbers of death and disability.

.... with high anxiety levels

Health visitors tend to find child abuse a particularly stressful aspect of their work. There has been a great deal of media attention focused on this problem, both in defence of parents where a child is thought to have been taken into care unnecessarily, and at the other extreme where a child has been harmed having been returned to his parents.

However, this was not mentioned in Valerie Weeks' (1982) study of the ways in which non-accidental injury caused professional anxiety. Health visitors who had been involved with actual or suspected cases reported most concern over their ongoing relationship with the family. Next came worries that their suspicion of child abuse might be unfounded and concern about legal proceedings. There was anxiety about insufficient training and information about procedures for dealing with cases, inadequate nurse manager support and problems with caseload size. There were several other worries, including those associated with borderline cases and children's behavioural

difficulties on being returned to their parents after having been 'in care'.

PREVENTING CHILD ABUSE

Both education and support have a part to play in promoting good child care. For example, learning about a child's development and basic needs may help engender good bonding and parenting skills. It can be useful to people to know about the services available to help parents under stress. Better understanding by the general public and more open discussion about taboo subjects such as child sexual abuse, may help prevent its occurrence. Support, for example in the form of having someone to turn to and trust, may help parents talk through their problems, lower stress levels and help avoid abuse of the child.

Health education

Both learning about child care in general and about child abuse in particular, may help to prevent the occurrence of child abuse. Some health visitors become involved in giving or advising on preparation for parenthood courses in schools and in teaching in antenatal sessions and other groups. Providing the opportunity to discuss and learn about babies' patterns of development and their emotional requirements, for example their need for attention and love, may help engender realistic parental expectations and good mother–child bonding. However, as we discussed in Chapter 3 (see pp. 47–48), there are no glib solutions to preparation for parenthood. It is difficult for people to visualise it in advance.

There are advantages if lessons in school also include discussions about child abuse. An understanding of the factors associated with this problem and knowledge of the facilities and services available, may help families with tensions and worries to recognise the need to seek timely advice and help. It might also lessen fears about seeking that support. A concise and very useful overview of child abuse has been written for the non-professional by Dana Ackley (1977). Molly Meacher (1982 p. 3) has sketched out a neat synopsis of current ideas on the nature, size and causes of the problem.

These same articles would also be useful as a general introduction for women's groups and other organisations. Some of the articles and books referred to in the next two sections of this chapter may be found useful in stimulating debate and discussion on general child abuse. It is a very wide subject. Child sexual abuse is provided here as an example.

Child sexual abuse

As in other aspects of child abuse, there is much to debate. Identifying the problem and finding effective and acceptable measures to deal with it are even more difficult than, for example, with physical abuse. Public and professional awareness of incest, for example, are said to be at a level roughly equivalent to that for physical abuse 15 years ago (Vizard, 1985).

Groups wishing to discuss this topic should be encouraged to read a variety of books and articles, in order to get a range of views. Four books written for the general public include a wide-ranging look at the subject by Forward and Buck (1981) and Jean Renvoise (1982) and a feminist point of view by Sarah Nelson (1982). *The last taboo* by Gay Search (1988) is now probably the best on the subject. It includes a chapter on prevention. A mothers' group might like to see the Child Sexual Abuse Prevention Education Project (CSAPEP) (1985) leaflet aimed at helping mothers identify the occurrence of sexual abuse in their own family.

Pamela Holmes (1986b) described a book specially designed to help children know how to cope with improper approaches.

There has been a proliferation of this type of literature in America. Commenting on this, Nicholas Tucker (1985) described some unfortunate side-effects of what he saw as an over-reaction to the problem. He said that in America there were examples of over-zealous accusations of incestuous behaviour, for example, in custody proceedings in the divorce courts. Walter Barker (1990b) is also apprehensive about over-reaction and provides a well-argued defence of children's need to experience physically expressed affection.

Group discussion of this topic is very likely to lead to questioning about local facilities and ways officialdom copes with the problem. Health visitors need to be sure they know exactly what the policy in their locality is on the management of child sexual abuse and how liaison between the relevant professionals is put into action (Vizard, 1985; Renvoise, 1982, pp. 166–216; Nelson, 1982, pp. 77–78; Forward & Buck, 1981, pp. 138–139). They need to know this both for their practice and in order to provide such a group with a clear picture of how cases are handled. It would also be useful to have made personal or telephone contact with the agencies willing to give adults and children confidential help (Pownall, 1985; CSAPEP & Driver, 1985), in order to be able to give an accurate account of the range and style of services available.

It has been suggested that 10% of adult Britons were sexually abused as children (Elliot, 1985). Widespread knowledge about confidential and supportive services for the sexually abused may do much more than encourage reporting of early cases. It could help discourage its occurrence in the first place, once potential, particularly incestuous, abusers were less certain they could rely on hiding behind a veil of secrecy.

General health visitor support

Supportive work is one of the basic mainstays of a health visitor's work. It involves, for example, telling mothers about local groups and schemes which offer help to young families. This was mentioned in Chapter 4 (p. 69). In Chapter 5 (pp. 95–98), helping people with loneliness, depression and stressful problems, such as having a persistently crying baby, were described. In some cases, this everyday work will help defuse and avert problems that might otherwise have led to child abuse. Support services more specific to child abuse are described in the next section.

In this section we have taken a brief look at some of the ways health visitors may be able to help prevent the occurrence of child abuse. Education, both on babies' emotional needs and on child abuse itself, was discussed, as was the preventive value of everyday support work in health visiting. Child sexual abuse was given as an example of the value of open debate on the subject.

IDENTIFICATION AND SELECTION

In this section we look at the means currently available to try to discover the people most vulnerable to the stresses and strains that can lead to them abusing their children. In essence the aim is to prevent the development of child abuse in families who have these difficulties, by providing them with the degree of extra care and support that seem to be required.

A form of screening?

The process of identification and selection of vulnerable people might loosely be considered screening. However, the process does not lead to the discovery of immediately verifiable early cases of child abuse, nor does it discover a presymptomatic phase which, if it received no attention, would inevitably result in child abuse. Many, or possibly most of the selected families will have no major problem. The purpose is to draw health visitors' attention to those most likely to be 'at risk'. These schemes provide a rather crude tool for selection. They need to be used with circumspection and to be given a great deal of thought about what is really being picked out.

Many health visitors are concerned about 'labelling' and the development of disparaging attitudes towards families selected by this type of scheme. This matter was touched on in Chapter 3 (p. 48). However, where health visitors are clearly able to provide the selected families with extra time and support, a feature incorporated, for example, in the Portsmouth scheme (Powell, 1985), or where facilities such as preferential day nursery places for families under stress are readily available, then concern will be less. The advantage of being able to channel help where it is most needed may be thought to outweigh the disadvantages of the system.

What and how extensive is the problem?

Some basic questions are:

- Exactly what is child abuse?
- How widespread is it?
- Who does it and why?
- Where is the borderline between physical child abuse and 'normal discipline'?
- To what extent is early discovery and support and/or therapy successful?

Answering these questions is difficult and in some cases impossible, basically because there is not and will not be a fully agreed definition of child abuse. Welfare professionals use the phrase to cover an enormous variety and range of notions and aspects of the problem. Agreed definitions, such as that for physical abuse quoted in governmental documents (Department of Health and Social Security, 1986, p. i), are generally stated in such broad terms that they could, if taken literally, include an enormous number of families. Another problem is that researchers using different definitions have necessarily come to a variety of conclusions so that studies cannot be compared and many questions inevitably remain inadequately answered (Parton, 1985, pp. 133–146). Either way, as ideas on child abuse are culturally defined and socially determined (Meacher, 1983, p. 3), definitions and ways of thinking about it are certain to continue to change over time.

A variety of basic approaches to the study of child abuse have been described by Nigel Parton

(1985, pp. 154–172) amongst them a national survey of family violence in the United States by Straus, Gelles and Steinmetz. Straus et al found that child abuse, far from being rare, was part of the normal pattern of a large number of children's lives. The lower the income level, the higher the rate and degree of violence tended to be. They found that amongst the poorest families, stress did not increase the likelihood of violence — high stress levels are part of normal life for them.

Many studies find a correlation between low socio-economic levels and child abuse. Professor Greenland's (1986) study of 100 child abuse and neglect deaths in Canada also found this tendency. As far as he could discover, only 6 out of 100 came from the white collar or professional classes. It is worth noting in passing that in a significant number of the cases (9) the suspected perpetrators were baby-sitters and not the parents.

An attempt was made by Elmer (Parton, 1985, pp. 166–167) to study the long-term consequences of child abuse by following up 17 children, abused under one year of age, eight years after they were originally examined, and comparing them with two other groups of children, matched for age, race, sex and socio-economic status. The children in one of the control groups had suffered accidents under one year of age; those in the other control group had had no record of either similar accidents or child abuse. To their astonishment the researchers found that *all* the children appeared fearful, anxious and depressed and demonstrated social and developmental problems. Subsequent work led them to feel that research into child abuse was discovering more about lower-class children in general, rather than specifically about abused children. There is an obvious need for further research using fully matched control groups.

Identifying those in need of support

A basic premiss of Kempe and Kempe (1978, p. 22) was that

abusive parents come from all walks of life.

Although this may be so, it looks, from the research quoted above, as if they are unevenly spread across the social classes. There seems also

to be an element of uneven selection and classification slanted towards lower class parents (Dingwall et al, 1983, p. 101).

The Kempes wrote the most influential of the early treatises on the subject. They described a cycle of abuse in which poorly-parented children grew up to become parents who cared badly for their children and so on through generations. In their work they had discovered four factors implicit in child abusing families, shown in Table 11.2, some aspects of which they said could be sensed from parental reaction to the newborn baby. These are listed in Box 11.1. A list of Lynch and Roberts' (1977) significant factors which they said could be gleaned from the midwifery notes will be found in Box 11.2. More recently, attention has been turning towards identifying parents during pregnancy too, in order to promote good bonding after delivery (Ounsted et al, 1982).

Table 11.2 Four factors implicit in child abusing families (from Kempe & Kempe, 1978, p. 24–38)

Factor	Features
Potential for abuse — acquired over the years	Lack of mothering imprint Isolated — cannot trust or use others Spouse passive — he/she cannot give support Unrealistic expectations of the child
Child appears different to parents	For example, hyperactive, retarded, suffers from a defect, appears similar to disliked person
Crisis or series of crises	Cannot cause, but precipitates abuse
Life-link lacking	No one to turn to in a crisis and to tell about feelings and problems

Research in Aberdeen took another approach. Dean et al (1978) studied health visitors' assessment of mother–child interaction to see if the more vulnerable families could be discovered this way. They found that health visitors could sense when families were having emotional difficulties, but tended to discount these and to concentrate on

Box 11.1 Parents' reactions in labour and delivery rooms (from Kempe & Kempe, 1978, p. 81)

Factors sensed	Reaction to new baby	Worrying signs
Potential for abuse	What mother said	Passive response to baby
How parents perceive child	How she looked What she did	React to him with hostility
Degree of tension	How father reacted	Seem disappointed over baby's sex
	Midwife's anecdotal information	Do not look baby in the eye
		Parents not loving towards each other

Box 11.2 A method for predicting bonding failure in the maternity hospital (from Lynch & Roberts, 1977)

Five factors from midwifery notes

Mother under twenty for first baby
Referral to maternity hospital social worker
Baby admitted to special care unit
Emotional disturbance recorded
Recorded concern over mother's inability to cope

Table 11.3 Health visitors' measure of mother–child interaction (from Dean et al, 1978)

Percentage of mothers	Coded	Description of situation by health visitor (coded later)
68	No concern	No stated environmental, behavioural or interactional difficulties
21	Mild concern	Any one word concerning environment or behaviour
7	Moderate concern	Prolonged separation Non-supporting situation Unrealistically high expectations of baby History of psychiatric illness — either parent History of prolonged marital discord
3	Great concern	Type of interaction between mother and baby (e.g. eye contact, physical contact) Presence of physically neglectful situation History of unstable/violent background — either parent (where description qualified, qualification discounted in coding)

the more physical 'mothering skills'. They felt that if health visitors had the courage of their own convictions, they could identify the families most likely to be in need of extra help. In the event, two thirds of the children in the family situations coded as causing the health visit or moderate or great concern (see Table 11.3), later suffered accident, injury or failure to thrive.

Spurred on by this sort of research, health visitors started to set up pilot schemes which attempted to checklist factors which would find the families most in need of help (Woods, 1981; Waterhouse, 1981; Fort, 1986). One example is Claire Johnson's (1985) scheme in Rochdale, in which 22 factors were selected. Special weighting was given to items shown by earlier research to be important. The scoring system chosen seemed to be successful in making it possible to identify the vast majority of parents who would need help.

Around two thirds of the families selected through this scheme had one or more episodes of suspected or actual non-accidental injury, neglect, failure to thrive or emotional deprivation during the year of the study. It follows that a third did not. They all had a yellow sticker on their file, including the third who never had any problems. It could be argued that there is an advantage to new or 'stand-in' health visitors if there is a systematic method of drawing attention to the families most likely to be suffering significant problems. However, there is also the disadvantage associated with the ethical problem of 'labelling' a family and, perhaps, not telling them they have been classified in this way. This 'labelling' should only be applied to families known to have abused or to have been suspected of it *and informed* of these suspicions.

This type of scheme is to some extent also useful from a planning point of view, making it possible to estimate the number of 'at risk' families in a caseload. It can help indicate the relative need for supportive services and levels of staff in and between areas. However, the Jarman (1989) scoring system would be a good deal cheaper and would probably provide an equally accurate indication of these needs. This all assumes that support services for these families are to be provided!

The whole idea of screening to discover potential child abusers is strongly called into question by Walter Barker (1990a). He argues lucidly and convincingly. He shows that no screening system is infallible and that there will inevitably be a high level of false positives. As he points out, this is not of concern in screening for developmental delay. Here the cases are selected out as those requiring further investigation and referred on to an appropriate clinic.

However, the situation is entirely different in child abuse screening. Here, the large number of false positives are parents thought likely to abuse their children at some time in the future, but who are and will remain, perfectly innocent. These families, especially the significant proportion continuing to be falsely selected by further 'more sensitive' screening tests, are likely to feel and to be, 'hounded' by the misinformed professionals responsible for follow up. Dr Barker feels that disadvantaged and less capable parents should have self-esteem boosting support, information and encouragement, which will help them find their own solution and reduce the chance of them abusing their children. This is much preferable to a system concentrating on 'search' that sees them 'as potential abusing "monsters".' Whatever the system, there is very little value in pin-pointing the families most likely to be at risk if there is no hope of offering them extra support.

Support services

There are self-help groups specially set up to help families finding it difficult to cope with stress and the tensions of parenthood. Anne Ashley (1980) described the history of the voluntary associations providing anonymous telephone counselling services and their subsequent proliferation. Some are able to provide group meetings too.

The work of the self-help groups in the Organisation for Parents Under Stress (OPUS) has been studied by the Mental Health Foundation (Meacher, 1982). A large number of people who had joined a group had benefited significantly. They were better able to talk about their problems and had changed their patterns of caring for their children.

Many of the volunteers had themselves experienced abuse as children. Many had had worries about their relationship with at least one of their children, which enabled them to empathise with the people they were trying to help. A 24-hour support service was felt to be important.

Few of the callers to OPUS suffered from unemployment or housing problems. Most were able to afford their own phone. Health visitors should remember that the families likely to feel most stressed, the low paid and the unemployed, are the least likely to use these self-help groups. They will need appropriate services organised locally.

Health visitors set up a walk-in unit in Hertfordshire (Butler, 1983). In that area, a great deal of time was spent in professional discussions about children 'at risk', and the unit was proposed as a way of providing a practical solution to some of the difficulties faced. It was a flexible facility, providing a place where:

- children could be left in safe hands for a short time
- mothers could
  — meet other mothers
  — discuss problems with the health visitor
  — join in activities with the children
- health visitors could observe
  — child behaviour
  — mother–child interaction.

The health visitors found it very helpful to be able to give the mothers reassurance and advice based on these observations, another example of the interlinking of health education and support in our work.

The success of the unit has led to a decision to amalgamate with a local play group to form a family centre. Several unemployed fathers have already shown an interest in it. It will be able to provide health education and support on a full family basis, increasing understanding and reducing stress, thereby helping to prevent child abuse and other problems.

In this section we have looked at schemes for identifying families thought to be 'at risk', with a view to providing them with extra care and attention, and at examples of special supportive services. The health visitor's aim is help minimise the degree of tensions, misunderstanding and other difficulties and so prevent the development of situations leading to child abuse.

WHEN PROBLEMS ARISE

The main thrust in this aspect of health visiting is in trying to prevent a crisis situation. However, we now turn to what happens when a crisis does occur. The decisions about what should be done are inevitably difficult and need to be child-centred and based on both medical and social factors. Support from nurse managers and inter-professional decision-making and action are very important factors.

Who is the client?

For some families the strains and tensions become too great and, to some degree, child abuse occurs. Where this has or seems to have happened, decisions have to be taken in order to help the family and to try to prevent further deterioration of the situation.

Deterioration for whom? Normally in health visiting each member of the family is considered a client. However, particularly in matters pertaining to child abuse, the child is seen as the primary client. Where parental interests conflict with those of their child, the child's welfare takes precedence.

What is normal and what is abuse?

The decision at one end of the scale might be, for example, to suggest a place for the child at the day nursery to ease family tensions by giving the parents and child a break from each other.

At the other extreme, it might be to encourage the parents to make immediate contact with the social services department and seek help or even for the health visitor to do so. The former decision would be based on the assumption that the problem was currently within reasonably normal limits but might get worse, the latter on the assumption that the situation seemed to be significantly more dangerous. Where is the borderline and how do we decide which conduct amounts to normal family behaviour and which to child abuse?

It is easy to classify as abuse a situation in which a parent or carer is clearly vindictive and cruel or has killed a child. However, most cases involve grey areas and therefore are not so clear-cut. There are guidelines but in essence the decision has to be based on a value judgement. It is interesting to note that a small study found the relative seriousness of various theoretical incidents of child mistreatment were categorised by health visitors and social workers in a remarkably similar way (Fox & Dingwall, 1985).

EARLY DECISIONS
Warning signs . . . . .

Sometimes non-accidental injuries come to the notice of health visitors because parents confide in them. In some cases, they are initially based on suspicions. This can be because:

- the child has bruises which show a particular pattern
- there is an inadequate explanation of the injuries, such as inconsistencies in the account
- there has been a delay in seeking care, perhaps the mother treated the injury and it was seen with another injury.

Additional warning signs can be apprehension by the child and disturbed parental behaviour (Ross et al, 1977) and the child being stunted in height and/or weight.

. . . . . and caution

There are traps for the unwary. Misunderstanding or, for example, inadequate knowledge of traditions amongst ethnic minorities can lead to mis-diagnosis of child abuse (Chan, 1985; Black, 1986). Inexperience in differentiating between non-accidental injury and accidental injury or failure to recognise certain medical conditions can lead to similar problems (O'Doherty, 1982; Oates, 1984).

Health visitors find themselves 'gate-keepers' to the system in which people become labelled as 'abusers' (Gelles, 1975). They are faced with inherent anxieties associated with attempting to decide the relative risks of physical injury, for example against the less immediately visible risks of emotional injury due to separation from the family (Moore, 1985).

A wide range of factors

Dingwall et al (1981, p. 21–22) found health visitors identified more cases than social workers confirmed because the former:

- combined social and clinical evidence
- were more particularly concerned with children, rather than the family as a unit
- were more concerned with the short term i.e. the pre-school years
- had greater concern for current symptoms than possible causes of the problem.

Both of the professions (and the parents) use 'justifications' and 'excuses', for example the particular cultural or economic circumstances of the family, to absolve parents to some extent. Assessments were made under a 'rule of optimism' in which, where possible, staff think the best of people.

This approach provides a solution to the problem of the tension in our society between its special regard for the privacy of the family and yet the need to inspect if children are to be protected. In exchange for free access, health and welfare services promise parents that they will think the best of whatever they find. This rule then, breaks down where parents resist inspection by these child protection agencies or where the family's circumstances have ceased to be private and have become public knowledge (Dingwall, 1983). Dingwall et al (1983, p. 101) suggest that this:

. . . . . would seem to filter moral character in such a way as to hold back some, upper-, middle-, and 'respectable' working-class parents, members of ethnic minorities and mentally incompetent parents while leaving the 'rough' indigenous working class as the group proportionately most vulnerable to compulsory measures.

Reports on how the system has failed (Department of Health and Social Security, 1982, p. 69) show that, amongst many others, these two factors are important, for example

many allegations of abuse by members of the public turn out to be well-founded. . . . . The child or children must be seen.

Professor Greenland's (1986) study of child abuse and neglect deaths showed, as has other research, the importance of continuous assessment of the progress of the child and the need to respond to warnings by neighbours and concerned relatives. An outline of the factors he showed to be key issues in helping to identify high risk situations are listed in Box 11.3.

More than half the victims in Professor Greenland's study died during their first year of life, a quarter died in their second year and fewer than 5% after the age of five. About half the victims were at or below the third centile for

Box 11.3 Some of the factors associated with deaths due to child abuse and neglect (from Greenland, 1986)

Child
Young baby, especially under one year
Already sustained broken bones/fractured skull
At or below third centile for weight and height
Severe behaviour disorder, difficult to rear
May express help-seeking behaviour

Parents
Already known to child protection agency
Underlying social and emotional stresses
Lack system of social, family or professional support
History of:
    criminal assaultive behaviour
    abuse of drugs and alcohol

Professionals
Inexperienced and unskilled professionals, such as medical/social workers
Poor interdisciplinary action and communication
Fail to respond to:
    warnings by neighbours and relatives
    help-seeking behaviour of parents

height or weight, and about the same number were already known to the child protection agency. Well over half had had previous injuries treated by a physician.

GUIDANCE

By nurse managers

It is clear that there are many factors to be considered in the decisions to be made. Health visitors, particularly the less experienced, need to have direct contact with and support from nurse managers in order to enable

- case discussion
- help with action planning
- preparation for case conferences
- preparation for court
- help to resolve allied emotional difficulties

from the earliest stages in this type of work (see Fig. 11.2). The local authority procedures manual on non-accidental injury to children is likely to encourage this (Department of Health and Social Security, 1986). An example of procedures for nursing staff is outlined in Box 11.4.

The Jasmine Beckford case highlighted the fact that although health visitors are responsible for their own actions, it is necessary for nurse management to provide support (Nursing Times, 1985; Jay, 1985). The health visitors in the Lucie Gates case were found in two reports to have acted conscientiously, but their managers were condemned for failing to provide adequate advice, support and supervision. It seems that the nurse managers failed to assess the problems and had not provided policies for nurses involved in child abuse cases. Neither of the nursing officers nor the senior nursing officer in the case had health visitor qualifications or experience (Nursing Times, 1982). Nurse managers without a health visitor background need to read widely about child abuse, and themselves need support until they have become experienced in this aspect of their work.

A graphic account has been given by Jane Schofield (1983) of the stress associated with setting up a good relationship with a couple and

DIRECT CONTACT AND SUPPORT

Fig. 11.2 Direct contact with and support from the health visitor nurse manager.

Box 11.4 Outline of an example of non-accidental injury to children procedures manual

Procedure for nursing staff
Aim: identification and regular surveillance to prevent occurrence of injury
1. *Where injuries*, established or suspected:
   Immediate action
   'Place of Safety' if necessary to prevent further injury
   Ensure:
   a. Seen by doctor
   b. Inform Principal Area Officer, Social Services (PAO)
   c. Inform Nursing Manager (NM)
   d. Plus written report to NM for PAO
2. *Where suspicion* but no immediate medical problem:
   a. Discuss with GP
   b. Inform NM
   c. Inform PAO
   d. Written report to Social Services
3. (i) Case conference:
      Convened by PAO — can be requested by others
   (ii) Previously notified cases:
      NM keeps file — submit regular report
   (iii) Legal services:
      Inform NM where legal involvement

then moving away from her usual non-judgemental approach on account of child mistreatment. Both parents were drug addicts. The mother, in particular, seemed very receptive to health visiting and talked about improving the children's welfare. However, the children's condition went from bad to worse while the parents' lives were dominated by the search for drugs, and the decision had to be made to protect the children. Miss Schofield said how lonely she felt and recounted the emotional confusion associated both with the decision to take the children into care and the experience in court. Later, an accidental fire at the flat when the parents were 'high' killed the father and nearly the mother too. This provided proof that it had been the right decision, but it had been and still was painful. She felt she had learned the hard way.

A six month trial in which a specialist nursing officer dealt only with child abuse was found to be particularly successful. The health visitors appreciated the accessibility at all times, the crisis support which helped to alleviate anxiety and the help with preparation for case conferences (Bailey et al, 1984). The trial was a small one but it increased enthusiasm for a specialist post amongst the health visitors taking part.

On violence to staff

One of the issues over which health visitors need particular support is associated with the degree of risk they run working in the homes of families in which violence is relatively commonplace (Cardwell, 1987; Health Visitor, 1987a; 1987b). Guidance has been given at health visitor meetings on how to look out for signs of approaching violence (Health Visitor, 1983d; 1986) and guidelines are outlined in Box 11.5. It seems that the arrival of the health visitor can become the 'trigger event' in a situation of rising tension. The health visitor can become a scapegoat and finish up as a 'lightning conductor' for the violence. The mere presence of professional people and the extra anxieties associated with the visit, can cause them to become the object of aggression.

Robert Dingwall (1984) suggested that economic stringencies have led to an increase in this danger for community nurses. He also said that, in a way, there has been a conspiracy of silence on the issue, perhaps to prevent exacerbating the problem by attracting public attention to it. In his research, however, he found that some employers were clearly not taking the problem seriously, even after an incident had taken place. He felt that an over-emphasis on training can lead to the misguided assumption that violence can be blamed on the failure of a nurse to use the proper techniques. This he felt diverts attention away from the need for an appropriate managerial response to the basic problem.

Box 11.5 Some signs of potential aggression and violence (from Health Visitor, 1983d; 1986)

Flushed face
Trembling hands
Sweating
Raised voice
Expression of anger/hate/excessive criticism
Excitable
Pacing around
Kicks furniture
Stands up to tower over visitor

Box 11.6 Outline of HVA guidance on staff safety (From Health Visitor Association, 1984, pp. 4–6)

Policies to:
- identify hazardous areas/times of day
- outline authority's actions to minimise hazards, e.g. working in pairs, visiting on priority occasions, at certain times
- provide guidance on reporting hazards/incidents
  — management discover scale of problem
  — to inform visiting staff of need for special care
- respect health visitor's opinion of advisibility of revisit by same health visitor
  — ensure safety if revisit to take place
- state procedures to be taken following an incident
  — immediately attending any GP/occupational health
  — report matter to police
  — complete report to line manager & health & safety rep
  — authority support of prosecutions

Precautions, where relevant:
- not visiting alone after dark
- visiting: on priority occasions; notifying colleague at end of visit; with colleague outside house; in pairs; with nurse manager; doorstep only; see only at clinic
- clinic work: with minimum levels of staff where isolated; security precautions
- use of special alarm equipment — value debatable

Training should:
- centre on health visitors most at risk
- ensure familiarity with authority's safety policy and procedures available to help avoid violence
- teach how to identify potentially violent situation; simple techniques to prevent/avoid physical aggression

Some student health visitors are given self-defence training during their course, others gain what information they can from books such as Pat Butler's (1982) *Self-defence for women* or Kaleghi Quinn's (1983) *Stand your ground*, though their value is questionable (Health Visitor, 1987c) It is most important to try to keep the situation as calm as possible to avoid having to use a physically defensive strategy and getting trapped, and to have a clear idea of possible exit routes (Health Visitor, 1983d; Finney, 1988; Leiba, 1987). An outline of the Health Visitors Association's (1984) health and safety guidance on staff safety will be found in Box 11.6. It is to be hoped that it is being widely discussed and instituted at field level. The Suzy Lamplugh Trust and Carolyn Puckett Memorial Fund can offer help and advice (Smith, 1988; see useful addresses).

On records

Nurse managers should aim to enable their health visitors to make up their notes contemporaneously, that is as near in time as possible to the visit, and certainly on the same day or within 24 hours. This is for accuracy and in case the evidence they contain should ever be needed in court (Godber, 1981). An audio-typing service is an obvious advantage.

Advice from tutors on recording information is no longer likely to be against making a permanent note of 'discrediting information', which is what Dingwall (1977) had found in his research in the early 1970s. If there is any suspicion of abuse, factual and pertinent evidence of what has been said, seen or done, both by the health visitor and/or family members, must be recorded. June Helberg (1983) described factors that need to be assessed and documented, some of which are incorporated into the list of important items for recording in Box 11.7

Borderline cases

It is difficult for health visitors to reach decisions when they come across what they feel are borderline cases. It is best if they can share their problem anonymously with a sympathetic co-professional

---

Box 11.7 Important items to record where child abuse is suspected

What has been *seen* by health visitor:
- traumata such as burns, cuts, bruising, noting location and appearance
- height and weight on percentile chart, noting changes in serial observation
- developmental attainments, if possible on a bar chart or step-ladder centile chart, noting changes in serial observation
- parent–child interaction, noting reactions to each other's initiatives e.g. by touching, visual contact

What has been *said* by parent(s) recounting:
- their viewpoint and explanations of the situation
- health history, particularly evidence of organic reasons for failure to thrive
- developmental milestones, e.g. aware of and responsive to bath, ability to sit unsupported, speech development (at appropriate ages)
- family history, e.g. alcohol, drugs and history of violence

What has been *done* by health visitor:
- appointments made with family, e.g. to visit GP or clinic and for further visits by health visitor
- co-professionals contacted, e.g. GP, social worker, NSPCC
- meetings attended
- dates
  — of home visits
  — notes left for family when not found at home
  — family seen but no access to child
- contact with nurse manager re problem, e.g. not able to see family and/or child

---

who is a good listener, perhaps a social worker, another health visitor, a GP or their nurse manager. A 'hypothetical case' presented in such a way that the family could not be identified, means the health visitor can speak freely and will 'label' no one. The process of explaining the pros and cons that make the case so borderline might trigger a decision one way or the other: either, for example, that there is no real problem, or that the suspicion seems justified and should be taken a step further and formally reported.

FORMAL PROCEEDINGS

The main purpose of setting in motion the formal procedures (see Box 11.4) is to protect the child through coordinated help to the family. Three agencies have a statutory investigatory role in the protection of children: the Social Services Departments, the NSPCC and, on occasions, the police. Health visitors have no statutory powers and are unable to undertake the prolonged and frequent visiting necessary for crisis management. The time it takes up would prejudice the preventive work for the rest of their caseload.

Reporting the problem to the social services department puts the process into action. Where there seems to be great and immediate danger, the child is taken to a place of safety such as a specially selected foster home. In all cases, a case conference will be called, and the urgency with which this is done will be determined by the apparent degree of risk to the child. If at the case conference the problem is confirmed, the child's name will be entered on to the Child Concern/Abuse Register and a plan of action for care and support of the family proposed.

Hazards

There has been considerable criticism of the system, for example that it can be protectionist and over-used (Buckle, 1979; Thomas, 1980). The case conference has been described as a blunt and expensive instrument, conducted like a secret trial, convened in haste and leading to ill-thought-out, ill-informed conclusions with a resultant lack of trust between social and health workers (Barrie, 1979; Moore, 1986). Communication between health visitors and social workers has been described as far too one-sided (Musanandara, 1984).

A governmental draft guide to inter-agency co-operation has made many suggestions which, if followed, should help overcome many of these difficulties. It should also help clarify where the responsibility lies for maintaining regular contact with and coordinating the work of the various agencies involved. These and other key matters, such as coordinating and ensuring a comprehensive review of the case at least six monthly, are clearly stated as the duty of a designated social worker from either the social services department or the NSPCC (Department of Health and Social Security, 1986).

It has been suggested that in certain rare circumstances a health visitor (or other nurse) might be nominated 'prime worker' to work with a 'case coordinator', a level 3 social worker, dealing with all the administrative arrangements which are the responsibility of the 'key worker' (see Fig. 11.3). Relevant circumstances might be if the health visitor were the only worker acceptable to a family with, for example, problems of emotional abuse and neglect. This arrangement could only be made if there were agreement between the line manager and the health visitor, who would be given relief from some other caseload work (Health Visitor, 1983a, 1983b; Fawcett-Henesy, 1986).

Continued contact

In line with the policy of providing extra help for families with greater problems, staffing levels permitting, a family with child abuse and neglect difficulties would be given an increased level of visiting. This would be for surveillance of child development and nutrition, health education and some emotional support for the parents. Very occasionally, health visitors become more involved (Cannon & Walker, 1985).

When the child has been removed into care, it is important that the health visiting service is still provided. From one point of view, the child still needs to be monitored and foster parents can be very grateful for support and advice (Health Visitor, 1983c). From another point of view, it is important both to support the parents and to help them talk through the situation, and to remain in touch in readiness for the child's return.

Health visitors would expect to write a report on the case or to attend every case conference. This would occur at least every six months. If health visitors can be as open as possible with the parents about, for example, the content of their reports, it gives the parents a chance both to discuss the criteria and the issues involved and to make appropriate moves to sort out the situation (Department of Health and Social Security, 1986, p. 18). Some will want to contact parents' organisations such as PAIN, Parents Against INjustice (Holmes, 1986a; Whitehouse, 1986), or the Family Rights Group for specific help and support (addresses at the end of the chapter). Parents Aid (1987) provides a useful

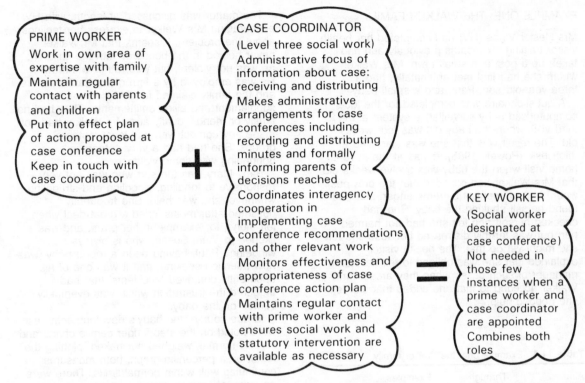

PRIME WORKER
Work in own area of expertise with family
Maintain regular contact with parents and children
Put into effect plan of action proposed at case conference
Keep in touch with case coordinator

+

CASE COORDINATOR
(Level three social work)
Administrative focus of information about case: receiving and distributing
Makes administrative arrangements for case conferences including recording and distributing minutes and formally informing parents of decisions reached
Coordinates interagency cooperation in implementing case conference recommendations and other relevant work
Monitors effectiveness and appropriateness of case conference action plan
Maintains regular contact with prime worker and ensures social work and statutory intervention are available as necessary

=

KEY WORKER
(Social worker designated at case conference)
Not needed in those few instances when a prime worker and case coordinator are appointed
Combines both roles

Fig. 11.3 Outline of functions of prime worker, case coordinator and key worker for cases where child abuse and neglect exists or is suspected.

booklet for parents with children in care or likely to be so.

A few health visitors are obliged to go to court and give evidence about their work with the family. Under these circumstances there is particular advantage if they have been open and truthful about their aims and opinions on how the family has been progressing, so that the parents learn nothing new in court. It is obviously an extremely painful experience for the parents, and is generally unnerving and distressing for the health visitor too. Peter Godber (1980a, 1980b, 1980c, 1981) has written lucidly and reassuringly on court procedure, and the Court Training Services offer pertinent advice on all the key aspects.

We have just taken a brief look at health visitors' work aimed at preventing a worsening of the situation when child abuse is discovered or suspected. Earlier in the chapter there were examples of the way health visitors aim, through

education, to prevent the occurrence of child abuse and, through selection and support, to prevent development of stresses and strains which can result in child abuse. The discussion has also provided yet another example of the use of the prevention framework proposed in this book.

EXAMPLES OF WORK IN THE FIELD OF CHILD ABUSE

The first example is of work with an exasperated young mother with an attention-seeking three-year old and a 'difficult to rear' baby. The second is of caseload-wide work aimed at preventing the occurrence and development of stresses and strains that can lead to child abuse. Outlines will be found in Tables 11.4 and 11.5.

EXAMPLE ONE: THE WALKER FAMILY

Mrs Hester Vines (HV) had completed her health visitor training six months previously and had taken up a post in a small town. Mrs Walker, whom she had first met antenatally, had a three-year-old son, Paul, and a small baby.

A questionnaire was completed for the local computerised baby surveillance system at the third visit, when the baby girl was four weeks old. The result was that she was classified as 'high risk' (Powell, 1985). It was at the seventh home visit when the baby was twelve weeks old that Mrs Walker had confided that the previous week, in a moment of extreme anger, she had found herself shaking the baby. She had checked herself and felt she had not harmed her, but was terribly distressed because she felt she might yet do that. The health visitor explained that she was obliged to tell her nurse manager of such cases when they arose. Mrs Walker acceded to that and added that she felt she needed help.

Table 11.4 Example one: the Walker family

Aim	Through	Examples
To prevent occurrence of child abusing situation	Teaching	Discussions at visits: babies' need for fondling and attention; tensions and child abuse
	Normal supportive services	Told about groups and agencies at birth visit, not followed up
To prevent development of stress & tensions leading to child abuse	1. Identifying those vulnerable 2. Enabling extra support for them	Computerised system indicated high risk baby More frequent visiting Discussion about difficulties; FIS and other entitlements
To prevent deterioration where child abuse seems to have occurred	Child-centred decisions with nurse management support	Use social and clinical evidence: naked weight and appearance; family history and social support Full, shared and contemporaneous records Multi-profession decision & action

The matter was discussed at length, with HV encouraging Mrs Walker to express her feelings about the problem. It seems that Mr Walker never helped in the house or with the children; he was not violent, but was rather withdrawn. He was employed by a firm of contract cleaners and the family claimed family income supplement and allied entitlements. They had no family or friends locally and Mrs Walker had not made any contact with any local mothers' groups. She had had a very autocratic upbringing with some violence.

Baby Mary was the sort who was not very responsive to fondling: wriggling and struggling whenever she was held. She frequently posseted after meals, cried a great deal when left alone, for example in her pram, and was likened to 'Aunt Susan, who is always wingeing'. Paul, having been a 'good baby' was now attention seeking, and it was one of his apparently contrived 'accidents' that had triggered the frustration which was eventually vented on the baby.

In due course, the baby's developmental tests were noted on the step-ladder centile charts and HV, as normal, weighed her naked, plotting the result on a percentile graph, both measures continuing well within normal limits. There were no signs of bruises, burns or weals.

Mrs Walker and HV discussed the idea of Paul attending a playgroup in the mornings and, if it were possible, getting a temporary place at a social services department day nursery two or three mornings a week. The health visitor explained she would need to tell the appropriate social worker about the problems Mrs Walker was having and that he/she might need to visit to assess for eligibility for these hard-to-come-by places. Mrs Walker said she was happy for that to be set in motion. They agreed too, that HV should contact the GP in order to ensure that an appointment be arranged for the baby to be checked over soon. A record of the visit was made before leaving the flat and HV arranged to return in two days' time.

Mrs Vines had phoned her nurse manager for an appointment and found Mrs Nora Major (NM) in her office that lunchtime as arranged. Just as Mrs Walker had found it helpful to pour out her heart to HV, HV was now grateful for NM's preparedness to listen sympathetically and to make practical suggestions. The health visitor reported that this family was not already on the Child Protection Register, and they discussed how the reports should be written. NM agreed that there would probably be playgroup and day nursery places for the children and asked if HV knew about the District 'Troublesome Baby Group' set up by some health visitors for such parents. They showed trigger films to stimulate discussion and found it had evolved into a good self-help group. She also asked if the GP knew about the problem, to which HV replied that he had undertaken to see the baby that morning.

In the event, the family was given the playgroup place for Paul and a two mornings a week nursery place for some months for Mary, which Mrs Walker found very therapeutic. She attended the 'Troublesome Baby Group' and found some good friends there. After a case conference, the family had been put on the Child Protection Register. Things went well and the name was removed at another case conference three months later. For some time after that, NM would enquire every few months how the family were progressing.

EXAMPLE TWO: STRATEGIES AIMED AT PREVENTING CHILD ABUSE

Miss Helen Voisey (HV) was reviewing schemes aiming to minimise the incidence of child abuse, both by working within her caseload and in the local community. Part of the caseload work involved trying to identify the people most vulnerable to this problem in order to offer extra support as it was needed, particularly through the first year of their baby's life. Work in the general locality involved trying to improve understanding about child care and matters associated with child abuse, to encourage open discussion, less apprehension about seeking help and greater knowledge of how to seek help, as well as better parent–child interaction.

In order to have some relevant support services, the West Seahaven District Health Authority had set aside some joint funding towards a family centre in the poorest part of town. The local authority social services day nurseries gave highest priority to cases involving actual or suspected child abuse.

It was a question of finding the families who most needed help. The previous year the health visitors had decided it would be a good idea to start an infant surveillance scheme similar to the one in Portsmouth in which both child abuse and sudden infant death factors were incorporated (Powell, 1985).

A working party had been set up and HV had been invited to join it. It had meant a great deal of hard work, looking up papers from the library and finding out how other authorities' schemes were working out. Now decisions were made

Table 11.5 Example two: strategies aimed at preventing child abuse

Aim	Through	Examples
To prevent occurrence of child abusing situation	Teaching	Parenthood courses in school: liaison with school nurse & teachers Group discussions on child abuse
	Normal supportive services	Tell about groups and agencies Normal 'therapeutic listening'
To prevent development of stress & tensions leading to child abuse	1. Identifying those vulnerable	Combined sudden infant death & child abuse surveillance scheme
	2. Enabling extra support for them	Tell of telephone crisis contact self-help groups More frequent visiting
To prevent deterioration where child abuse seems to have occurred	Child-centred decisions with nurse management support	No recent experience of suspected or actual child abuse

and the scheme they had instituted was running smoothly.

Some 5% of HV's caseload were rated as 'high risk', and so far she had had none rated 'very high risk'. Very few needed the sort of supportive help that was required in the areas nearer the centre of town. Many of the women in her caseload were able to afford babysitters to give them a break, had mothers or sisters living nearby, or had joined a specially organised self-help babysitting circle. She had just introduced two new mothers to a newly developing group and had been invited to lead a discussion on child abuse at one of their monthly evening meetings. It seems they had heard about her talks at the women's groups of the local churches.

At a recent meeting of community health nurses and teachers at the local school there had been a great deal of interest in health educational aspects of child abuse. The school nurse, HV and the general studies teacher had spent a good deal of time discussing various aspects of the topic, and had swapped ideas and given each other leads on relevant articles and pamphlets. The other two had not known of the Ackley (1977) paper; HV heard about pamphlets specifically for children, about which some of 'her mothers' might like to know. The teacher had asked if HV knew a mother who would be prepared to come and bath her baby and to talk about what it really feels like to be a mother — the difficulties as well as the joys. One mother, an ex-teacher, had since offered to go.

It seemed to HV that working together with other professionals had helped improve all their contributions towards health education over child abuse. She had worked with the priests and vicars and was now working with the teachers and, as ever, with the school nurse. Working with other health visitors had helped bring in a useful new infant surveillance scheme.

However, Miss Voisey concluded, child abuse could never be thought about or dealt with in isolation, but was necessarily an aspect of wider considerations. For example, in health education it is just one part of any discussion on parentcraft, in caseload work a relevant part of wider infant surveillance and, for the individual parent, part of and influenced by their social situation.

USEFUL ADDRESSES

Court Training Services
79 Merton Hall Road
Wimbledon
London SW19 3TX
Tel 081 540 7487

Family Rights Group
6–9 Manor Gardens
Holloway Road
London N7 6LA
Tel 071 272 4231/2
071 272 7308

PAIN, Parents Against Injustice
Conifers
2 Pledgeon Green
nr Henham
Bishop's Stortford
Herts
Tel 0279 850545

Sue Weston
Carolyn Puckett Memorial Fund
c/o Oxford Regional
Health Authority
Old Road
Headington
Oxford OX3 7LF

The Suzy Lamplugh Trust
14 East Sheen Avenue
London SW14 8AS

REFERENCES

Ackley D C 1977 A brief overview of child abuse. Social Casework 58: 21–24

Ashley A 1980 Voluntary self-help for parents under stress in Britain. Midwife Health Visitor and Community Nurse 16: 244–246

Bailey J, Ramm K, Warner U 1984 The nursing officer's role. Nursing Times Community Outlook 80, 11: 102

Barker W 1990a Practical and ethical doubts about screening for child abuse. Health Visitor 63, 1: 14–17

Barker W 1990b The aetiology of child sexual abuse. Nursing Times Community Outlook 86, 14: 25–26

Barrie H 1979 Personal opinion — on case conferences. Midwife Health Visitor and Community Nurse 15: 188–192

Black J A 1986 Misdiagnosis of child abuse in ethnic minorities. Midwife Health Visitor and Community Nurse 22: 48–53

Borkowski M, Murch M, Walker V 1983 Marital violence — the community response. Tavistock Publications, London

Buckle J 1979 NAI registers: a substitute for communication. Social Work Today 10, 30: 23

Butler A J 1983 A walk-in unit for pre-school children and their mothers. Health Visitor 56: 411–412

Butler P 1982 Self-defence for women. New English Library, London

Cannon D, Walker J 1985 Getting off the treadmill. Health Visitor 58: 192–193

Cardwell C 1987 Victims of violence. Health Visitor 60, 11: 355

Chan M C K 1985 Chinese and Vietnamese families (letter). British Medical Journal 290 1588

Child Sexual Abuse Preventive Education Project, Driver E 1985 Have your children been sexually abused? CSAPEP, c/o Hungerford House, Victoria Embankment, London WC2

Dean J G, MacQueen I A G, Mitchell R G, Kempe C H 1978 Health visitor's role in prediction of early childhood injuries and failure to thrive. Child Abuse and Neglect 2: 1–17

Department of Health and Social Security 1982 Child abuse. A study of inquiry reports 1973–1981. HMSO, London

Department of Health and Social Security 1986 Working together. A draft guide to arrangements for interagency cooperation for the protection of children. DHSS, London

Dingwall R 1977 The social organisation of health visitor training. Croom Helm, London, p. 108

Dingwall R 1983 Child abuse — the real questions. Nursing Times 79, 25: 67–68

Dingwall R 1984 Who is to blame, anyway? Nursing Times 80, 15: 42–43

Dingwall R, Eekelaar J, Murray T 1981 Care or control? Decision-making in the care of children thought to have been abused or neglected. A summary of the final report. Social Science Research Council Centre for Socio-Legal Studies, Wolfson College, Oxford

Dingwall R, Eekelaar J, Murray T 1983 The protection of children. State intervention and family life. Basil Blackwell, Oxford

Elliot M 1985 The child assault prevention programme. Health Visitor 58: 187–188

Fawcett-Henesy A 1986 Who is the key worker? Community Care 605: 20–21

Finney G 1988 One false move. Nursing Times Community Outlook 84, 15: 8–9

Fort A 1986 The spider's web. The Health Service Journal 96: 558–559

Forward S, Buck C 1981 Betrayal of innocence: incest and its devastation. Pelican Books, Harmondsworth, Middlesex

Fox S, Dingwall R 1985 An exploratory study of variations in social workers' and health visitors' definitions of child mistreatment. British Journal of Social Work 15: 467–477

Gelles R J 1975 The social construction of child abuse. American Journal of Orthopsychiatry 45, 3: 363–371

Godber P 1980a The health visitor in court – 1. Health Visitor 53: 83–84

Godber P 1980b The health visitor in court – 2. Health Visitor 53: 162–164

Godber P 1980c The health visitor in court – 3. Health Visitor 53: 206–209

Godber P 1981 Confidentiality of case records. Health Visitor 54: 193

Greenland C 1986 Preventing child abuse and neglect deaths: the identification and management of high risk cases. Health Visitor 59: 205–206

Health Visitor 1983a Child abuse: a step forward. Health Visitor 56: 41

Health Visitor 1983b Health visitor's role in child abuse clarified. Health Visitor 56: 43

Health Visitor 1983c Children in care: HVs should be more involved. Health Visitor 56: 115

Health Visitor 1983d Violence: coping strategies for HVs. Health Visitor 56: 442

Health Visitor 1986 Violence to health visitors: health authorities must have safety policies. Health Visitor 59: 27

Health Visitor 1987a Violence towards NHS staff. Health Visitor 60, 6: 208

Health Visitor 1987b Violence against staff: an increasing risk. Health Visitor 60, 9: 305

Health Visitor 1987c Health visitors at least risk. Health Visitor 60, 11: 375

Health Visitor Association 1984 Health and safety in the community — some guidance on safety policies from the Health Visitors' Association. Health Visitors' Association, London, p 4–6

Helberg J L 1983 Documentation in child abuse. American Journal of Nursing 83, 2: 236–239

Holmes P 1986a Innocent parents. Nursing Times 82, 3: 16–18

Holmes P 1986b It's OK to say no. Nursing Times 82, 3: 18

Jarman B 1989 General practice. In: While A (ed) Health in the inner city. Heinemann Medical, Oxford

Jay M 1985 The Jasmine Beckford case. Death of a child in care. The Listener 114, 2931: 6–7

Johnson C 1985 Identifying children at risk: a system for health visitors. Health Visitor 58: 195–196

Kempe R S, Kempe C H 1978 Child abuse. Fontana, London

Korbin J E 1980 The cross-cultural context of child abuse and neglect. In: Kempe C H, Helfer R E (eds) The battered child 3rd ed. University of Chicago Press, London

Laurance J 1985 Collating information to prevent child abuse. Primary Health Care 3, 11: 6

Leiba P A 1987 Violence: the community nurse's dilemma. Health Visitor 60, 11: 361–362

Lynch M A, Roberts J 1977 Predicting child abuse: signs of bonding failure in the maternity hospital. British Medical Journal I: 624–626

Meacher M A 1982 Self-help groups for parents under stress: a contribution to prevention? Mental Health Foundation, London

Moore J 1985 For the children's sake. Nursing Times 81, 42: 19–20

Moore J 1986 All in the family. Community Care 609: 22–23

Musnandara T 1984 Communication between workers: the key in cases of child abuse? Health Visitor 57: 233

Nelson S 1982 Incest: fact and myth. Stramullion Co-operative Ltd, Edinburgh

Nursing Times 1982 New team to look at Gates death. Nursing Times 78: 2010

Nursing Times 1985 The Beckford case has shown it is vital to have sufficient clinical managers to back up community staff. Nursing Times 81, 50: 3

Oates R K 1984 Overturning the diagnosis of child abuse. Archives of Disease in Childhood 59: 665–666

O'Doherty N 1982 The battered child. Recognition in primary care. Bailliere Tindall, London

Ounsted C, Roberts J C, Gordon M, Milligan B 1982 Fourth goal of perinatal medicine. British Medical Journal 284: 879–882

Parents Aid 1987 Guide for parents with children in care: 101 questions and answers. 4th ed. Parents Aid, 66 Chippingfield, Harlow, Essex CM17 ODJ

Parton N 1985 The politics of child abuse. Macmillan, London

Powell J 1985 Keeping watch. Nursing Times Community Outlook 81, 2: 15–19

Pownall M 1985 A family affair? Nursing Times 81, 43: 58–61

Quinn K 1983 Stand your ground: a woman's guide to self-preservation. Orbis, London

Radbill S X 1980 Children in a world of violence: a history of child abuse. In: Kempe C H, Helfer R E (eds) The battered child 3rd ed. University of Chicago Press, London

Renvoise J 1982 Incest: a family pattern. Routledge and Kegan Paul, London

Ross K R, Smith E S, Williams E O, Bradley S J, Wright J D 1977 Frozen awareness. A guide to diagnosis and management of non-accidental injury to children. Wolverhampton Area Review Committee, Wolverhampton

Schofield J 1983 Visiting can be stressful, too. Nursing Mirror 157, 13: 20–21

Search G 1988 The last taboo. Sexual abuse of children. Penguin Books, London

Smith S 1988 Take care, be aware. Nursing Times Community Outlook 84, 15: 10–12

Thomas T 1980 Blinded by the light when the red button is pushed. Health and Social Services Journal LXXXX: 950–951

Thorneley N 1986 Child abuse lessons from the past (letter). Nursing Times 82, 2: 12

Tucker N 1985 A panic over child abuse. New Society 74: 96–98

Vizard E 1985 Facing the facts. Nursing Mirror 161, 17: 14–15

Waterhouse I 1981 A bar on abuse. Health and Social Services Journal XCI: 1302–1303

Weeks V 1982 Health visitors, stress and non-accidental injury to children. Health Visitor 55: 75

Whitehouse A 1986 The anguish of the parent. Community Care 597: 20–22

Woods J 1981 A practical approach to preventing child abuse. Health Visitor 54: 281–283

FURTHER READING

Child sexual abuse

Anna, Founder of Incest Crisis Line 1989 (letter) Sex abuse sufferers. Nursing Times 85, 34: 14 — Provides address for help for any mother whose partner has sexually abused her child.

DSS 1988 Diagnosis of child sexual abuse. Guidance for doctors. HMSO, London

DHSS 1988 Report of the inquiry into child abuse in Cleveland 1987. Chaired by Elizabeth Butler-Schloss. HMSO, London

Dingwall R 1987 A parental perogative? Nursing Times 83, 17: 51

Dingwall R 1987 The new language of care. Nursing Times 83, 29: 19–20

Dunn M 1988 Breaking the silence. Health Visitor 61, 8: 258–260 — Cleveland child sexual abuse crisis, a personal perspective.

Dunn M 1989 Realities of Cleveland. Nursing Times 85, 10: 28–31

Fillmore A 1987 Sexual molestation of children: becoming aware. Health Visitor 60, 10: 325–327

Johnson R A 1985 Incest Crisis Line. Health Visitor 58: 187

McFarlane K, Waterman J 1986 Sexual abuse of young children. Guildford Press, New York

Mills J 1985 Breaking the last taboo. The Listener 114, 2933: 11–12

Roberts J, Dundee Royal Infirmary Child Sexual Abuse Team 1987 How to cope when your child has been sexually abused. A guide for parents. The Child and Family Trust, 21 Bath Street, Glasgow G2 1HX — Copies provided free for parents.

Trowell J 1985 Working with families where incest is actual or feared. Health Visitor 58: 189–191

Vizard E 1984 The sexual abuse of children. Health Visitor 57: 234–236

Vizard E 1984 The sexual abuse of children — part 2. Health Visitor 57: 279–280

Wild N J 1986 Sexual abuse of children in Leeds. British Medical Journal 292: 1113–1116

Zeitlin H 1987 Investigation of the sexually abused child. The Lancet 2: 842–845

Decision-making and evidence

Hall J G, Mitchell B H 1978 Child abuse — procedure and evidence in Juvenile Courts. Barry Rose, Chichester

Vernon J, Fruin D 1986 In care. A study of social work decision making. National Children's Bureau, London

Emotional abuse

Gath A 1984 Emotional abuse. Maternal and Child Health 9: 229–232

Gath A 1985 Recognition and treatment of emotional abuse. Update 31: 445–452

Trowell J 1983 Emotional abuse of children. Health Visitor 56: 252–255

Ethical dilemmas

Community Outlook 1988 Cinderella on the doorstep. Nursing Times Community Outlook 84, 6: 3

Taylor S, Tilley N 1989 Health visitors and child protection: conflict, contradictions and ethical dilemmas. Health Visitor 62, 9: 273–275

Emery J L 1987 (letter) Preventing child abuse. Health Visitor 60, 2: 36

Emery J L 1987 The ethics of intervention in child abuse and sudden infant death. Health Visitor 60, 10: 332–334

Taylor S, James D 1987 Children at risk: the changing role of the health visitor. Health Visitor 60, 10: 329–330

General

Appleby F 1989 Essential reading. Health Visitor 62, 9: 286 — There are also many reviews and articles on child abuse in this copy of the journal.

Carver V (ed) 1978 Child abuse, a study text. Open University Press, Milton Keynes

DHSS 1987 Access to children at risk CI(87)4. DHSS, London

DSS 1988 Child protection: guidance for senior nurses, health visitors and midwives. Prepared by Standing Nursing and Midwifery Advisory Committee for Secretaries of State for Social Services and Wales. HMSO, London

DOH 1988 Protecting children: a guide for social workers undertaking a comprehensive assessment. HMSO, London

Jones D N 1982 Understanding child abuse. Hodder and Stoughton, London

Kempe C H, Helfer R E 1980 The battered child. 3rd edn. University of Chicago Press, London

Lee C M (ed) 1978 Child abuse, a reader and sourcebook. Open University Press, Milton Keynes

Renvoise J 1978 Web of violence. A study of family violence. Penguin Books, Harmondsworth

Rogers W S 1989 Child abuse and neglect. Nursing Times Community Outlook 85, 10: 21–22

Rogers W S, Iskander R 1990 'You did everything possible'. 'What if I got it wrong?' Dilemmas of child protection for health visitors and school nurses. Health Visitor Association, London

The law

Bailey J M 1980 The law and the community nurse. Nursing Department, Cumbria Area Health Authority, Caldcotes, Caldewgate, Carlisle CA2 5TT

Burr M 1982 The law and health visitors. Edsall, London

Department of Health and Social Security 1985 Review of child care law. Report to ministers of an interdepartmental working party. HMSO, London

Health Visitors' Association 1982 The law and health visitors. Health Visitors' Association, London

Health Visitors' Association 1989 Appearing in court as a witness. Health Visitors' Association, London

Mother–infant bonding

Robson K M, Powell E 1982 Early maternal attachment. In: Brockington I F, Kumar R (eds) Motherhood and mental illness. Academic Press, London

Valman H B 1980 Mother–infant bonding. British Medical Journal 280: 308–310

Chapter 12 develops the health visitor cycle model for a community-wide view of the work, looking at background knowledge, liaison work, client perspective and evaluation, as the different levels of information that help decision-making in community health development.

12

Inner city work

This chapter moves on to a community perspective in health visiting. It starts with a brief description of some of the difficulties in inner city work. This is followed by real-life examples of community health development, an increasingly popular and effective way of providing health promotion services in these and other deprived areas. There is a discussion, presented through the health visitor cycle format, of some of the matters associated with this work.

FINDING SOLUTIONS

It is well known that special attention is needed in many inner city areas. Multiple problems including poor environmental conditions, families on low income, high levels of unemployment and mobile populations from a diversity of backgrounds and cultures, mean specially tailored solutions need to be devised.

Acceptability of schemes

Recent reports on primary health care in the London inner city areas were reviewed by Alison While (1982). Each had suggested more resources and improved staffing levels. She questioned whether this would prove to be the solution to the problems and suggested that a change of approach might be more important. She felt there was a need for more sensitivity to the acceptability of the services offered to inner city dwellers. The present 'middle class medical model' seemed inadequate and a more flexible approach was advocated. Examples of good practice and useful ideas have been brought together in *Health in the inner city* (While, 1989).

A study by Downham et al (1980) which looked at the provision of child health services in Newcastle upon Tyne, showed that services were not concentrated in the parts of the city where they were most needed. Downham et al also felt that the most important factor is the *quality* of the services and that it is this that affects the extent to which they are used. However, they said that improving the quality of services is very difficult whilst they remain quantitatively inadequate.

Three examples of inner city initiatives aiming to improve the health of the local people, were described by Elizabeth Watson (1984). One at the Thomas Coram Research Unit set up experimental 'walk-in' clinics, which adopted a wide view of child health surveillance and included concern with the mothers' mental health. 20% of the children attending were found to have special problems. The mothers appreciated the broader approach and continued to attend as the children got older. This was in contrast to the normal, shorter pattern of clinic attendance in which the initial frequent visits with a new baby tail off sharply, with few people returning to discuss the care of toddlers and young children.

Parental involvement

Child health surveillance programmes were rejected in the Riverside project in Newcastle upon Tyne, in favour of giving parents common clinical information which research had shown was ill-understood. In this way, the project enabled parents to make their own decisions, to take responsibility for their children's health and motivated them to do something about it.

In a third example of inner city initiatives described by Elizabeth Watson, one in Nottingham, the number of routine examinations was reduced. The emphasis was changed towards dealing with the problems identified by parents, nursery teachers and others in contact with the child. Health

visitors, of course, had a key role. It had been suggested that they should refer children to a named doctor. Dr Nicoll (1983) described how this more flexible system was both more efficient and effective in detecting new problems, by concentrating doctors' skills where a problem is already suspected and by using other people's skills in recognising that something needs to be looked at.

Concern over scoring system

A birth scoring system for identifying 'at risk' babies was implemented in Nottingham. It showed around 5% of the babies in the more affluent areas were classified as high risk, as opposed to 30% in some inner urban wards. Here the health visitors' workload was increased because, not only was there a large number of high scoring babies, but the birth rate was also higher. It had been decided to allocate new staff, as they became available, to these inner city wards and to maintain the level of health visitor services in the more affluent areas. The scheme would be dependent, though, on attracting staff to work in these inner city areas (Madeley & Latham, 1979).

After seven years' experience with this system, Madeley (1988) now advises health authorities against setting up a scoring system. He is concerned about disproportionate resources being poured into such schemes to the exclusion of others and suggests concentration on improved standards of responsiveness to parents' requests and active professional education. Wendy Hull (1989) graphically pointed out that a rigid schedule is not compatible with a responsive, needs-led service.

Work with local people

One health visitor accepted the challenge of inner city work in a very positive way. Sue Phillips (1986) found herself working on a historically under-resourced housing estate, with high levels of social deprivation. The estate was on the edge of two local authorities, neither of whom was keen to accept responsibility for providing facilities. She decided that some part of her time must be spent campaigning for increased services, working as a 'catalyst' behind a community based project to set up a family centre. This activity was undertaken in partnership with parents, local residents and local workers. She was allowed to work on her own initiative and received encouragement over the project from her managers.

The question was raised as to whether health visitors should be involved in 'political action' of this nature (Phillips, 1986). Health visitors, like other workers, face the problem that where change is sought, this is recognised as a form of political activity. However, deciding to take no action to change things and supporting the status quo, is just as much 'political action'. The difference is that the inactivity associated with tacit acceptance makes it less noticeable.

Acceptance of things as they are can have derogatory effects. When searching for possible failures in the child care services associated with infant deaths, Jepson et al (1983) concluded that health visitors should not work in grossly deprived areas for too long. This was on account of the likelihood of their eventual acceptance of conditions that would be considered abnormal by an outsider. A health visitor busily engaged in background help aimed at improving the local situation, is less likely to be so accepting and immune to the reality. Sue Phillips provides a good example of what *can* be done in the face of gross social deprivation and we shall return to her work in the concluding pages of this book.

Planning positively

A common dilemma facing health visitors working in inner city areas, is associated with expectations that they will fill in the gaps created by the lack of social services and staff. Working in Southwark during the strike by social workers brought this fact into sharp focus for Jane Schofield (1984). She described how easy it is to respond to people's crisis situations and to slip into a social work role. Other, more routine visiting suffers as a consequence, and the risk of missing important health problems in other families is increased. It is important, she says, to be clear about what we are employed for, and that it may help to remember that other workers would not step over into our nursing role if there were a shortage. In essence, each authority must be held responsible for its own obligations — and health visitors should undertake health visiting.

These inner city pressures can also crowd out time to plan logically to change from our traditional approach towards a consumer approach, which identifies and responds proactively to local need (Fatchett, 1989).

However, there are some health authorities who are taking positive steps towards ensuring health visitors are free to perform their proper function in inner cities and large housing estates, particularly in those with multiple deprivation.

COMMUNITY HEALTH DEVELOPMENT: FOUR REAL-LIFE EXAMPLES

One approach to health visiting in areas of deprivation is community health development. In the rest of this chapter, we shall concentrate on this particular aspect of inner city work. Four examples demonstrate the style of work and each is outlined in the health visitor cycle framework, slightly modified to accommodate this wider perspective of health visiting. One example also includes a modified family health needs model and two examples include a modified prevention model. The health visitor cycle provides the format for the second half of the chapter in which we look at some of the important issues involved in this work.

Each of the examples highlights a particular aspect of community development. The first looks especially at the processes and outcome and the next at the specialist health visitor's influence on other health visitors. The third looks more closely at the project users and in the final example, the health visitor has a particular remit for 'Under-fives'. In this and the following three chapters, half the space is given to real-life examples, to enable the reader to have a better picture of what is actually happening in practice.

EXAMPLE ONE: HEALTH-HUT-BASED COMMUNITY DEVELOPMENT

The work of Christa Wynn-Williams in a Scottish inner city housing estate, goes right to the heart of client-centred health visiting. Christa's aim is to enable people to understand and to take control of their health — on their own terms. It is a catalytic role and is outlined in Figure 12.1.

The project has been developing over the past five years, starting for the first two with only one worker. It has recently moved into 'The Health Hut', a building that was, up until recently, the health clinic. A community development worker and a part-time worker from the local community are the other members of the project team. Their remit is to encourage people's strengths and enable them to use their own skills. The project uses a collective rather than an individual approach.

Employing this perspective in health visiting has paid off. We can demonstrate this by taking the 'Women and Food Group' as an example. The group grew out of work with one woman, who after some visits on other issues, poured out her worries about compulsive eating. A medical approach looking at physical factors, cutting food and regular weighing, had failed. The next step, 'victim-blaming', would have labelled her as recalcitrant and non-cooperative. Fortunately, Christa is very aware that this sort of problem involves much wider issues, such as self-image and a variety of interlocking social and emotional factors. She wondered how to

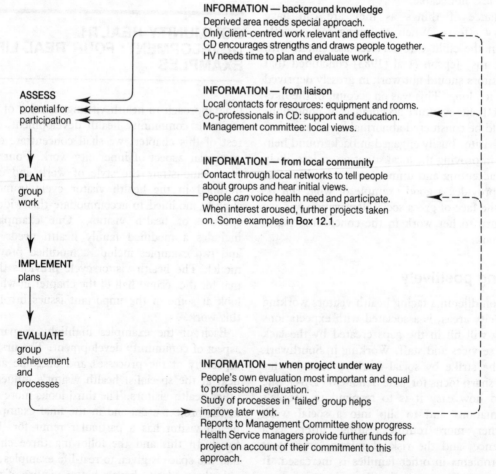

Fig. 12.1 Health visitor cycle outlining Christa's catalytic approach to group work, enabling community development (CD) in an inner city housing estate.

respond. Her remit to take a community perspective led Christa to ask if her client knew of other people with this difficulty and suggested the woman got them together, perhaps in her own home.

Twelve people came to that first meeting. The group grew. Members gradually trusted and then confided in each other. As their basic problems came to light they were able to talk them through and to support each other. A deeper understanding evolved and they are now much better able to cope.

The team is involved in many aspects of care. Some of the projects are listed in Box 12.1. Their policy is to provide child care, as necessary, whenever meetings are held. These new premises have a crèche room. Funding includes money to pay a crèche worker part-time. This will mean that the mothers will be able to concentrate better on the discussions of health and welfare issues in the Health Hut group work.

A significant success is the Elderly Forum, an organising group of pensioners, which meets in the members' homes. It takes up any issue pertaining to the health of the elderly. This group sets up 'Away Days' when about 80 pensioners are taken to pleasant surroundings and have a choice of fun and discussion workshops. These outings broaden social contacts and experience, as well as a wider understanding of health. They include:

- art
- keyboard music
- dream workshop
- creative writing
- discussing death, coping with change
- aromatherapy
- gentle exercise
- massage
- relaxation.

This pensioner 'ginger group' arranged a conference to find out what older people felt is needed. Three of the needs identified at the conference are being met through setting up an Urban Aid Elderly Project employing four workers. In another project, the group found their chiropody services inadequate. After this campaign, local clinics were doubled and the campaign continues throughout Lothian.

It is hard work enabling people to organise things themselves. It would be much quicker for Christa to do much of the work herself. But it would not have anything like the same result, either in the increased self-confidence of the participants or in the further projects taken up. This 'empowering' approach is clearly necessary.

On the face of it, sitting and drinking tea with old people appears an easy job. However, what the casual observer will not see is, for example, Christa's helping to:

- monitor group processes
- develop group work skills

Box 12.1 Family health needs model showing some examples of the local problems in an inner city housing estate and local people's solutions, enabled through Christa's endeavours

Environment	Physical health	Mental/emotional health	Social aspects of health
Problems			
1. Poor uptake of available services	4. Nutrition poor. Fruit and vegetables expensive	7. Many emotional problems	9. Many isolated people
2. People's view unknown and unsought	5. Weight difficulties	8. Children distract in group work	10. Child care provision for under 2's is minimal
3. Health service provision inadequate	6. Elderly: many foot problems: chiropody waiting list closed		
Solutions			
1. Group work approach improves participation in health work	4. Fruit and vegetable cooperative set up by local people	7. Group work provides mutual support and self-help counselling	9. Local social networks increased by group and campaigning activities
2. Conference & questionnaires glean views and encourage activism	5. Women and Food Group established	8. Crèche enables concentration on work at group sessions at Health Hut	10. Project supportive of a child care group which is working on this issue
3. Campaigning improved service provision	6. Chiropody service doubled		

- pick up group members' particular interests
- encourage client evaluation and
- find leadership qualities.

Talking with Christa, it is easy to see how her personality and her approach provide the necessary background support and sensitively measured encouragement. She has written about how she was drawn into group work and has provided some useful hints on what makes it successful (Wynn-Williams, 1988).

People working in community development have themselves a special need for support. A social work trainer now acts as Christa's consultant and they regularly discuss her work. The project team reviews its work weekly. Full reports are written for the project's management committee, which is mainly made up of local people.

It is clear that this style of health visiting is extremely valuable in a deprived area. It is an approach of which we will hear more.

EXAMPLE TWO: HEALTH-CENTRE-BASED COMMUNITY DEVELOPMENT

There are some important potential advantages in working from a health centre base. Firstly it is easier for a health visitor specialist in community development, such as Yvonne Ashley, to maintain close contact with the profession. Secondly, she and the team of health visitors (HVs) can build up a two-way support and education system.

Yvonne came into this Edinburgh inner city post after three years researching women's health in relation to group work. Yvonne was very aware of the lack of tuition in group skills during her health visiting training and at first was forced to rely on the expertise she had built up on women's health both during her research and from her earlier career. Later, she formed a management group to help guide her work and training. This group was composed of workers from health education and community education as well as health visitors from management and from within the Health Centre team. Initially, they met three-monthly to consider Yvonne's written report on her work. In between these meetings she saw individual members for guidance and support.

There are many advantages in assigning a post such as this within an inner city health visiting team. The other health visitors are either GP attached or work in a very wide geographical area. This prevents them from developing an intimate knowledge of the people and the locality

in which they are based. Yvonne has been able to pass on to the rest of the team her increasing knowledge of the area: its strengths as well as its health needs. Working with other health visitors so closely means that they get absorbed into many of the projects Yvonne is involved with, either directly, or through referring clients to groups. This has stimulated interest and drawn many of the team towards working in a community development way.

Yvonne works closely with community development workers from other disciplines. This helps with her 'education' and allows them to make use of her health visiting expertise. She has worked with them on various projects including women's groups and a festival for older people. She 'networks' within the community, constantly visiting community centres, church halls and places where people collect, such as bowling clubs, old age pensioner groups, women's organisations and schools. She gets around by bike and finds it a very good way to travel as she sees so many people on the way.

Discovering local health needs and local people's feelings about the suitability or otherwise of the services available, is central to the work. The aim is to encourage involvement and participation in health decisions through promoting self-confidence and increasing access to health knowledge. An informal approach is used to help individuals articulate their health needs and to help them to meet these needs in ways that are comfortable for them. For example, as an alternative to parentcraft classes, the health visitors have set up groups called 'Becoming A Parent'. Here health visitors do not give talks and invite a response, but act as facilitators to encourage expectant parents to discuss their fears and hopes with one another. This helps them begin to acknowledge their own expertise and knowledge in this area and so increases their self-confidence as prospective parents. They also get support and advice from each other and develop friendships which continue into the postnatal period. The informality of the sessions encourages parents to see health visitors as friends and not figures of authority.

Yvonne and other health visitors have been working with a group of local people to open a Health Shop. This will provide open access for the local population to obtain health information and get help with problems. It will be staffed and managed by local volunteers who will be trained in information giving and may go on to do counselling training if they wish. They will work alongside health visitors and other nurses. In this way, more equal relationships between professionals and lay people can be formed and different kinds of knowledge be seen as complementary.

Good results have come from all this client-centred work, which is outlined in Figure 12.2. There is plenty of evidence of improved self-esteem amongst the participants and this is reflected in an increased take-up of other opportunities that exist. These include activism in other local projects, furthering general education and joining in health related activities such as swimming. Many people were too shy before, and gained confidence through the health groups.

Local people are grateful for the health contribution brought to both the newly created and the established groups. This is being reported back from a variety of sources. Yvonne

has provided greater access to health promotion and has significantly raised the profile of health visiting locally. There are now frequent requests for her involvement in health related activities. The cooperation of local newspaper journalists enables people to be informed about what is going on. There is a great deal of interest in the plans for the Health Shop.

The exchange of ideas between Yvonne, as a health visitor doing community development within a health visiting perspective, and the other health visitors within the team looks a very good formula for improving inner city health and welfare. The mutual support is essential as working together on the Health Shop and in the 'Becoming a Parent' group has shown. It is evident that a symbiotic relationship can develop from health-centre-based community development health visiting.

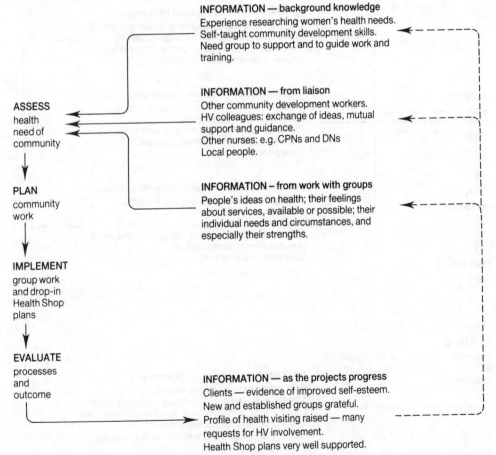

Fig. 12.2 Health visitor cycle outlining Yvonne Ashley's community group work and plans for a Health Shop in an inner city area.

EXAMPLE THREE: MULTI-DISCIPLINARY TEAM COMMUNITY DEVELOPMENT

The housing estate of about 4000 inhabitants where Dorothy Robbie works, has been designated an area of multiple deprivation. A multi-disciplinary team was established to increase the community's access to a wide range of professional skills, and Dorothy applied to become the team's health visitor.

Health visiting through locally based initiatives certainly appealed. This approach, outlined in Figure 12.3, is useful to get through to people with the greatest need and poorest health. It can discover how these people view their own health needs and the requirements of their neighbourhood and respond, using whatever opportunities happen to arise. An informal setting allows professionals to be seen primarily as people and helps to encourage active involvement of the local residents.

Under the current GP attachment arrangements, 27 health visitors visit families on the estate. The service is therefore very fragmented and it would not be easy for so many to work together using a community perspective. Having worked as a GP attached health visitor, Dorothy was very aware of the limitations of the system.

The multi-disciplinary approach provides a wide variety of experience and skills for special initiatives. The team is based in a Family Centre, the old health clinic. Besides the health visitor, there is:

(from the Health Board)
- health education officer

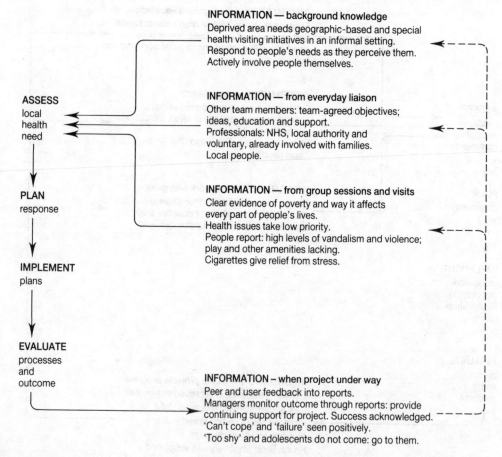

Fig. 12.3 Health visitor cycle outlining Dorothy Robbie's community development health visiting in an area of multiple deprivation.

(from the Education Department)

- home economist
- teacher
- educational psychologist (one day a week)

(from the Social Work Department)

- nursery nurse
- clerical assistant with a knowledge of welfare rights
- project coordinator with a social work background.

Despite a wide variety of working conditions and different salaries, members of the team work together very harmoniously. However, special efforts are needed when new staff join. Objectives for the project are regularly discussed and agreed by the whole team. Team members are able to develop their own special interests and abilities.

A great deal is achieved at the Family Centre (see Table 12.1). It provides a 'drop-in' facility and a supportive 'holding effect' for people until they are able to be seen by the appropriate service. Local services are very limited. One example is that there is no chemist. Another is the many women with significant stress

Table 12.1 Prevention model providing some examples of how Dorothy Robbie's health visiting aims are achieved

Aim	Through	Examples
Prevent occurrence of problems	Health education and promoting awareness	Individual awareness heightened: specific health issues in group work Managers and policy-makers: reality of problem for people who have inadequate resources and services
Prevent development of problems	Search and early care	Discover use of service preferred: e.g. group attended for cervical smears Try to fill in gaps in services: counselling for depressed, liaison for the Homeless Unit
Prevent deterioration where problems already exist	Support	Much of the work is 'drop-in' and 'holding effect' Act as advocate, using knowledge of system and contacts, to get help for very needy: e.g. patients admitted to psychiatric unit

symptoms — and an eight month waiting list for a psychologist. Dorothy is able to use her special knowledge of the health services to get help for people who need immediate attention, such as when she has enabled urgent cases to be admitted to a psychiatric unit.

Many of the people who come to the Family Centre are self-referrals or have been told about it by their neighbours. A wide range of regular sessions is held, for example mother and toddler groups and a playgroup for children over two, and parents can attend two sessions a week. There is a crèche provided for parents coming to activities like the health economist's food workshop or the women's health group. At the latter, topics such as

- pre-menstrual tension
- menopause
- gynaecological matters
- female anatomy and physiology
- basic health and
- exercise

are chosen. They have taken a trip to the local sports centre and have gone as a group to get a cervical smear test.

Conversations in the group sessions bring clear evidence of poverty and the way it affects every part of people's lives. Day-to-day living is very hard. For example, there are high levels of vandalism and violence and there are no safe child-play amenities. Health issues take low priority. Cigarettes provide a means of relief from stress. The health workers have to accept and to understand factors such as the high levels of smoking and other health-inhibiting behaviour. There is nothing to be gained, and a great deal to be lost, by appearing to be judgemental about such issues.

In order to help to find out people's wishes, the health education officer devised and circulated a questionnaire. Local people have acted as interviewers. The forms are just coming back now. This activity will make it much easier to pinpoint the areas of health of concern to the local community. Early feedback shows that the problem of dog fouling and lack of local chemist and GPs are prominent issues.

Working in this deeply client-centred way is by no means easy. Trying to cope in the face of an almost total lack of services at the local Homeless Unit, provides a good example. The team's mutual guidance and support system for each other is very important. Feeling 'a failure' and 'unable to cope' are seen as permissible and perfectly normal, a factor not widely understood in nursing.

On account of being allowed so much professional freedom, the health visiting post has in fact been developing well. The Health Board will therefore be continuing to finance it when the project's urban aid funding runs out.

Half of the project's management committee of ten is from higher echelons of the Health Board and half from local authority management. Through this contact, they have become more aware of the gap in the services to very vulnerable families. There has been an improved link through to the policy makers, especially in the social work and housing departments, which have subsequently planned for more interdisciplinary strategies offering supportive services. There are no local people on this management committee, which would have ensured even clearer awareness and impetus for change.

Looking to the future, Dorothy is hoping to become better known in the community and to meet people too shy to come to the Centre. She hopes to go out to where the problems are and has tentative plans to help young girls who are pregnant and those who have young babies and do not use the clinic. Detached youth workers, community education workers, trained to use unorthodox methods to reach young people, will probably be able to help her make contact.

It is clear that special initiatives are necessary in areas of multiple deprivation. Health visiting from within a multidisciplinary team is yet another effective way to provide the scope, support and encouragement, planning and evaluation necessary for this work.

EXAMPLE FOUR: COMMUNITY DEVELOPMENT: COMBINED POST

The huge 1930s Midland city council housing estate where Angela Pardo has worked ever since she qualified, was clearly identified in the 1981 Census statistics as an area of multiple deprivation. A programme of improvement was undertaken from 1984. Community and family centres and various community workers were provided. Much of the housing has been modernised.

Two years ago, in 1988, Angela took up a joint-funded health visiting post which forms part of this programme. The funding is specifically for families with under-fives, but apart from that, the post has a very broad remit for preventive health care on the estate. Figure 12.4 and Table 12.2 outline the work.

Being at the forefront of any professional field

has its challenges. It was difficult to find role models or to know where to turn for advice. Vari Drennan's (1984) project report was very helpful and now further relevant literature has become available. Angela would dearly have liked to have met other health visitors undertaking similar work.

Every four to six weeks, Angela meets her health visitor manager and they talk about what has been achieved and what should be planned as future projects. Angela finds these very supportive meetings. She is preparing a report on the first year's work. The first six months was spent without a regular caseload. More recently the decision was made to combine the community approach with two days a week acting as a family visitor, using the Child Development Project for twenty families on the estate, and taking a baby clinic.

These activities keep Angela in close touch with her colleagues, from whom she has a great deal of support. She is based with them in a health centre. Each day they all have coffee

Table 12.2 Prevention model showing examples of Angela Pardo's community approach to health visiting in a large council housing estate

Aim	Through	Examples
Prevent occurrence of difficulties	Health education	Many organisations request 'Look After Yourself' courses
		Regular work in schools; with mother and toddlers planned
	Promote awareness	Newspaper articles and items effective
Prevent development of difficulties	Monitoring/ search	Women's health clinic: accessibility to lady doctor popular
		Local volunteers — valuable contribution
		Campaigns with HV colleagues to follow up non-attendance at clinics, e.g. hearing test in the home
Prevent deterioration where difficulties already exist	Support	Yellow car well known: it shows Angela's whereabouts
		Accessible — approached for guidance and support
		Regular 'market place' venue
		Counselling by local volunteers increases service and its acceptability

together away from the 'phones. This is the time when Angela is able to float ideas for campaigns, such as chasing up hearing clinic defaulters (with many subsequent referrals) and organising to find out what prevents antenatal women from coming to parentcraft sessions. The team then sets about planning to provide something that suits the women. These coffee-time meetings provide a regular opportunity to give the other health visitors feedback on their clients and for Angela to receive informal support from her colleagues. This exchange of ideas and information is very valuable.

Having worked for five years as a GP associated health visitor in this same housing estate, Angela was already well known when she took up this new post. In those early days, she spent time consolidating relationships with other workers on the estate, and in planning

how they could work together. Angela had a great deal of guidance and support from the community workers at the family centre. She also went on some courses.

The 'Look After Yourself' tutors' course has proved to be very useful. Angela has provided four full courses in response to popular demand. A local course on 'Making use of the media' gave her courage to write articles and news items for the neighbourhood and the city newspapers. Special group-work training has proved invaluable.

A pregnancy testing and counselling service has been set up. Angela now takes part on a rota basis with locally recruited volunteers. There is a women's health clinic with a (lady) family planning doctor in attendance. Angela wrote an article about it in the neighbourhood newspaper. Many young women have come for cytology tests, family planning supplies and matters such

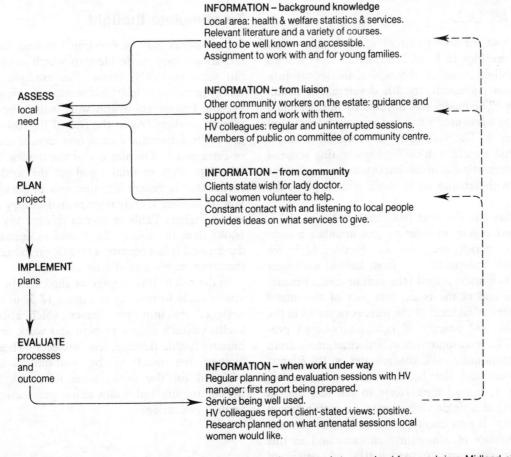

INFORMATION – background knowledge
Local area: health & welfare statistics & services.
Relevant literature and a variety of courses.
Need to be well known and accessible.
Assignment to work with and for young families.

ASSESS
local
need

INFORMATION – from liaison
Other community workers on the estate: guidance and support from and work with them.
HV colleagues: regular and uninterrupted sessions.
Members of public on committee of community centre.

PLAN
project

INFORMATION – from community
Clients state wish for lady doctor.
Local women volunteer to help.
Constant contact with and listening to local people provides ideas on what services to give.

IMPLEMENT
plans

EVALUATE
processes
and
outcome

INFORMATION – when work under way
Regular planning and evaluation sessions with HV manager: first report being prepared.
Service being well used.
HV colleagues report client-stated views: positive.
Research planned on what antenatal sessions local women would like.

Fig. 12.4 Health visitor cycle outlining Angela Pardo's community approach to caseload-free work in a Midland city huge council housing estate.

as counselling on personal relationships. Older women are often interested in health checks, such as for lumps and bumps which they have avoided taking to the local (male) GPs. Pre-menstrual tension, sexual problems and many other matters are raised and discussed at these sessions.

There is a market each Wednesday morning in the community centre car park. Angela has set up a regular stall, in order to make herself clearly accessible. A different health topic is highlighted each month. There was one for example, for National No Smoking Day and for National Smile Week. A Drink-wise Day is planned for June and 'accidents' will be part of the winter theme.

The work involves a great number of health educational sessions, including some with school leavers in the local school for children with special problems. Their contact with Angela means they get to know and trust a friendly professional person to whom they can turn, should they face difficulties as many do, during the years after leaving school.

In the future she hopes to have more work in the local schools, particularly with the mother and toddler groups in the nurseries there.

In this post, Angela is able to do the sort of work that the other health visitors would like to do, if only they had the time. She feels that the work that she is doing is just what Shirley Goodwin (1988) was describing in her 1988 Keynote Speech, 'Whither health visiting?'. Angela enjoys using this forward-looking approach.

THE MODEL

In each of the above examples, the health visitor cycle (see Figs 12.1, 12.2, 12.3 and 12.4) is used to highlight some of the behind-the-scenes processes in community health development health visiting. The model was introduced in Chapters 1 and 2 and was used again in the records section of Chapter 8. The version in these earlier chapters provided a useful vehicle for highlighting some of the information sources important in one-to-one work with families or in work with a particular group.

In this and the next few chapters the model is modified slightly in order to accommodate a community perspective. As in Figure 12.5 for example, 'Information — from liaison' no longer refers to matters prior to the visit or contact made. At this end of the book, this part of the model concentrates on some of the teamwork issues in the planning and practice of community-based projects. The level underneath, 'Information — from local community', still concentrates on the clients' viewpoint and the health visitor observations. However, it no longer refers to the information available at a single visit or meeting with a family or group. It now encompasses information from a wide variety of community contacts and in this chapter concentrates particularly on issues of perspective.

To stimulate thought

Some readers may be concerned to find that it is not always easy to decide into which category to put some particular factor. For example, something pertaining to the community view may become known via liaison work with other community workers. As in the rest of this book, it is not really important *exactly* how data is classified or categorised. The aim is that the models help to stimulate ways of thinking about the work. The model that is generating questions is working for you. If lists are merely regurgitated as they appear in the Figure, Table or Box in this (or any other) book, then the use of the model is limiting and dangerous. It has become a muzzle on thought and therefore on practice. Please take care!

In the rest of this chapter we shall use the health visitor cycle format, as in Figure 12.5, to look at some of the important issues which affect the health visitor's ability to plan and work on community health development projects. These will include the need to be well-motivated and educated for the work, some teamwork issues, the community and health visitor perspectives and finally, evaluation.

Fig. 12.5 Health visitor cycle highlighting some aspects of information which guide and help decision-making in community development health visiting.

DISCOVERIES

INFORMATION — from background knowledge

New approaches needed

Health visitors are becoming increasingly aware of the limitations of the traditional perspective which concentrates on the individual family. The urgency to improve practice and to take up the new ways of working were brought out very clearly in the debate at the Health Visitors' Association Annual Study Conference in 1987 (Health Visitor, 1988). Health visitors tend to be very inno-

vative, although they may not rate themselves as such (West, 1989). The energetic debate stimulated by Shirley Goodwin's (1988) Keynote Speech is bringing this creativity into greater profile.

Various people work most comfortably in different ways. To make best use of resources, it is important to maximise on individuals' skills and interests. Diversity in the provision of the service would enable full use of health visitor talent and motivation. It has been recommended that a health visitor concerned with community health development should work with a health visitor team (Drennan, 1985, p. 73; Orr, 1989). For example, family visitors, first parent visitors and community health visitors could plan together and support each other. With each using their special skills and remit, they could provide for a wide range of need.

It is likely that there will be more health visitors coming into community health development because it is:

- cost effective — much of work undertaken voluntarily by the people of that community
- responsive — local people's views and willingness to work on particular issues guide the service provision
- positive — working with people's strengths and with those who want to get things to happen
- enabling development — increasing people's self-esteem and levels of confidence
- practical — bringing greater levels of effective self-care
- targeted — at particular communities with low levels of health and few health care facilities
- efficient — improving people's access to health information and existing resources
- informal — so the professional is seen foremostly as a friend
- versatile — a great variety of schemes implemented.

Community health development is no easy option. It needs a health visitor with a strong enough character to be able to cope with the inevitable moments of loneliness and doubt associated with being at the sharp end of the arrow, spearheading new initiatives. A great deal of time and support is needed for learning about, planning and evaluating the work. A basic requirement is willingness to experiment. Another challenge is explaining about the work to 'unbelievers' in management and amongst colleagues and, indeed, being motivated to educate oneself.

Self-education

Few health visitors have formal education in the knowledge and particular skills necessary for community health development. It has not normally been included in the course. Most of those cur-

rently in this work are self-taught, having turned to other workers in the community for advice and support.

Health visitors are finding a wide variety of ways of responding to personal and community health need, and in describing many schemes, Jean Orr (1982; 1983) regretted that so few write about what they are doing. One exception to this has been Vari Drennan (1984; 1985; 1987; Drennan & McGeeney, 1985) who was employed specifically to work with groups in the community and freed of the normal commitment to individual families. She was involved at different levels and in varying ways with 25 of the 40 community groups and organisations with whom she made contact. She worked evenings and weekends to fit in with the groups' needs and also took part in five public events during her 15 months in this post.

The project was backed by a steering group, some members of which Ms Drennan met regularly. This group provided constructive support over the planning, the practical work and evaluation. The report of this research project (Drennan, 1985) and a book specifically for health visitors on group work (Drennan, 1988) will encourage the use of this approach and will provide guidance.

A handbook about the experiences of the Nottingham Community Health Project (Perkins, 1988) is also particularly helpful. It notes the inadequacies for this work of the health visitor's traditional experience and training. The book is written primarily for managers and trainers, outlining the principles and many of the practicalities involved in community health development. It gives much valuable advice on how to help staff and on how to avoid the pitfalls.

Guidelines on how to set up community health projects will be found in the Community Health Initiatives Resource Unit's (1987) *Guide to community health projects*. This guide also includes information on funding and grants, together with an outline of many examples of the work.

Ideas for community health initiatives can be found in Sue Dowling's (1983) *Health for a change*, the Community Projects Foundation's (1988)

Box 12.2 Some of the literature particularly useful regarding work with self-help groups

Book	Date & author	Publisher	Available from
Unemployment and health. Resource pack (2nd edn)	1987 Black D, Laughlin S (eds)	Health Education Department, Greater Glasgow Health Board	Belvedere House 1362 London Rd Glasgow G31 4QY
Age well. Ideas pack	(two packs) 1985 & 1988 Health Education Council	HEC and Age Concern	60 Pitcairn Rd Mitcham Surrey CR4 3LL
Women and health. Activities and materials for use in women's health courses and discussion groups	1986 Curran M Pleaner M Black J	Workers Educational Association (North West District) and Health Education Council	WEA 9 Upper Berkeley St London W1H 8BY
Working with parents. A training resource pack	1986 De'Ath E Pugh G. (eds)	National Children's Bureau	8 Wakeley St London EC1 7QE
Working towards partnership in the early years	1989 De'Ath E Pugh G	National Children's Bureau	8 Wakeley St London EC1 7QE

Action for health, and Caroline Smith's (1982a) booklet describing some 60 schemes. Guidance on how to set up voluntary groups and promote health (see also Box 12.2), where to look for help and how to apply for funds is also available (Smith, 1982b). The Department of the Environment 1970s research into self-help groups in inner city areas of London, showed there were fewer groups in these areas than elsewhere. This research enabled some useful advice to be given on how groups in inner cities might be encouraged (Knight & Hayes, 1981).

Keeping up to date

Making contact with the National Community Health Resource (NCHR) library (see useful addresses), and if possible following this with a visit, is a good way to keep up to date on the latest literature. This library has a large number of reports of community health projects. The librarian may well be able to tell health visitors of projects and of community workers active in their area. Taking up membership of the NCHR would

enable health visitors to remain abreast of current ideas and the Unit's activities.

A newly launched Health Visitor Association special interest group is providing the opportunity for the exchange of information and support for a fast growing network of health visitors interested in community initiatives (O'Gorman, 1989; see useful addresses). The group is expanding rapidly and by the time this chapter is printed, it will be providing a valuable and active background resource.

GUIDANCE AND SUPPORT

INFORMATION — from liaison

Guidance, ideas and support for those venturing into community health development come from many sources. Here we look at aspects of liaison with regard to a steering group, co-professionals, other health visitors and local workers.

A steering and support group

A steering group or management committee is a basic necessity (McCarthy, 1985; Community Health Initiative Resource, 1987, pp. 103–105). It can provide a secure foundation for the project and help to clarify its aims and objectives. This is an important factor because every project is different. There is an infinite variety of possible ways for the work to be undertaken, so no blueprint can be available. Mark McCarthy argued that the steering group should include local people, the funding agency and the participants, and that they should develop a built-in evaluation to enable development of ideas as the project progressed. Dunford and Hughes (1988) highlight many of the issues associated with drawing in local participants.

The members of the management support group need to understand the rationale and purpose of the work and have appropriate experience and open minds. Sympathetic and well-informed backing for the health visitors, with regular planning sessions, is essential. For example, a manager who does not know about community development work may, without first having discovered local feeling, seek to prescribe particular tasks. The result is that negative measures and inappropriate objectives could be imposed. Traditional goals such as increasing immunisation, high levels of breastfeeding and/or the discovery of early deafness could muzzle a project's success. The local people may have completely different priorities. The work *must* respond to the public view and the health visitors need to have the freedom to respond to the client-led opportunities as they arise.

Contact with health visitors . . . .

Community development health visitors not based in a health centre with other health visitors, need some system to ensure free flow of ideas between themselves and their caseload colleagues. This sort of two-way support and education is invaluable for mutual encouragement and for sparking off ideas and using each other's knowledge. There is an obvious advantage all round if, for example, community development health visitors are drawn into management committees for the caseload workers or into in-service support groups.

. . . . and other professionals

It is important to spend a good deal of time networking (Pugh & Woodward-Smith, 1989, pp. 80–82) to get to know all the other people who are working in the same patch. Dr Perkins (1988, pp. 19–22) points out that although health visitors tend to have many contacts, the network in community development needs to be much wider and of a different quality. Time to establish these contacts and relationships is a key requirement and, with all the other demands of this work, is only effective in a caseload-free post (Community Projects Foundation, 1988, pp. 30–31; 64–66). Networking goes side by side with building up a written patch profile and allied activities, such as discovering useful equipment and facilities for use in future groupwork.

There is an obvious advantage in getting to know and to maximise on services already in an area, be they health services or any other. For example, if contacts with the media are good, it helps to get a higher profile. A local newspaper may be prepared to run an article or an advert on what is proposed and seeking the involvement of the public.

There are innumerable workers with whom contact might be made (see also Chs 13 & 15). It is essential to work in close liaison with:

- other community development workers in the patch and
- professionals already involved with the families.

Others might range from a paid consultant employed to help extend the health visitor's skills and ability and to give support (Perkins, 1988, p. 40), through to tutors for groupwork specialist teaching, such as for the Alexander technique (Daisley, 1986; Potrykus, 1989), aromatherapy (Westwood, 1986; Tisserand, 1987; Wise, 1989) or massage (Byass, 1988; Wyatt & Dimmer, 1988; Trevelyan, 1989).

Workers from the community

Links with members of the community who have become local workers become increasingly likely. There have been some important moves towards encouraging women in a locality to take some training and then provide help for a particular family or families. There is very little difference between client and helper in some of these schemes. The idea is a little reminiscent of a strategy mentioned in the introductory chapter, where the Manchester and Salford Ladies Sanitary Reform Association trained and employed 'respectable working women' to visit homes (Owen, 1983). It is possible they were more acceptable to and empathetic towards working-class mothers than had been the earlier volunteer 'lady' visitors.

An excellent example of this approach is the scheme in Dublin, which is under the auspices of the Child Development Project (1984). Here some women who have demonstrated a particular aptitude in bringing up their own children, have been trained as 'Child Development Aides' (CDA). They have then worked under the guidance of Irish health visitors, visiting and supporting first-time mothers. In due course, some of the mothers who were visited in this scheme, have themselves become CDAs. Other examples of this approach are those of the Lisson Grove Health Centre (Wood, 1985) and Newpin (Mills & Pound, 1986; Potrykus, 1989) schemes.

PERCEPTIONS

INFORMATION — from the community

In this section we look briefly at how information is gleaned from the community and consider some differences between professional and client perspectives. Patch profiling and building up a written picture of the community, will be considered in greater depth in Chapter 15.

Health visitor findings

Besides being caseload free, the work needs to be applied to a geographic patch. In inner-city work, GP attachment can tend to lead to fragmentation and overlap. 'Patch work' enables the health visitor to concentrate totally on the community perspective and to respond to any opportunities that may arise within that area.

Local social networks are used and contact is made with people who have a finger on the pulse of that community. The aim is to find out people's ideas about health and feelings about the services that are, or could be, available. The basic remit is to respond to people's stated perceptions of their neighbourhood and their own health needs, and to enable the active involvement of the people themselves. It is a very positive approach, working with and maximising people's strengths. As local interest is aroused, more and more activities can be undertaken that are based on clients' ideas, feelings and willingness to act on them.

Professional perspectives

Some staff rigidly trained in the traditional system may find it difficult to accept the client-view as appropriate and what the client says as most important. Even if that is accepted, there can be some subtle but significant differences between how the client and the observing professional perceive a given issue. There are innumerable possible variations and Table 12.3 provides an example. The professional habit of looking at people 'with problems', a supposedly 'scientific' approach, can narrow matters down to the relatively unimportant. The people themselves see the whole picture. For them, other qualities and aspects of life are not blocked out.

Table 12.3 An outlined example of subtle but significant differences in professional and client perspective that could occur when an issue or tendency that concerns a client is being considered. It shows that inevitably the client has the best-informed perspective

Issue:	View of issue needing attention	
	by professional	by client
called	problem	difficulty
extent	greater degree	more medium degree
presents	task	obstacle to be overcome
tenor	negative	more optimistic
seen as	label?	one aspect of person
conclusion:	limited view	informed view

A small inner city study provides an example. The mothers interviewed saw their life with their small children in the context of their income, social networks, housing conditions and (non-existent) child day care facilities. With some notable exceptions, the health visitors tended to concentrate on mother:child interactions and on establishing 'good' social habits for the children (Mayall & Foster, 1987).

Experience can change views. Two years' working with the parents at 45 Cope Street changed the professionals' attitudes (Billingham, 1989a; 1989b). Newpin, the New Parent Infant Network, wishes to help health visitors cross the 'professional divide' and become more on an equal footing with their clients. Training is being offered (Potrykus, 1989; see useful addresses) and it will be interesting to see how many take up the challenge.

Advantages

Health visitors' special professional perpective can be very useful in community health development. For example, their knowledge of illness means they can differentiate between people with problems, identifying those with a clear need for direct clinical care. They have a foot in the door of the health services, are acceptable to and talk on equal terms with doctors, managers, and other nurses, thereby providing a very good bridge between the community and the health service. As ever, they are a helpful source of information about existing health service provision.

Client view

The Child Development Project has emphasised the need to listen to parents as the experts on their own children. In the same way, we are now learning to listen to the local people, the experts on their own locality, facilities and needs.

In order to learn people's opinions, it is necessary to be accessible to them. The choice of a base for the project can be crucial. For example, a community hall or neighbourhood centre may be seen more as community territory and bring in more people than a physically distant or a more formal

health centre. Travelling by bicycle is another way of maximising availability.

A questionnaire is one way of gleaning public opinion, but the genuineness of responses can be debatable when the survey is conducted by the professional (Cubbon, 1987). This problem was overcome by the West Pilton Clinic Users Group. The two parent members on this group, along with a couple of the professionals, created a local questionnaire. The parents recruited a few more volunteers and some 100 questionnaires were completed. They published their results (Alexander & Beagley, 1988). User participation in this community health project has been very influential and creative.

Self-help health groupwork is an excellent source for discovering the consumer viewpoint. Yvonne Ashley (1987) found consumer perspectives were very different from the health professionals'. The participants' feelings about touching themselves for breast self-examination were that it was 'a bit dirty' and that they could not do it. More recent research showed the sort of factors preventing large numbers of women from attending for cervical screening. They had feelings of embarrassment over, for example, the much reported association between cervical cancer and promiscuity, or shyness about their own bodies (Swaffield, 1989). A service can only be successful if it takes people's feelings into consideration, and groupwork can do this. Leathar and Roberts (1985) concluded that emotional support is crucial and that trying to educate through the mass media will only increase anxiety.

At a very different level, client views can be gained from activities that draw people in from the general community. Examples are a women's health shop (Robinson and Roberts, 1985), a health fair (Begg, 1989) or festival (Drennan, 1988) and a health market stall (Brierley et al, 1988). As in all health visiting, there is constant learning about other people's perspectives. In family-caseload health visiting it affects face-to-face decisions and interaction. In community health development the client view comes into even higher profile as it provides the basis for future groupwork and other projects or experimentation. It is the key to turning the latent possibility into actual self-help amongst people whose health needs are greatest.

REPORTING

INFORMATION — as the work progresses

This section considers reporting on progress. We look at some important features of evaluation, basic to the reporting process, and start with where to find help and guidance.

Literature

There is now a range of books providing relevant advice on evaluation (Drennan, 1985, pp. 18–22, pp. 55–74; Graessle & Kingsley, 1986; Feuerstein, 1986; Community Health Initiatives Resource Unit, 1987, pp. 107–109; Meadows & Turkie, 1988; Perkins, 1988, pp. 16–18, Appendix 3). From these, health visitors can draw together the ingredients that will help them create an assessment scheme most suited to their particular situation. Mog Ball's (1989) *Evaluation in the voluntary sector* describes behind-the-scenes issues which are also relevant to community development and provides practical checklists and guidance.

Guidance for future work

Graessle and Kingsley (p. 7) demonstrate that good evaluation

assesses what has been achieved
against what was intended and
explains why this happened in order to
derive some lessons for future work.

They show (p. 9) that the two most common approaches to evaluation in the medical world, epidemiological research and carefully controlled studies, are inappropriate for community health development. Client perspectives and influence upon the work, interactions between participants and the evaluation itself, are all part of a dynamic process. This needs an entirely different method of assessment.

There is no need to be afraid of value judgement or the 'unscientificness' of the client view or health visitor assessment. Alternative systems of evaluation concentrating on easily quantifiable factors, need choices to be made on what should be measured. These decisions also involve value judgements.

Basic information for the reports mainly comes from:

- notes from the health visitor's daily diary detailing events
- meetings and observations of the underlying processes
- allied professional and service-user views.

Examples of key issues to be discussed are how:

- clients are involved in group's
  — aims and objectives and
  — evaluation
- the work is improving participants'
  — self-esteem and confidence
  — ability to initiate health services
  — support for each other
- processes within groups and personal interactions are studied
  — to maximise learning from difficulties and produce new ways of working.

'Failed' groups are now recognised as a part of progress and of learning through experience. Equally, health visitors' feelings of inadequacy and inability to cope should also be seen in a positive light. It is a necessity for workers to be able to grieve, in order to adjust to the difficulties and challenges of the work. Any evaluation should take a critical look at the quality and effectiveness of support being provided for the staff.

Regular reports . . . .

All the issues mentioned above can be discussed by the steering group. There are normally regular meetings with this committee, generally three-monthly, when written reports submitted by the health visitor are discussed and future plans proposed. In between these sessions, contact with particular individual members may be made for discussions and support.

. . . . showing work developments

The reports may at first seem a daunting task. There is so much that could be included and choices have to be made. Much will depend upon how long the post has been established. For example, in the early stages there may be more need to discuss what contacts have been made and to describe preparations for teamwork. A little later, priority might be given to the sort of issues raised by Christa Wynn-Williams (1988) on establishing work with groups such as:

- discovering resources in the area — equipment and rooms
- knowing the local networks for informing clients
- a reliable and regular commitment by the health visitor
- group members setting objectives and measuring results
- awareness of group processes and
- advice, support and experiential learning for the health visitor.

Once the post is well established and many activities are under way, the report might concentrate on, for example, the relevance of the work to an area's high level of child abuse. As social workers are cut back, caseload health visitors find themselves increasingly pressured into taking on a policing role (Kent, 1988; Jones, 1988). All this concentration of health visitor effort offers nothing positive, no support, no elucidation and no break in the cycle. On the other hand, community development type of groupwork is able to offer a positive approach, it uses the community's latent resources in people's ability to support each other and to gain increased understanding, self-esteem and ability to cope (Potrykus, 1989). It is a good example of a cost effective use of health visiting.

Wide application

Many of the features of community health devel-

opment could also be applicable to family health visiting. For example, setting up appropriately representative steering groups, making a clear written statement of aims and achievable objectives, taking positive steps to discover client perpectives and regular written reports could all help health visitors clarify and demonstrate the basic issues of their work (see Fig. 12.6).

This chapter has concentrated mainly on community development health visiting and has provided four real-life examples. The health visitor cycle model has been used to draw attention to some important features of the work. It is likely that more and more health visitors will become involved in community health development, thereby helping to provide an increasingly effective service in deprived areas, such as those in our inner cities.

Fig. 12.6 A senior manager tells another decision-maker about health visiting achievements described by health visitors in their report about their recent initiatives.

USEFUL ADDRESSES

HVA Community Development and
Initiatives Special Interest Group
Ms Fedelmia O'Gorman
Health Visitor,
12–22 Linenhall Street
Belfast BT2 8BS
Tell 0232 321313

National Community Health Resource
(NCHR)
75 Charlton Street
London NW1 1HU
Tel 071 383 3841

NEWPIN
Sutherland House
Sutherland Square
London SW17 3EE
Tel 071 701 2660

REFERENCES

Alexander K, Beagley M 1988 West Pilton Clinic Users
Group. User participation in practice. Granton
Community Health Project, The Health Hut, West Pilton
Park, Edinburgh EH4 4ET — Succinct and well
presented.
Ashley Y 1987 Sharing and learning: the experience of
health education in women's self-help groups and its
implications for nursing, midwifery and health visiting. A
report of a day conference for senior nursing managers.
Scottish Health Education Group, Edinburgh. pp 34–40
Ball M 1988 Evaluation in the voluntary sector. The Forbes
Trust, Forbes House, 9 Artillery Lane, London E1 7LP
— Essential reading.
Begg E 1989 Planning a health fair. Nursing Times
Community Outlook 85, 41: 19–22
Billingham K 1989a 45 Cope Street: working in partnership
with parents. Health Visitor 62, 5: 156–157
Billingham K 1989b 45, Cope Street. Nursing Times
Community Outlook 85, 50: 8–10
Brierley H, Goddard P, Wildbore A 1988 Yes, we have no
bananas, but plenty of health care today. Health Visitor
61, 12: 369–370
Byass R 1988 Soothing body and soul. Nursing Times 84,
24: 39–41
Child Development Project 1984 Child development
programme. Early Childhood Development Unit, Senate
House, University of Bristol, Bristol BS8 1HT, pp 25–28
Community Health Initiatives Resource Unit 1987 Guide to
community health projects. Community Health Initiatives
Resource Unit, London. Available from National
Community Health Resource, 15 Britannia St, London
WCIX 9JP — Outlines many projects. Much valuable
advice in Part 4.
Community Projects Foundation 1988 Action for health:
initiatives in local communities. Community Projects
Foundation, London — Essential reading.
Cubbon J 1987 Consumer attitudes to child health services.
Health Visitor 60, 6: 185–186
Daisley J 1986 The Alexander technique. Health Visitor 59,
7: 212–213
Dowling S 1983 Health for a change. The provision of
preventive health care in pregnancy and early childhood.
Child Poverty Action Group, London — Many useful
ideas.

Downham M A P S, White E McC, Moss T R 1980 A
study of childhood morbidity and mortality in relation to
the provision of child health services in Newcastle upon
Tyne, 1975 and 1976. Health trends 12: 96–98
Drennan V 1984 A new approach. Nursing Mirror HVA
Supplement 159, 14: x–xi
Drennan V 1985 Working in a different way. A research
project examining community work methods and health
visiting. Community Nursing Service Paddington and
North Kensington Health Authority. Available from the
Health Promotion Unit, Green Lodge, Barratts Green
Road, London NW1O 7AP — Essential reading.
Drennan V 1987 Working in a different way. Senior Nurse
6, 1: 11–13
Drennan V 1988 Celebrating age. Nursing Times
Community Outlook 84, 23: 4–6
Drennan V (ed) 1988 Health visitors and groups: politics
and practice. Heinemann Nursing, Oxford
Drennan V, McGeeney S 1985 Menopausal support.
Nursing Mirror 160, 23: 27–28
Dunford H, Hughes J 1988 Pimlico Patch Committee. An
experiment in locality planning. Primary Health Care
Group, King's Fund, London.
Fatchett A 1989 Alternative approaches. Nursing Times
85: 42, 64–65
Feuerstein M T 1986 Partners in evaluation. Evaluating
development and community programmes with
participants. Macmillan, London — Intended for third
world: contains many practical ideas.
Goodwin S 1988 Whither health visiting? Health Visitor 61,
12: 379–383 — Essential reading.
Graessle L, Kingsley S 1986 Measuring change, making
changes. An approach to evaluation. London Community
Health Resource, London — Essential reading.
Health Visitor 1988 Are health visiting policies perpetuating
the health problems associated with poverty? Health
Visitor 61, 1: 24
Hull W 1989 Measuring effectiveness in health visiting.
Health Visitor 62, 4: 113–115
Jepson M E, Taylor E M, Emery J L 1983 Identification of
failures in the child health services by means of
confidential enquiries into infant deaths. Maternal and
Child Health 8, 1: 26–31
Jones M 1988 (letter) Health visiting: the time has come to

define the job more clearly. Nursing Times 84, 3: 11 — Key issue discussed.

Kent A 1988 Health visitors or police? Nursing Times 84, 1: 18 — Key issue discussed.

Knight B, Hayes R 1981 Self help in the inner city. London Voluntary Service Council HMSO, London

Leathar D S, Roberts M M 1985 Older women's attitudes towards breast disease, self examination, and screening facilities: implications for communication. British Medical Journal 290: 668–670

McCarthy M 1985 Understanding health needs. Health and Social Services Journal XCV: 133 — Well written and concise, re-evaluation and steering groups.

Madeley R 1988 Preventing sudden infant death syndrome: future strategies. Health Visitor 61: 8, 241–243

Madeley R J, Latham A 1979 Management aspects of high risk strategies in child health. Community Medicine 1: 36–39

Mayall B, Foster M C 1987 Mothers' lament. Nursing Times 83, 42: 64–66

Meadows A, Turkie A 1998 How are we doing? An introduction to self-evaluation for voluntary groups. National Council for Voluntary Organisations Inner Cities Unit, London – Well written and presented.

Mills M, Pound A 1986 Mechanisms of change: the Newpin Project. Changes 4, 2: 199–203

Nicoll A 1983 Community child health services — for better or worse? Health Visitor 56: 241–243

O'Gorman F 1989 (letter) Special interest group for community development. Health Visitor 62, 7: 229

Orr J 1982 Health visiting in the United Kingdom. In: Hockey L (ed) Primary care nursing. Churchill Livingstone, Edinburgh

Orr J 1983 Is health visiting meeting today's needs? Health Visitor 56: 200–203

Orr J 1989 The blueprint already exists. Health Visitor 62, 8: 238

Owen G 1983 The development of health visiting as a profession. In: Owen G (ed) Health visiting, 2nd edn: Baillière Tindall, Eastbourne, p 5

Perkins E R 1988 Working with the wider community. A handbook for managers and trainers. Health Education and Promotion Unit, Memorial House, Standard Hill, Nottingham NG1 6FX — Essential reading.

Phillips S 1986 A centre for change. Nursing Times Community Outlook 82, 7: 15–17 — Was presented a Bard award: well deserved.

Potrykus C 1989 A brand Newpin. Health Visitor 62, 9: 282–283 — Important scheme: Newpin address above.

Pugh J B, Woodward-Smith M A 1989 Nurse manager. A practical guide to better employee relations. W B Saunders, Philadelphia.

Robinson S E, Roberts M M 1985 A women's health shop: a unique experiment. British Medical Journal 291: 255–256

Schofield J 1984 A health visitor's dilemma. Nursing Times 80, 23: 21

Smith C 1982a Directory of community health initiatives. National Council for Voluntary Organisations, London

Smith C 1982b Community based health initiatives. A handbook for voluntary groups. National Council for Voluntary Organisations, London

Swaffield L 1989 Wasted lives. Nursing Times 85, 18: 22–23

Tisserand R 1987 Aromatherapy for everyone. Penguin, London

Trevelyan J 1989 Relaxing with massage. Nursing Times 85, 39: 52

Watson E 1984 Policies for child health in inner cities. Maternal and Child Health 9: 123–128

West M 1989 Innovation in health visiting. Health Visitor 62, 2: 46–48

Westwood C 1986 Aromatherapy. Health Visitor 59, 8: 251

While A 1982 Primary health care in the inner city: time for a new approach? Health Visitor 55: 116–117

While A (ed) 1989 Health in the inner city. Heinemann Medical Books, Oxford — Essential reading.

Wise R 1989 Flower power. Nursing Times 85, 22: 45–47

Wood T 1985 Formal and informal support systems for mothers with newborn. Midwife Health Visitor and Community Nurse 21: 42–49

Wyatt G, Dimmer S 1988 The balancing touch. Nursing Times 84, 21: 40–42

Wynn-Williams C 1988 Coming to grips with groups. In: Drennan V (ed) 1988 Health visitors and groups: politics and practice. Heinemann Nursing, Oxford

This chapter continues the wider view of health visiting, this time concentrating on the perspective of the prevention model. Five real-life examples of work for homeless families each include this model, highlighting the value of aiming to prevent the occurrence, development and deterioration of health problems by taking the broader approach.

13

Homeless families

The basic framework in this chapter is a prevention model with a community perspective. A brief introduction to health visiting homeless families is followed by five examples of a very positive approach to the work. The second half of the chapter looks more closely at the three aspects of the model outlined in Table 13.1. In the first aspect, health promotion is seen as sharing information, not only with clients, but also with decision-makers. In the second, the discussion moves on to the need to take positive steps to assess the type and extent of the problems involved. The final aspect is about support for and cooperative effort over common problems.

A HIGH PRIORITY

In the past few years, health visitors have been meeting increasing numbers of families in bed and breakfast temporary accommodation. These families' circumstances and their consequent health problems make them high priority for health visiting. Often they are not registered with a GP locally and are many miles from their home local authority, to which they must return to apply for social services. The daunting task of trying to provide an appropriate and adequate health visiting service is made worse by frequent changes of address and late (if any) notification of these moves (Lovell, 1986) and overburdened caseloads (Conway, 1988, pp. 96–99).

These families with very high health needs tend to have the greatest difficulty in gaining access to primary health care (Hadley, 1988). This has been the subject of a joint committee of the Health Visitors' Association (HVA) and the General Medical Services Committee (GMSC) of the British Medical Association (Cross et al, 1989). The committee's recommendations included proposals that, where there were a large number of homeless families in an area, a health visitor should act as coordinator, should have clerical support and should not have responsibility for more than 50 families at a time. It was pointed out that care has to be taken to ensure that the workload does not lead to a poor service for other people on GP list or health visitor caseload. There were also proposals to improve both access to GP lists and systems of notification.

Learning about homelessness

Until recently, the problem has had a distinctly low profile. It is gradually becoming less hidden. The recent publication of several booklets is making it easier to find out the essence of the problems involved in homelessness. Concise and well written introductions draw together relevant research and references for further study, for example, in the context of inner-city health (While, 1989) and the HVA/GMSC booklet mentioned above (Cross et al, 1989). One report looks specifically at the effects on children's health (Furley, 1989) and another describes the actual situation for the families and the concern of the professionals involved (Conway, 1988). A study pack specifically for health visitors has been drawn together by members of the HVA Special Interest Group for Homelessness (SIGH) (1989). It includes a huge list of references for further study and much useful information, for example, an outline of welfare benefits. Other features, such as the diagram showing patterns of information-giving, planning and action, will generate useful ideas and discussion.

There are many obstacles to being able to provide an adequate service for families in temporary accommodation. However, in this chapter we shall concentrate mainly on what health visitors *can* do and show five examples of health visitors taking positive steps to provide a good and appropriate service.

THE MODEL

Each example includes a Table in which aims and activities are outlined in the prevention model format. This model, used many times earlier in the book, is now slightly changed in order to demonstrate a wider perspective of our work. This modified model is also used in Examples Three and Four in the previous chapter (Tables 12.1 and 12.2. See also Tables 14.1, 15.1, 15.2 and 15.3).

The main points are summarised in Table 13.1.

Table 13.1 Prevention model outlining some aspects of health visiting work in the field of homelessness, showing the importance of taking a proactive, community-oriented approach

Aim	Through	Examples
Prevent occurrence of problems mainly by helping to influence decision-makers	Health education	Early access: notification & records.
	Increasing awareness of actual potential problems	Listening to clients; taking initiatives
		Regular reports to nurse managers
		Meet with involved dept/agencies
		Work with co-professionals & others active in homelessness locally
		Media: letters to influential people
		Take office: become more influential!
Prevent development of problems by gathering information for report	Monitoring/ search	Who and where are homeless families, what are their particular circumstances and why? Discover local dilemmas
	Aiming at early care	Relevant, acceptable, accessible and flexible services, avoiding stigma
		Health authority initiatives
Prevent deterioration where difficulties already exist	Support	Listening, groups, drop-in refuges, helping others help homeless
	Positive action	Cooperative effort — select major problems and work together with e.g.: education welfare officers, lawyers, environmental health officers

In the first section of the model, the notion of health promotion is widened. As before, it includes health education in which individuals and families are helped to gain useful information and understanding. However, space in this model is also given to the aspect of health promotion in which health visitors help to increase the awareness of decision-makers. Often, the health visitor is the only professional with access to, and knowledge of, the actual circumstances of homeless families. It is imperative that reports be made available, to enable *informed* decisions on how to revise services and reallocate resources to prevent the occurrence of health problems for future as well as present families with accommodation problems.

The second section of the model now looks at monitoring and search on a scale well beyond the interests of the individual family. A community-wide picture of the scale and type of difficulties being met by homeless families is an obvious prerequisite to the provision of accurate reports for decision-makers, mentioned above. This data is also required by health·visitors and their colleagues for themselves. They need to plan local health care and other services, which will help prevent the development of health problems by making the services relevant, acceptable and accessible.

In the third section, positive action through teamwork is added to the armoury of individual and group-type supportive services, which aim to help prevent deterioration where problems already exist.

In reality, all the issues in the model overlap and interact. As in the earlier models, an artificial separation has been created in order to highlight and provide a way of analysing certain important aspects of the work.

FIVE REAL-LIFE EXAMPLES

Once again we give about half the chapter to real-life examples. The first and second examples are of family health visitors who stepped outside their day-to-day role, one to undertake in-depth research and the other to help a charitable trust which provides a refuge for single parents. Next come two specialists in homelessness. The first of these health visitors works with a team and visits the homeless families within a 'patch'. The second is mainly caseload free, with a coordinating role. The last example is of health visitors who formed a group to investigate housing issues and difficulties.

In addition to the prevention model, each example has at least one health visitor cycle which outlines the planning processes. The third and last examples also include a pair of family health needs models.

Some readers may prefer to go on at this point to the general discussion which makes up the second half of the chapter, and to come back to the examples.

EXAMPLE ONE: DETAILED RESEARCH INTO HOMELESS FAMILIES

Poor uptake of developmental screening services by homeless people, made Veann Helyger curious to know more about the health and circumstances of these families and about the particular problems they face. She was coming across increasing numbers of families in temporary accommodation in the south coast provincial town where she works. Believing in a proactive approach to health visiting based on full and reliable information, Veann decided to undertake her own research. She was encouraged in this by her manager. He helped in a practical way by assigning Veann 80 days free of other work to do the project. The head of the health research unit at the nearby university undertook to be her supervisor, thereby ensuring scientifically-based, reliable research findings. Figure 13.1 and Table 13.2 provide an overview of the work.

The first thing was to find where the people were. A list of addresses of families in temporary accommodation from the housing department turned out to be completely out of date. However, local health visitors provided addresses of homeless families of whom they knew and also helped to get the questionnaires completed.

INFORMATION – background knowledge
Value of research to improve practice.
Need to clarify local homelessness problem
and discover most important elements.
HV research requires time and supervisor.

ASSESS
knowledge
needed

INFORMATION – from liaison
Manager: enthusiastic re research.
Housing Dept: provided list (outdated).
HV colleagues: addresses of homeless and
helped with questionnaire.

PLAN
own
research

INFORMATION – from daily work
Clients: concerned re housing, not HV agenda.
HV: observes frequent 'no access' visits and
clinic non-attendance; clients are 'problems'.
Post research: real difficulties discovered;
engenders new approach to work priorities.

IMPLEMENT
plan

EVALUATE
outcome

INFORMATION – from research findings
Firm understanding of homelessness issue,
e.g. homeless mothers remarkably stressed and
reporting that they were depressed.
Research well received by study day HVs and
at Rcn research conference.
Influence of publication .... to come ....

Fig. 13.1 Health visitor cycle outlining Veann Helyger's research into homelessness.

Determined to make a thorough investigation, Veann chose to study 169 variables in 65 families. Sorting out the data and writing it up has been a huge undertaking. Veann wistfully regretted not having had help available from a support/clerical worker able to work creatively with a computer. Such a service would have meant that much more information could have been available. Also, the report could have come out much sooner.

The results of the work that has been processed is very interesting. Veann's research has shown similar features to those in *Prescription for Poor Health* (Conway, 1988) but with one main exception. In this coastal town, homeless clients are mainly registered with a GP.

There were 102 children in the 65 families

surveyed. Similarities in the two research studies were found in the proportion of children who were underweight, underheight and had delayed development. Poor nutrition, poor speech and behavioural problems were also similarly very common, as was poor parental health.

The Rutter et al (1970) Malaise Inventory Score was used by Veann to provide a crude indicator of levels of maternal stress. These scores were compared with those of control groups; clinic attenders who have homes. 40 out of the 65 homeless had high scores, indicating they suffered high levels of stress. They were being constantly harassed by a multiplicity of problems.

A series of scoring systems was devised in order to discover some of the difficulties faced.

Table 13.2 Prevention model of Veann Helyger's research work into the health and circumstances of families in temporary accommodation

Aim	Through	Example
Prevent occurrence of homelessness problems	Promoting awareness	Information on actual circumstances and health profile of children and parents now available to managers, co-professionals, colleagues and eventually the public
		Able to influence decision-makers
Prevent development of problems due to homelessness	Monitoring/ search	Housing Dept information inadequate: shows need better system for early health visitor contact with families
	Early care	Poor health of children and parents highlighted: shows need for special health visiting endeavours
Prevent deterioration where homelessness problems established	Support	Research shows clear need for supportive services for parents and for efforts to be concentrated in this direction

Questions were asked about facilities such as:

- two rooms available?
- sink in bedroom?
- heating?
- laundry facilities?

⎫ 'comfort score'

- kettle?
- sink in bedroom?
- two rooms available?
- breakfast?

⎫ 'privacy score'

- kettle?
- sink in bedroom?
- refrigerator?
- access to kitchen?

⎫ 'food preparation score'

A 'complaints score' based on some open questions, when cross-referenced with the above, showed that complaints were soundly based and were always accounted for by lack of these very basic facilities. Accommodation was exceedingly poor. Taking the 'comfort score' as

an example, only 14 of the 65 got more than half the possible total score and 20 families failed to get even a quarter of the points.

The questionnaire had been made as simple as possible. For example, inquiry about anaemia status asked whether they were on 'double iron'. Aspects of health in the most recent pregnancy at this time of being homeless, were compared with health associated with previous pregnancies. The chosen indicators showed a very much greater incidence for the homeless of, for example, anaemia, hypertension, urinary tract infection and premature birth.

Veann discovered these people to be really vulnerable right across the whole spectrum. Previously she had thought of them more as 'problems who took up a lot of a health visitor's time.' She had been preoccupied with ineffective (no access) visits, the families' failure to respond to invitations to hearing tests, vaccination, etc. and their constantly wishing to talk about housing — thereby obstructing, she added tongue in cheek, the real delivery of care! But joking apart, Veann feels that her attitudes towards these families have changed. She is much more aware of the potential trap in a health visitor-centred approach tending to pay only lip-service to the client's view. This research has made Veann sure that we should concentrate on responding to the needs of the mothers or parents. It is missing the central point to be so overwhelmingly preoccupied by developmental assessments and child-centred care.

Another of the conclusions from the project is that even when we treat the homeless the same as others, our services are not good enough. That is, in order to achieve equal access to care and treatment, we need to offer unequal and improved service as they are a group with special needs.

Many other useful recommendations are coming out of this work. The report of Veann's research was well received by health visitors at a study day. Veann's description of her work at a Royal College of Nursing research conference on 14 April 1989, was received with warmth and hearty congratulations. At the time of writing, the report (see useful addresses) is very close to being completed. It has already influenced her own practice and when published will be sure to influence many others.

This project clearly demonstrates the value of time being set aside for good quality study, planning and evaluation. Many families will benefit.

EXAMPLE TWO: WORK WITH THE HAVEN TRUST

Sue Chew is another health visitor who has found the value of stepping outside the day-to-day health visiting role. Her work in a Gloucester family centre in a provincial city convinced her that regularly working alongside other professionals and lay people and pooling and sharing ideas, leads to a more acceptable and helpful service. This view and her special interests in single parent families and in homelessness led her to call and offer help at The Haven, an aptly named refuge in the centre of the city, where young families in bed and breakfast (B & B) could visit or spend the day.

Sue soon found herself on the support committee which helps the centre's workers. Then she was asked to join the main committee. Some years before, a centre on the edge of the city had been set up by a church organisation, but it was too far from the bed and breakfast area. The accessible central site, which had been run for a while by the Manpower Services Commission, was delapidated and far from ideal.

It was decided to form a charity, The Haven Trust, in order to buy a suitable centrally placed property. An enormous amount of fund raising was undertaken by very hardworking and well-connected members of the committee. Financial support came from innumerable organisations and charitable foundations. The property has been bought, decorated and furnished by volunteers, and is now open. There

INFORMATION – background knowledge
Special interest in homelessness and single-parent families.
High rate of homelessness in city.
Knowledge of local facilities,
including The Haven centre.

ASSESS
committee's
and client
health need

INFORMATION – from liaison
Committee work: able to explain about homelessness, lone parents, B & B etc.
Law centre, social workers and others.

INFORMATION – from many visits
Bed and breakfast addresses gathered.
List enables questionnaire discovering client-view of priorities.

PLAN
how to help
committee
and staff

IMPLEMENT
plan

EVALUATE
effect of
action
taken

INFORMATION – from work with committee
Committee grateful for guidance: changed policies.
Staff grateful for support.
Increase in use of service by mothers showing work with others benefits clients.

Fig. 13.2 Health visitor cycle view of Sue Chew's work with The Haven Trust.

are laundry, cooking, a variety of play and many other facilities supervised by Judith, a nursery nurse with experience of inner city work.

In committee Sue has been able to explain about the reality of being in bed and breakfast accommodation, of homelessness and the plight of lone parents. Some of the other committee members have little or no experience of these things. Sue arranged for health visitor colleagues to inform her of addresses at which they had clients in B & B. This provided useful factual information and has also enabled Judith to take a questionnaire round to the young parents in bed and breakfast accommodation and to ask them what sort of service and facilities they would prefer. So the committee is provided with a very good understanding of its clients'

Table 13.3 Prevention model of Sue Chew's work with The Haven

Why	How	Examples
Prevent occurrence of homelessness problems	Promote awareness	Inform councillors through their contact with The Haven Inform public through the media interest in The Haven
Prevent development of problems due to homelessness	Monitoring/ search	Sue asked HVs to provide information on whereabouts of bed and breakfast accommodation Constructed questionnaire to find out what problems met and client views of what needed
	Accessible & acceptable services	Helped committee provide social contact, washing facilities, safe play and sleep Helped increase awareness of rights and benefits to enable full uptake
Prevent deterioration where homelessness problems established	Support	Helping the committee to provide: • relaxed atmosphere where Judith and other helpers able to listen and to understand • mutual support amongst parents • support for staff

feelings, needs and wishes and has accordingly modified its views. For example, where it was originally thought that The Haven should provide a hive of activity for the mothers, it is now realised that a place to relax and talk is more valuable.

Other agencies are also involved in the Haven. For example, the local Law Centre has an advice worker who is willing to visit and explain about rights, such as those under the Homeless Persons Act. Social workers and others are happy to call in for discussions and help. It may not solve all the problems, but working with others has helped to develop relevant provision for the health and welfare of these young families. Figure 13.2 outlines aspects of the planning and monitoring of this work.

Table 13.3 shows under primary prevention how it is hoped to influence policies by promoting awareness of the current crisis situation and, under secondary prevention, to provide appropriate practical help early. Local councillors' involvement and media interest in The Haven project both help increase public awareness of the extremely high rate of homelessness. Knowledge of the whereabouts of the families in temporary accommodation and the questionnaire seeking their view of priorities, led to relevant facilities to help prevent some of these people developing major problems. Where major difficulties do already exist, a listening, supportive atmosphere is available and mutual self-help facilitated.

EXAMPLE THREE: A SPECIALIST HEALTH VISITOR

There are advantages in providing specialist health visitors for homeless families. An expertise can be built up. Also, time and effort can be concentrated on trying to improve the circumstances and welfare of these families. Sylvia Scott felt their unmet health needs should be given special priority. It was three years ago when she took up this inner city post.

No special training was offered, so Sylvia learned as she went along. All aspects of her broad education and training helped provide a good basis for her self-tuition. For example, her mental health training has made it easier to understand people's feelings and their response to being homeless. It has also helped her with her own stress management, a very important factor for this sort of post. Figure 13.3, Table

13.4, Box 13.1a and Box 13.1b provide an outline of the work.

The team currently has four full-time workers. There are two health visitors. A Bengali worker/translator is employed, as a very high proportion of the clientele do not speak English. The fourth worker, a clinic clerk, is able to take over time-consuming tasks such as:

- telephoning many Boroughs' Housing Departments
- finding records
- phoning hospitals and
- dealing with transfers and forwarding addresses.

When there is a child under one year, the new health visitor to whom the family will be going, is contacted personally.

The activity given highest priority is visiting the families in their hotel or hostel. Sylvia generally visits about four times a year, but more frequently as the need arises. She quickly built up an expertise in offering relevant advice and in boosting these families' confidence in their parenting skills. Each of the health visitors has a caseload of around 150 families, so they cannot give the service they would like to. As homelessness gets worse, the team has to put a limit on the number of families it can take on. Increasingly generalist health visitors are also visiting families in temporary accommodation. The team can act as an advisory resource. It is very special work. 'Health' as a priority for homeless families, often comes well after 'housing' and 'money' and this can be disorienting for health visitors. However, the

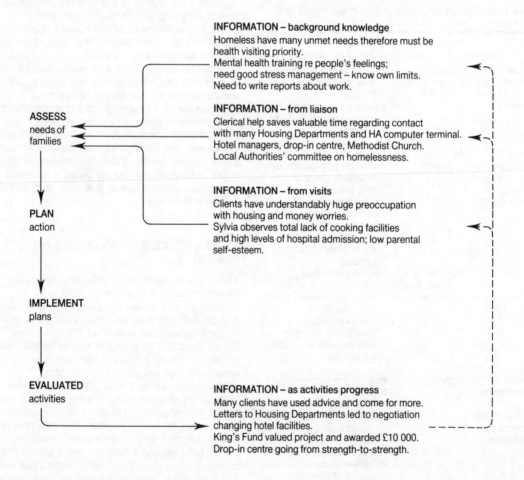

Fig. 13.3 Health visitor cycle outlining some features of Sylvia Scott's approach to work with families in temporary accommodation in a London inner city area.

problems are real. Some of the families have been in 'temporary accommodation' for more than three years!

Proactive help has been given. Seeing a need for a place where the mothers could get together, Sylvia worked in conjunction with a sympathetic GP, and set up a drop-in centre, for which she was later granted a £10 000 King's Fund award. Since then the centre has developed significantly. Children can be left twice a week in the mornings and it becomes a family centre in the afternoons. They have weekly health, English language and welfare rights sessions and hope soon to set up an after-school homework club.

In the early days a mobile clinic bus was provided outside the drop-in centre to give easy access to health facilities. However, the bus lacked space, privacy, and a telephone to check immunisation records. It came to be considered a second class service. The clients gained the confidence to walk past it and go on to the ordinary health clinics. It had outlived its usefulness and is no longer used.

Outreach workers have a base in a local Methodist church. Sylvia and the Bengali worker go along to give a programme of health sessions on topics such as:

Box 13.1a Family health needs model showing examples of the more pressing difficulties for homeless families identified by Sylvia Scott

Environment	Physical health	Mental/emotional health	Social aspects of health
For the parents Inadequate and temporary accommodation	Poor nutrition and hygiene	Inadequate contact with social workers	Poor social network, especially families from outside Borough
Unemployment	Lack access to general practitioner	Lack of knowledge of coordinating services and local health and social services	Few support workers
Decreasing benefits	Uptake of local health services and facilities use poor		Living circumstances lead to disruption of marital relationship
Overcrowding: e.g. large family in one room		Most have language problems	
Lack of cooking facilities even to boil water!	Low level of child immunisation	Ignorance about welfare rights	Non-participation in local activities
	Family planning problems	Poor access to health education	Too few crèche places
			Few accessible meeting places
Inadequate contact with Housing Departments		Low self-esteem	
		Emotional stress and depression	
		Lack of motivation	
In addition, for the children Lack safe play space	Nutritional inadequacies	Lack of stimulation and motivation	Poor socialisation
Unsafe stairs and windows	Delays in walking and coordination	Cognition poor	Delayed speech
Cramped play conditions	Frequent accidents: burns and scalds	Difficulty over school places	Inadequate play experience
	Gastroenteritis endemic		Poor access to toy libraries, play groups, play bus, mobile crèche
	Many admissions to hospital: vomiting, eczema and asthma		
	Coughs, colds & minor illnesses very common		

Box 13.1b Family health needs model showing a few of Sylvia Scott's responses to the more pressing problems of homeless families. (NB. There are obvious limitations on what can be achieved by one small homelessness team.)

Environment	Physical health	Mental/emotional health	Social aspects of health
Activities using a community perspective			
Letters to Housing Departments re hotel facilities	Membership of committee: increases awareness of health needs	Health sessions in Methodist Church	Drop-in centre set up and increasing number of clients using it
Activities for individual need			
Home visiting as frequently as possible, assessed on relative priority	Supportive encouragement to attend clinics	Individually tailored advice for families re coping	Much advice about child play and stimulation
	Advice on nutrition, safety, etc.	Much morale boosting	Encouragement to use local crèche and attend social facilities
		Work with translator	
		Family planning a speciality	

- family planning
- nutrition
- play and stimulation
- immunisation
- footcare
- teeth and dentistry
- cervical smears.

A special survey undertaken by this health visitor revealed a great need for information about family planning. The Bengali mothers appreciate the translations and the fact that she brings along the various contraceptive devices to improve understanding of the choices available. This topic is requested time and time again.

Access to the families in the hotels has changed significantly. A special relationship has been built up between Sylvia and the hotel managers and receptionists where she visits. At first some refused to tell their 'guests' about the health visitor calling, thinking she might be a nuisance in some way. Once they became aware of what health visitors do, they were very helpful. Now they will even phone to tell her of their concern about a family. When there is a new manager, it is necessary to start this process all over again. This liaison is very valuable. It facilitates earlier access to health services.

When the post was taken up, there were hotels accommodating bottle-feeding mothers who had no access to cooking facilities and no fridge. They were not even allowed a kettle. Mothers consequently did the best they could in the circumstances — and babies went to

Table 13.4 Prevention model outlining some aspects of Sylvia Scott's work with inner city homeless families

Aim	Through	Examples
Prevent occurrence of problems	Health education	Sympathetic one-to-one work in hotels
		Group work with translator
	Increase awareness	Letters to Housing Departments
		London Boroughs' committee work
		Talks to students — future managers
Prevent development of problems	Monitoring/ search	Opportunistic child screening
		Clinic clerk helps find families and relevant information
		'Notification' from hotel managers
	Acceptable services	Confidence gained to attend ordinary clinics — mobile bus no longer needed
Prevent deterioration where problems already exist	Support	Sympathetic one-to-one work in hotels
		Drop-in centre and other services
		Group work enables mutual support
		Hotel managers also enable early support

hospital with diarrhoea and vomiting. Sylvia wrote letters to the Housing Departments requesting improved facilities. This action led to negotiations with the hotels and now some have converted a bedroom into a kitchen, some rooms have a microwave and others access to cooking facilities where earlier there were none. Kettles are now permitted.

The Association of London Authorities and the London Boroughs Association has a working party on homelessness where workers from housing, social services, environmental health, health and education come together. Sylvia is a member of this committee. Aspects of health discussed are those such as:

- access to general practitioners
- need for female general practitioners
- access to hospital services
- health consequences of hotel conditions
- need for interpreters
- some health workers' lack of access to families
- need for a key worker for homeless households
- a code of practice on provision of social services where the child is at risk of non-accidental injury
- inadequacy of health care for children in hotels
- health visitors' need for support and low caseloads.

This health visitor is able to give a very realistic description of hotel life.

Often Sylvia is the only person visiting 'her families'. Few enough workers are so well informed. She has had many congratulations from important people that she has shown around her 'patch'. Although she can see much more still to be done, she can also see that she is, in her own words, 'slowly chipping away at the problem'.

EXAMPLE FOUR: A HEALTH VISITOR FOR HOMELESS FAMILIES

It is quite evident that Teresa Murray enjoys the challenge of her work as health visitor for homeless families in Haringey. The post arose out of the local Community Health Council's concern about the health care of families in temporary accommodation in their District. A health visitor spent six months working alone on the problem and in her reports recommended that it should be tackled jointly with the local authority (LA). This resulted in joint funding for an extra health visitor post, which has the additional benefit of enabling the other health visitors (HVs) to continue with their normal workload.

The purpose of the post is to investigate delivery of health care to homeless families, not to take up a caseload. This means Teresa can take a broad approach and has time to coordinate and plan (see Fig. 13.4). Her main problems were:

- who and where are the homeless families;
- which is the placing local authority responsible for them;
- what was preventing access to and take-up of health service;
- which specific problems encountered by these families should be tackled first.

First priorities for Teresa were reading up as much as possible, joining the Health Visitors' Association Special Interest Group on Homelessness to meet other HVs in this field and getting to know other people working with homeless families in her area. She met weekly and twice weekly respectively with the local:

- housing officer and
- social workers.

Teresa instigated a monthly group meeting with the LA

- social worker for the homeless
- group worker from the LA Homeless Persons Unit
- education welfare officer for homeless children,

where they pooled their knowledge and experience and started to tackle the problems outlined above.

A Housing Support Group grew out of this and a working party for Bangladesh homeless families, drawing together representatives from all the local community groups such as

- Asian community groups
- Welcare
- Youth and Community Services
- women's health groups
- Citizen's Advice Bureau
- Legal Aid

bringing an even greater wealth of understanding and cooperation. It also links in with other authorities, cross-fertilising ideas and information.

The group wanted to find practical solutions to the difficulties encountered by homeless families. They have drawn up an information pack on the services in their area able to be contacted directly, that is, needing no referral by a third party. These services include:

- health

INFORMATION – background knowledge
Major problem needs full-time assessment,
planning and coordination.
Need for practical solutions.
Special interest in children 'at risk'.
Need to write report.

ASSESS
problem

INFORMATION – from liaison with
Housing officers: own and other authorities.
Other specialists for homeless – pooled
knowledge and experience.
Health visitors.

PLAN
solutions

INFORMATION – from many visits
HVs report:
– difficulties in contacting and caring for
  homeless
– records get lost.
Clients encounter:
– strange environment and extra tensions
– prejudice and unknown system.

IMPLEMENT
ideas

EVALUATE
result
of work

INFORMATION – after system set up
HVs report:
– more time for proactive work;
– earlier contact with homeless.
Pooling expertise very creative.
Ideas from Homeless Support Group:
– positive response.

Fig. 13.4 Health Visitor cycle outlining Teresa's work in investigating and planning access to health care for homeless families.

- educational
- social
- housing
- community groups
- advice centres.

The pack is currently being printed and arrangements are being made for its distribution by placing authorities and for someone to explain about it. There will be a translation available in Bengali. The effect of the pack will be monitored.

As the group has direct contact through to influential levels of every local institution involved with homelessness, several practical problems

have been able to be solved. For example, families in bed and breakfast accommodation were being told there was no room in the schools, even though places were available. Joint action enabled this problem to be nipped in the bud.

Health visitors have indicated where help is needed, reporting for example:

- out of date information on families' addresses and much time wasted tracing them
- records often lost
- families with enormous problems, needing extra visiting
- families with 'at risk' children in caseloads

where no HV is employed
- children needing the service, not being referred to child guidance.

Many of their clients find themselves:

- moved into a new area, away from family
- ignorant of the locality and its services
- under great strain with their children and
- facing prejudice.

Through her housing contacts, Teresa has been able to provide early notification of temporary accommodation placements and changes of address. Also, support groups and appropriate child guidance services are being planned and client-held records will be tried out.

Table 13.5 Prevention model of Teresa's work planning access to health care for homeless families.

Aim	Through	Examples
Prevent occurrence of homelessness problems	Education	Homeless Support Group: • ideas influencing policy • institutional problems tackled Teresa's student teaching increases awareness
Prevent development of problems associated with homelessness	Monitoring and early care	Group discovering: • who, where and why homeless enabling practical solutions • institutional problems
	Acceptable & accessible services	Care will be facilitated by: • early notification of placement • client-knowledge of services • accessible child guidance
Prevent deterioration of established problems	Support	Visits for some homeless families • 'at risk' in 'empty caseload' • encountering multiple problems Support groups planned Joint action on school entry

Teresa is able to visit 'at risk' homeless families where no health visitor is employed and also certain families encountering a multitude of problems. Her suggestion that young antenatal mothers remain in their own LA is receiving favourable attention. She used *Prescription for poor health* (Conway, 1988) to illustrate the women's needs.

The Housing Support Group is increasingly turning its attention to why it is that people are becoming homeless, and are proposing practical solutions as to how it might be prevented. For example, making a contract with a family to maintain a single parent for a couple of extra months whilst appropriate accommodation is found and provided. Table 13.5 shows a prevention model of the work.

The report that Teresa is writing will describe much more fully what she is achieving than space allows here. It is exciting work and a very effective use of health visiting for the homeless.

EXAMPLE FIVE: A GROUP STUDYING THE HOUSING PROBLEM

Health visitors (HVs) working in Southampton became aware of a huge and increasing number of young families in bed and breakfast accommodation. General discussion about housing at a staff meeting, led to the decision to take time out to study the problem. A group of interested HVs, mainly from the city centre, met approximately six-weekly. They started by planning how best to tackle the investigation and whom to contact in order to discover the local facts and figures. They aimed to find out about the difficulties and explore possible solutions. Figure 13.5a outlines their planning process.

The group adopted a democratic structure. Having no chairperson or secretary meant that all members were responsible for helping to organise it and equally entitled to express their views and suggestions. This format has worked well.

Meetings were arranged with agencies working on various aspects of housing. These meetings proved to be very informative. They learnt about the Housing Department policies and of the existence of the Southampton Housing in Multiple Occupancy Group (SHMOG). This is a group of representatives of statutory and voluntary organisations with an interest in housing and homelessness problems. Group members subsequently attended and brought back a great deal of information and some very

INFORMATION – background knowledge
Must set aside time to increase knowledge
of who and what available locally.
Liaison to learn, inform and influence.
Group work provides mutual support.
Need to keep reading up to date and
to share new experiences by writing.

ASSESS
potential
for improved
understanding
and influence

INFORMATION – from liaison
LA Housing Dept policy, schemes,
limitations and medical applications.
Environmental Health Dept policy, legal
powers and staffing shortages.
SHMOG: co-professionals and volunteers.

PLAN
group work
and liaison

INFORMATION – at many visits
Clients: increasing numbers with poor
housing and reporting health hazards.
Many health visitors' observations and
deep concerns gathered in the SCUF
questionnaires, then survey report.

IMPLEMENT
activities

EVALUATE
effect of
action
taken

INFORMATION – after 1st stage of project
Health given higher profile by EHOs.
Improved knowledge of health visiting by
other workers.
No simple solution and don't work alone!

ROBERTSON

Fig. 13.5a Health visitor cycle outlining Southampton health visitors' group work on housing difficulties: first stage.

helpful contacts, addresses and telephone numbers.

At another HV group meeting, a Nurse Advisor for Child Health described her research project for the Southampton Children Under Five (SCUF) group. She showed the group her questionnaire for health visitors. This project was designed to discover the conditions for families with very young children living in housing in multiple occupancy (HMO). The nurse advisor later came to a staff meeting and presented her completed report. This showed a very high number of children in HMOs. The health visitors' responses in their questionnaires highlighted their many concerns about the families' health

(Box 13.2a) and listed suggestions as to what could be done (Box 13.2b). The picture in this unpublished report was similar to that in *Prescription for poor health* (Conway, 1988).

The Principal Environmental Health Officer (EHO) (Housing in Multiple Occupancy) described her department's legal powers, policy and limitations. She outlined how EHOs and HVs can cooperate. This meeting was particularly productive. The group's many examples of lack of safety and poor hygiene led to a change of Environmental Health Department policy. They had been concentrating on overcrowding and moved on to giving greater attention to cases with direct health implications.

Box 13.2a Family health needs model showing some of the more common problems faced by families in bed and breakfast accommodation (B & B) and noted in the Southampton health visitors' questionnaire, which they completed for the nurse advisor's SCUF report

Environment	Physical health	Mental/emotional health	Social aspects of health
Lack of privacy Lack of space, and overcrowding Damp building Faulty appliances Inadequate heating Insufficient money Unemployment	Shared kitchens and bathrooms Poor hygiene and nutrition Lack of storage space for food and equipment Inadequate clothes washing facilities Unsafe playspace: child accidents — burns, scalds and falls Children passive smoking — all family in one room	Noise from other tenants: family rows Harassment from landlord Hassle from other residents Poor self-esteem and depression Marital breakdown Child behaviour problems Other people's attitude to their B & B status	Lack of play space and toy storage Moved away from family support Obliged to go out in the day Not on local waiting list for nursery or playgroup: no places available Children sharing parents' room, observing sexual intercourse

Box 13.2b Family health needs model listing some of the suggestions made by Southampton health visitors, who had listened at length to their clients' views on what needed to be done to help with the very varied needs of families in bed and breakfast accommodation (B & B)

Environment	Physical health	Mental/emotional health	Social aspects of health
Many suggestions regarding: 1. increase in council housing stock 2. improved availability of reasonably priced rented accommodation 3. improved surveillance and supervision to promote and maintain high standards of temporary accommodation Financial help	Safer and more sanitary conditions Facilities for preparation of own food — and that are hygienic Appropriate fixtures and fittings Ability to stay in room during the day	Support groups, especially self-help, and not associated with 'imposed officialdom' Respite care for families particularly in school holidays Fair and considerate treatment by Local Authority and landlords	Provision of temporary accommodation in own area Communal rooms for child and group activities Day 'drop-in' centre for families in B & B Nurseries and day minders where children can be left for short periods

The group showed the EHO the SCUF Report. This new information, being very relevant, was taken to the Housing Sub-committee (HMO), to inform the members and help form policy decisions.

Amongst other speakers were medical assessment officers from the housing department. The members of the group became more aware of other agencies' and departments' systems of work. They were more able to understand the problems experienced by these agencies. Other workers discovered the role of HVs and health issues were brought to the forefront. As one member of the group pointed out, previously there had been 'not so much *low-profile* as *no-profile* health visiting!'

After meeting for about a year, the group members wanted to produce a report for their managers and colleagues, but found it too daunting a task, given the amount of information obtained and the complex issues involved. Fortunately, it was at this point that voluntary help became available from a support worker with access to a word processor. Even so, although each member of the group undertook to prepare a section of the report, it still took a number of meetings over some months to complete. Figure 13.5b provides a health visitor

INFORMATION – background knowledge
Must keep managers informed.
Need to spread knowledge gained to
health visitor and other colleagues.
Need *time* to write/clerical support.

ASSESS
managers' and
colleagues'
needs

INFORMATION – from liaison
Address and telephone list of relevant
voluntary and statutory workers.
Useful information such as housing dept
points system.
Feedback to agencies: send report.

PLAN
report and
recommendations

INFORMATION – anticipated
From meetings with colleagues:
– other health visitors' experiences
– their clients' suggestions.

IMPLEMENT
plan

EVALUATE
outcome of
activities

INFORMATION – during 2nd stage of project
Managers very supportive over group's
activities, report and recommendations.
Report received positively by E H dept.
Time made available for sessions to
inform and discuss issues with colleagues.

Fig. 13.5b Health visitor cycle showing second stage of Southampton health visitors' group work: writing report and discussion sessions with colleagues.

cycle perspective of this second phase of activity and Table 13.6 a prevention model overview of the group's work.

A summary, and later the full report (Davies et al, 1989) were well received by managers, as it kept them up to date with this important and creative work and presented them with recommendations on how they could help this process. The group was encouraged to continue both to build up liaison contacts and to add to their knowledge of the local situation.

The group is now considering the next stage which is to compile lists of information for local health visitor and other colleagues. For example, relevant and useful names and telephone numbers and an explanation of the housing

department points system. The group plans to maintain its interagency work. Major changes on government legislation have been made in the time that the group has been meeting. The outcome of these changes will need to be monitored. Also if the group's recommendation for a research project is funded, the momentum will be continued. Meanwhile, temporary accommodation problems continue to increase both locally and nationally.

Whatever decisions are made next, this is an example of group work which clearly shows the value of taking a few hours outside the day-to-day role of the health visitor in order to identify health issues of the local community.

Table 13.6 Prevention model showing the purpose of the formation of the Southampton Health Visitor Housing Group.

Aim	Through	Examples
Prevent occurrence of homelessness difficulties	Education	Improved HV knowledge of special services available — to give families appropriate & early advice
	Promoting awareness	Of Local Authority decision-makers re health threatening aspects of temporary accommodation — group's observations and SCUF report Summary & Report to Health Authority community unit managers and discussions with colleagues
Prevent development of problems due to homelessness	Monitoring/ search	Use of information available through health visitors (SCUF report) to demonstrate size of problem, geographical location and health needs Recognition of necessity to monitor effects of recent Housing and Social Security Acts
Prevent deterioration where homelessness difficulties established	Support	Create list of agencies discovered to be helping families: circulate information to enable HV colleagues to work with and tell families of support services

SHARING INFORMATION

HEALTH PROMOTION

Following the pattern seen in Table 13.1, we start by looking at some of the ways that health visitors can help prevent the occurrence of difficulties and health problems. These are firstly, by ensuring that homeless families have access to useful infor-mation and secondly, by sharing knowledge of the actual situation experienced by these families with local decision and policy-makers.

For the families

Early access

Families in temporary accommodation need very early access to information about health and welfare services in the locality in which they find themselves. For example, they need to know about:

- play facilities
- local GP services
- health clinics and other health services
- access to welfare rights
- social work arrangements and
- relevant voluntary agencies.

Information is being provided in some places in the form of a printed pack in an appropriate range of languages. It can be made available at hotels, or given out, with relevant explanations, by health visitors or the housing department officer placing the families in the hotels. Posters can also be useful.

Early notification to health visitors of in-coming families is very important. Arrangements vary considerably. They range from being the responsibility of a Health Authority Homeless Persons Liaison Officer (Cross et al, 1989, p. 18) through to health visitors' systematic enquiries into whether there are young families living in the hotels, by talking with the hotel managers and receptionists. Although effective, this is very time-consuming (Nursing Standard, 1987).

Records

Much time can also be wasted in trying to trace and to send on health visitor records (Jackson, 1989). Josephine Boyer (1986) and her colleagues decided not to send for records except in exceptional circumstances. In Tower Hamlets, a group of health visitors devised a form to improve efficiency of transferring homeless families' health information on to the receiving health visitors (Furley et al, 1988).

Client-held records provide a possible solution (Cross et al, 1989, p. 18; Jackson, 1989). However, families in temporary accommodation tend to be very sensitive about the stigma associated with being labelled as 'homeless' (Cross, 1986; Hadley, 1988). Care has to be taken in case holding their own cards causes them to feel singled out. This will no longer be a problem when holding one's own cards becomes a normal feature of health care.

Staffing

Inadequate staffing levels can prevent early and adequate contact (Lovell, 1986; Davies, 1987). In some areas, health visitors simply have not answered advertisements for the posts. The grading system can now change that. Health Authorities really serious about providing the service for this high priority group, can attract appropriate staff. They can now reward with a relevant grade and income, higher than that of the average health visitor, the expertise and breadth of responsibility in the specialist work with homeless families.

Another important factor in the equation is staff support: regular contact with managers and time set aside for health visitor mutual support groups, perhaps with others working with the homeless. The issue of support groups was raised in Chapter 2.

Learning from experience

Sometimes young, newly qualified health visitors are assigned to work with homeless families. This was the experience of Claire Johnston (Nursing Standard, 1987). It is a daunting task. Normally our work is mainly discussing health promotion issues. However, this is very low priority for these families who have, for example:

- no cooking facilities
- no food storage facilities, either shelving or refrigeration
- no safe place for the babies and children to play
- no privacy
- no right to be in the room in the day

- no break from the children
- no GP and
- a minimal income.

Sensitivity to the families' situation is crucial. For example, many have a reasonable knowledge of what is needed for a nutritious diet. However, they are locked into making compromises (Conway, 1989, pp. 62–73; Health Visitor, 1989). It is the same with the fire hazard associated with portable gas fires and also their potential for condensation and mould problems (Institution of Environmental Health Officers, 1985; Lowry, 1989). The alternative heating system supplied can cost as much as £25 a week. It leaves no option. This particular issue is a worry because the fire risk in houses in multiple occupancy (HMO) is about ten times higher than that in normal dwelling houses (Health Visitor, 1987a).

Confusions

It is common for the visiting professionals to feel guilty about their own homes and to feel very stressed (Fry, 1987a; 1987b). There are frequently misunderstandings at first about health visitors' influence with the housing department. These add to the feelings of frustration on both sides (Cross, 1988). Ann Cross recommended that where re-housing is an urgent priority and preoccupation for the family, health issues should not be discussed at the first meeting (Hicks, 1985).

Ways to help

Perfect solutions do not exist (Parsons, 1987). However, by taking a very positive approach and by being seen to be helpful, practical and sympathetic, health visitors can help. They might for example, take portable scales into the hotel and run a monthly or weekly clinic session. They might be able to take in toy library equipment on a regular basis and may know, for example:

- a volunteer who would run a mother and toddler group and/or a crèche service while the mothers were occupied with health promotion.

- a solicitor willing to discuss the families' rights and other issues.
- an environmental health officer skilled in HMO work.

Examples of other approaches include the Bayswater Family Health Care project's group for parents and under fives (Cross, 1988) and the project's publication of a much needed booklet, *What can we eat?* (Thomas et al, 1989a; 1989b). Lizzie Hibbitt's (1990) approach is to actively seek from young mothers, descriptions of how they coped in bed and breakfast accommodation. In her work as a midwifery parentcraft co-ordinator, she hands on tips such as;

- rigging up a washing line for the room
- having two dustbins — one for food, the other for nappies
- bathing the baby in the sink
- having two sterilising units — one for normal use, one for what has fallen on the floor.

Lizzie has also found young mothers willing to come and share their experiences with antenatal mothers.

Listening carefully to these families and willingness to take positive initiatives over the provision of information are important aspects of our work. However, these cannot change the fundamental problem.

For a wider audience

In planning and policy-making

It is by informing others of the families' situation that we can help to bring about the adjustments necessary in health and welfare services and in housing. Health visitors are often the only public service employees actually to see the families in the hotels. As the main people with knowledge of the health data on which policy decisions need to be based, it is imperative that we make it available by writing reports. These reports are likely to be better if we work closely together and pool knowledge with other local workers in homelessness.

In the context of homelessness, it is particularly easy to see the importance of this aspect of health education, that is increasing the awareness of

policy-makers (Draper et al, 1980). This aspect is one of the five, categorised and neatly outlined by Coutts and Hardy (1985). The four others are:

- medical
  — a clear and simple message
- educational
  — based on learning needs
- media
  — impact on public opinion
- community development
  — using people's strengths.

Field-level information is essential for management planning and policy-making. A well intentioned project in Bloomsbury failed because planners were unaware of the scale of the problem (Lovell, 1986; Health Visitor, 1987b).

Writing reports for nurse managers takes time, but is far better than providing a verbal report or the Körner statistics (see Ch. 8: Quantification). A written report makes it much easier for the managers to formulate their own plans of action on homelessness (Brown, 1987; Health Visitor, 1987c). It also makes it easier for them to pass on an accurate account of the health visitor findings to a higher level of management. This would be particularly helpful for District Health Authorities setting out to plan and to set clear, relevant objectives for the health of homeless families (Cross et al, 1989, p. 17).

Community Health Councils are also becoming more interested in the size and extent of the problem (Association of Community Health Councils for England and Wales, 1989). June Thompson (1986) suggested that information and relevant articles could be sent to such people as:

- the district general manager
- the health authority chairman
- local councillors
- the director of social services
- local GPs and
- the MP and party leaders.

She also suggested that offers should be made to take members of the health authority and councillors to visit the homeless.

The HVA Special Interest Group for Homelessness (see useful addresses) has been particularly active and successful in increasing awareness of homelessness issues. Georgina Ray (1988) has described how to provide objective data and positive suggestions on what should be done, in a letter to your MP.

Some misunderstandings about nurses' rights to 'speak out' were described in the *Nursing Times* (1987; Lyall, 1987), but these were later resolved in an explanatory letter (Williamson, 1987). The Health Visitor Association provides media training days and advice. It has also published a useful booklet (Health Visitors' Association, 1989). In the unlikely event of attempts by management to imply threats or in any way to limit this side of the work, then advice can also be sought from the professional staff in the Standards and Ethics Department of the United Kingdom Central Council (UKCC) for Nursing, Midwifery and Health Visiting (see useful addresses). The UKCC advisory document is quite clear about the need to seek remedies and not simply to accept minimum standards for our clients (Pine, 1988; United Kingdom Central Council for Nursing, Midwifery and Health Visiting, 1989).

Working together

Meeting with others working in the same field makes it possible to exchange information about each other's roles and experiences, to draw together relevant information and to seek practical means of collaboration. The Bayswater project has a coordinating group which includes people from:

- voluntary agencies
- several local churches
- education welfare
- various health workers
- social services
- Community Health Council
- local advice agencies
- Committee for Racial Equality
- schools
- homeless families themselves and
- from the local community.

This group sends statistical information and a newsletter to many people and has invited key local authority decision-makers to their meetings (Cross, 1988, pp. 85–87).

Take office

One way of being more influential is by becoming a local councillor or by taking up membership of committees in which the relevant decisions are made. The Women into Public Life campaign (see useful addresses) offers advice and some training (Sturt, 1989).

SEARCHING QUESTIONS

MONITORING TO PLAN FOR HEALTH CARE

In this version of the prevention model, we look at monitoring from a community perspective, highlighting the part of our work in which we set out to discover and to build up a picture of local health needs. The aim is to provide an improved basis for planning appropriate preventive health care, in this case from the point of view of homelessness. We shall take a general look at community profiling in Chapter 15.

Who and where?

When any sizable problem seems to be emerging, it is important to work with others to obtain a clear picture and then to make a report. First suspicions of a problem tend to be introduced through anecdotal stories. The accumulation of data needed to demonstrate the actual situation, for example on the number and location of homeless families, requires a cooperative effort. A health visitor or multi-professional working party may be able to draw it all together. Alternatively, specialist health visitors' contact with the appropriate homeless persons unit or units may provide the data.

Problems associated with discovering the number and the whereabouts of homeless families have been touched on at several points earlier in the chapter. Another issue is that of the confidentiality of families' personal information. Cross et al (1989, p. 17) feel that most homeless people would give their consent for the transfer of information, for example,

- names
- birth dates
- current address
- recent previous addresses

if, as part of their counselling, it were explained why it is needed.

Systematic mapping of where families are living in temporary accommodation and of the location of health facilities could help to clarify trends and show where new services would be valuable.

Inexpensive computers

It takes time and a great deal of paperwork to draw together the information needed. Josephine Boyer (1986) and her colleagues in Ealing requested a computer to help with this type of work. The request was refused on account of shortage of money, which is surprising in the light of the inexpensiveness of second-hand computers and software. These are advertised every week, for example in *Micro-Computer Mart*. Also, the cost of learning how to use a computer can now be very reasonable. Disk and tape sets obtainable from organisations such as Headline Communication (see useful addresses) make it both cheap and easy.

What problems?

It is not enough just to know where the people are. It is important to find out what particular problems they are facing. Health visitor research, an added dimension for the computer, will help improve both the health visitor's own, as well as a wider general understanding. Readers will recall Veann Helyger's excellent work in Example One.

There is no lack of issues to study. A survey by Drennan and Stearn (1986) showed that many health visitors all over the country are involved with homelessness and are seeing its effects on health. The health visitors were particularly concerned about:

- mental health — depression is commonplace
- the high incidence of infectious disease
- safety — many accidents to small children and
- the level of malnutrition.

Immunisation rates tend to be poor (Parsons, 1987).

With or without original research, health visitors' reports about homelessness can include copies of articles on relevant surveys and reports. Good examples are Janet Hadley's (1988) neat summary of the *Prescription for poor health* research (Conway, 1988) and Sheila Falconer's (1988) small survey of the eating patterns of bed and breakfast families in seven King's Cross hotels. The reports can also present local information in the context of national trends and statistics.

An even fuller picture can be gained if it is possible to get to know about the difficulties faced locally by such departments as housing and environmental health, and about the way their services are organised. The health visitors in Example Five discovered a great deal about local housing issues and planning, through their meetings with officers from departments such as

- housing
- environmental health
- medical applications for housing

and their regular meetings with a group of professionals and volunteers working with the homeless.

How to provide care?

Schemes for providing relevant, acceptable and accessible services for homeless families will vary considerably between areas and differing circumstances. Many of the basic issues have been discussed in earlier chapters. Strategies for families in temporary accommodation need to be flexible (Parsons, 1987) and can benefit from groupwork (Cross, 1988). It has been suggested (Conway, 1988, pp. xviii–xx) that health authorities should arrange, for example:

- appropriate staffing levels
- locally based outreach services
- mother and baby centres
- food and health policy
- health visitor referral to antenatal clinics
- self-referral to services by homeless people.

The aim is to provide services before problems develop.

BOLSTERING ACTION

PREVENTING DETERIORATION

This last section looks briefly at some of the ways in which health visitors can work with others, firstly to help provide effective support for homeless families and secondly to target selected recurring problems.

Support

Large numbers of homeless families face significant and multiple difficulties. Contributory factors (Cross, 1986; Conway, 1988) include those such as:

- delays regarding a permanent home
- squalid conditions in temporary accommodation
- ignorance of rights
- marginal income and isolation.

Health visitors' therapeutic listening, referral to appropriate services and other supportive work with individual families, is of course relevant. However, it is limited in this context to reacting to people's problems as they arise.

Another and very important part of the role is to act in a proactive way, working with others in local supportive services. The aim is to increase the ability to provide an appropriate service and to improve the potential for mutual support between the families. This approach may for example, lead health visitors to get together with others to set up a group similar to the Bayswater parents and under-fives group (Cross, 1988).

So much depends on local circumstances. There may be opportunities for behind-the-scenes advice

and support for a drop-in day centre similar to that described earlier in Example Two. This refuge offers facilities for washing, cooking, relaxing, talking with friends, safe play and sleep for babies and children and naps for parents. Basically, it provides a place where in the daytime, young families in bed and breakfast accommodation can follow the same pattern of activities that everyone does in their own home. The sustaining atmosphere of this centre facilitates mutual support between the families and provides a nurturing atmosphere for self-help.

In a similar way, close work with staff and families at the local family centre can be valuable. Even such a simple gesture as drawing attention to recent literature, such as on accommodation rights (Campaign for Bedsit Rights, 1989) and benefits information (Chapman et al, 1989; Kennedy et al, 1989), can help others enable families to receive a better supportive service. The Glasgow Health Education Department's *Unemployment and Health* resource pack for use by and with groups, covers many relevant basic issues. Understanding them can help people feel less isolated (Black & Laughlin, 1987).

Positive action

There are many advantages to regular meetings of a group of professionals and volunteers working with homeless families. Such a group might involve a range of workers similar to that mentioned above from the Bayswater coordinating group. It might also include:

- environmental health officers
- lawyers interested in homelessness
- Citizens Advice Bureau workers and of course
- health visitors.

Some advantages have already been mentioned. Another is that, as members of the group discuss and compare their experiences, they may see some patterns emerging in the difficulties that the families encounter. Where these problems are due to inadequacies, misunderstandings or failures in local services, they may be able to be dealt with through cooperative effort within the group.

For example, several group members may discover that parents of school-age children in temporary accommodation are being told that the schools have no places. If at the same time, newcomer parents with permanent addresses report no difficulty about school entry, a pattern is seen. Education welfare officers would be able to find out whether or not there was a lack of places. A positive strategy could then be adopted by the group, using their contacts to discover the extent of the problem. The matter could then be sorted out, for example, via the education welfare officer and the higher echelons of the education department.

One recurring problem for some health visitors is the dilemma they face when they wish to press the local council to improve conditions of bed and breakfast accommodation over issues such as

- fire precautions
- safety of equipment in rooms
- overcrowding
- extent of sharing of facilities
- food storage and kitchens
- safe and well-equipped play areas
- accessible public telephones
- general safety and cleanliness
- the families' privacy,

but want to maintain a good relationship with the hotel managers to facilitate access to homeless families (Conway, 1988, pp. xvi; 39–40).

Regular discussions within the group may throw light on the problems faced locally by the environmental health department (Conway, 1988, pp. 113; 105–115) and inspire positive schemes, such as those undertaken by Southampton and Brighton environmental health departments' Housing in Multiple Occupancy Teams (Douglas, 1989).

Whatever priority is chosen, there is a clear advantage in aiming to direct energies towards particular targets of selected issues, rather than only reacting to individual cases. This cooperative effort has the benefit of helping to prevent deterioration of the situation and its effect on other families.

This chapter has shown some of the ways health visitors can help homeless families, and has provided various examples. The three main themes have been health promotion, assessment of the local situation and teamwork for supportive work, using a prevention model with a community perspective. Homelessness engenders high stress levels for the families and for the workers. Health visitors need a supportive and enabling management approach, the subject of the following chapter.

USEFUL ADDRESSES

Headline Communications Limited
PO BOX 22
Hereford HR4 8UW
Tel 0432 271598

HVA Special Interest Group for Homelessness
c/o Health Visitors' Association
50 Southwark Street
London SE1 1UN
Tel: 071 378 7255

Ms Veann Helyger
Baker Road Clinic
Cheriton
Folkestone
Kent
Tel 0303 275100

Standards and Ethics Department
United Kingdom Central Council for Nursing, Midwifery and Health Visiting
23 Portland Place
London WlN 3AF
Tel 071 637 7181

Women Into Public Life
c/o 300 Group
9 Poland Street
London WIV 3DG
Tel 071 437 2728

REFERENCES

Association of Community Health Councils for England and Wales 1989 Homelessness: the effects on health. Association of Community Health Councils for England and Wales, London

Black D, Laughlin S (eds) 1987 Unemployment and health: resources, information, action, discussion, 2nd edn. Greater Glasgow Health Board, Health Education Department, Glasgow — Recommended. Available from Belvedere House, 1362 London Road, Glasgow G31 4QY Tel 041 556 2201

Boyer J 1986 Homelessness from a health visitor's viewpoint. Health Visitor 59, 11: 332–333

Brown P 1987 A vulnerable minority: homeless families. Senior Nurse 7, 4: 33–35 — Advice and ideas for nurse managers

Campaign for Bedsit Rights 1989 Bedsit rights. A handbook for people who live in bedsits, flatlets, shared houses, lodgings, hostels and 'Bed and breakfast' hotels. Campaign for Bedsit Rights, London — Very useful, clearly written and well presented. Available from 5/15 Cromer Street, London WC1H 8LS Tel: 071 0598/9

Chapman V, Lakhani B, Read J, Wood P 1989 National welfare benefits handbook 1989–90, 19th edn. Child Poverty Action Group — Very useful, clearly written and well presented. Available from CPAG (Pubs), 4th Floor, 1–5 Bath Street, London ECIV 9PY

Conway J (ed) 1988 Prescription for poor health. The crisis for homeless families. London Food Commission/Maternity Alliance/SHAC/Shelter, London — Essential reading.

Coutts L C, Hardy L K 1985 Teaching for health: the nurse as health educator. Churchill Livingstone, Edinburgh, p 24

Cross A 1986 The scandal of B & B hotels. Maternity Action Jan/Feb: 7

Cross A 1988 Improving health care for the homeless. In: Drennan V (ed) 1988 Health visitors and groups: politics and practice. Heinemann Nursing, Oxford — Essential reading.

Cross A, Holden M, Iskander R, Rumney S, Chisholm J W, Eastham D G, Lynch J B, Wilks D M 1989 Homeless families and their health. A joint report by the Health Visitors' Association and the General Medical Services Committee of the British Medical Association on access to primary health care by homeless families. General Medical Services Committee — Essential reading. Available from BMA House, Tavistock Square, London WCIH 9JP

Davies A, Cartwright A, Percy L, Baylis S, Pope E, Davies R and Buchan M 1989 Report from the Southampton Health Visitors Housing Group. Southampton and South West Hampshire Health Authority — Available from Community Nursing Office, Aldermoor Health Centre, Aldermoor Close, Coxford, Southampton S01 6ST

Davies P 1987 Health risks for the homeless. Health Service Journal 97, 5068: 1069

Douglas J 1989 HMOs: a problem multiplying. Municipal Journal 97, 46: 34–36 — An environmental health team approach to difficulties associated with houses in multiple occupation.

Draper P, Griffiths J, Dennis J, Popay J 1980 Three types of health education. British Medical Journal 16th August: 493–495

Drennan V, Stearn J 1986 Health visitors and homeless families. Health Visitor 59, 11: 340–342 —Influential survey of health visitor activity with families in temporary accommodation.

Falconer S 1988 Biscuits for breakfast. Maternity Action 33: 7–8 — Provides clear picture of catering difficulties in temporary accommodation.

Fry A 1987a London like a large refugee camp for homeless claims Howarth. Community Care 682: 1

Fry A 1987b An impossible task for those working with homeless people. Social Work Today 19, 14: 7 — Report of a conference on homelessness.

Furley A 1989 A bad start in life. Shelter, London — Essential reading.

Furley A, Martin J, Crosby M, Pengelly M, Yeang J, Prior J, Pollard L, Gardner S 1988 Homes for Eastenders. Health Visitor 61, 1: 23

Hadley J 1988 Health care for homeless people. Health Service Journal 98, 5120: 1122–1123

Health Visitors' Association 1989 Hitting the headlines. An HVA guide to working with the media. Health Visitors' Association — Well written guide. Available from 50 Southwark Street, London SE1 1UN Tel: 071 378 7255

Health Visitor 1987a Multiple occupation homes. Health Visitor 60, 2: 57

Health Visitor 1987b What is the best approach? Health Visitor 60, 2: 57

Health Visitor 1987c What is the nurse manager's role? Health Visitor 60, 2: 57

Health Visitor 1989 HEA refuses to publish report linking unhealthy diet to poverty. Health Visitor 62, 12: 359

Health Visitor's Association Special Interest Group for Homelessness 1989 Health visiting and homelessness. Pack 1 Families in bed and breakfast accommodation. Health Visitors' Association — Excellent introduction, available from 50 Southwark Street, London SE1 1UN Tel: 071 378 7255

Hibbitt E 1990 Health promotion with homeless families — extending the role of the midwife. Midwives Chronicle and Nursing Notes 103, 1224: 8–10

Hicks C 1985 Life in the B & B. Nursing Times 81, 20: 17–19

Institution of Environmental Health Officers 1985 Environmental health professional practice. Mould fungal spores — their effects on health, and the control, prevention and treatment of mould growth in dwellings. Institution of Environmental Health Officers, Chadwick House, Rushworth St, London

Jackson C 1989 When traditional health visiting becomes impossible. Health Visitor 62, 4: 129–130 — Strategies for care in London and Manchester.

Kennedy C, McMullen J, Rowland M 1989 Rights guide to non-means-tested social security benefits, 12th edn. Child Poverty Action Group — Very useful, clearly written and well presented. Available from CPAG (Pubs), 4th Floor, 1–5 Bath Street, London EC1V 9PY

Lovell B 1986 Health visiting homeless families. Health Visitor 59, 11: 334–337 — Influential article on problems encountered by health visitors.

Lowry S 1989 Temperature and humidity. British Medical Journal 299: 1326–1328 — Discusses cold rooms, dampness and health.

Lyall J 1987 Brent's big brother. Nursing Times 83, 36: 21–22

Nursing Standard 1987 Help for homeless. Nursing Standard 2, 4: 30

Nursing Times 1987 Avenues must be offered within the health service so that professionals have less need to seek redress elsewhere. Nursing Times 83, 34: 3

Parsons L 1987 Flexible care strategies. Health Service Journal 97, 5038: 214–215 — Action taken by City and Hackney Health Authority.

Pine R 1988 On being accountable. Health Visitor 61, 6: 173–175

Ray G 1988 Dear Mrs Thatcher. Nursing Times Community Outlook 84, 19: 6–11

Rutter M, Graham P, Yule W 1970 A neuropsychiatric study in childhood. Heinemann Medical, London

Sturt J 1989 A woman's place . . .. Nursing Times Community Outlook 85, 24: 12

Thomas D, Moore C, Nelson J 1989a Living in bed & breakfast, What can we eat? Parkside Health Authority — Practical and attractive leaflet. Available from Parkside Health Promotion Department, Green Lodges, Barratts Green Road, London NW10 Tel: 081 965 6566

Thomas D, Moore C, Nelson J 1989b (letter) Eating in B & B. Health Visitor 62, 12: 388

Thompson J 1986 Homelessness: a priority for political action. Health Visitor 59, 11: 325

United Kingdom Central Council for Nursing, Midwifery and Health Visiting 1989 Exercising accountability. A framework to assist nurses, midwives and health visitors to consider ethical aspects of professional practice. United Kingdom Central Council for Nursing, Midwifery and Health Visiting, London

While A (ed) 1989 Health in the inner city. Heinemann Medical Books, Oxford pp 6–10; 70–72

Williamson L 1987 (letter) Finding avenues for communications about district problems. Nursing Times 83, 38: 14

FURTHER READING

Travellers

Community Outlook 1987 Travelling right. Nursing Times Community outlook 83, 19: 3

Cornwell J 1984 Improving health care for travellers: report of a conference organised by Save the Children in collaboration with the King's Fund, held at the King's Fund Centre, 29th February, 1984. Kings Fund, London

Crout E 1987 Trailer bound. Nursing Times Community Outlook 83, 19: 12–14

Dopson L 1990 Black Country care. Nursing Times 86, 1: 60 –61

Hussey R M 1988 Travellers and preventive health care: what are health authorities doing? British Medical Journal 296: 1098

McCann V K 1987 Health education for a traveller community. Health Visitor 60, 9: 293–295

Morris M 1987 Stopped in their tracks. Nursing Times Community Outlook 83, 19: 16–19

Patel R 1988 Traveller Families. Association of Metropolitan Authorities, London

Thompson J 1987 Providing care for travellers. Health Visitor 60, 9: 283

Wilson G 1988 On the road. Nursing Times 84, 3: 26–27

Windness B 1987 One year working with travellers. Health Visitor 60, 9: 289–291

General

Special issue of the Health Visitor 1990 On the margins: homeless people and health. Health Visitor 63, 6: 186–205

This chapter returns to the health visitor cycle format. An enabling style of management is discussed from the point of view of background knowledge, health visitor participation, professional development and support and lastly, evaluation.

14

Management style

Some research and ideas from industrial management, relevant to management style in health visiting, are described. A brief introduction to some of the salient factors is followed by four health visiting examples of good practice. The second half of the chapter is divided into the now familiar four sections of the health visitor cycle. A variety of relevant practical issues is discussed.

An enabling management style is the main key to innovation and to taking a broader perspective in health visiting. Both the health visitors and their managers need to understand the strategies involved. It is an interactive process in which both 'sides' contribute. In addition, health visitors can apply these same basic principles to their work with clients.

In this introduction to the subject, many overlapping issues such as management structure and managers' health visiting background or otherwise, have sadly not been able to be included. The main aim has been to increase awareness of the ways that health visitors and their managers can help each other achieve a more participative way of working. Many examples are available of the way this approach helps to overcome the various difficulties currently having to be faced.

THE ESSENTIAL PROBLEM

Managers are being caught in a dilemma. Low and often decreasing levels of resources are coinciding with an increasing need for the service. There is no simple formula for how to respond. There are difficulties, for example, in trying to provide the necessary universal health visiting cover while at the same time concentrating effort where it is most needed. Various approaches are being tried out and solutions are emerging (Orr, 1989). However, every locality is different and the service has to be able to be responsive to these variations.

A management style is needed which maximises on health visitors' and their co-professionals' skills, motivation and knowledge. The aim is to enable staff to plan and implement a high quality, flexible and well-thought-through service, which is responsive to local people's requirements.

THE BASICS

Observations on how to make the most of organisational and staff potential has become available through the research and book, *In search of excellence*, by Peters and Waterman (1982). They were seeking the key elements of success in American industry and found eight basic features. They also found that where most of these features were present together and enthusiastically pursued, there was a correlation with success. These basics can be summarised as:

1. A bias for action — analytical approach to decision-making in which analysis does not impede action; reports and other documentation kept to a minimum.
2. Close to the customer — best ideas from customers, acquired by concentrated and regular listening. Customers specifically courted.
3. Autonomy and entrepreneurship — fostering many leaders and innovators in the organisation, encouraging practical risk-taking and supporting good tries. Small groups of 'pragmatic bureaucracy-beaters' provide a source of much innovation.
4. People more productive when noticed/ involved — attention to employees produces 'an endless stream of Hawthorne effects' (p. 6). Needs small units. Effort put into supporting, training and trusting staff.

5. Explicit attention paid to short, simply stated values on what the organisation stands for, creating an exciting environment; personal attention by management at grass roots level.
6. The organisation stays reasonably close to the core business for takeovers. In the time it takes the new top managers to learn a new industry, key parts of it can be destroyed through bad management.
7. Simplified organisation with few top senior level staff — limiting bureacracy and facilitating creativity, adaptation and concentration on key values.
8. Maximum individual autonomy, but insistence on maintaining key values.

The researchers point out that many institutions *say* they pursue these attributes: the 'excellent' *live* them!

Peters and Waterman regret that a 'numerative rationalist' approach to management has dominated business education, bringing with it a concentration on quantitative analysis. They observe that man is not a rational being; for example, he deludes himself and lives by myths and stories. Staff motivation, participation and self-esteem in management/staff and staff/customer relationships are key factors. In the rationalist approach there is a tendency to guidance by rule-book: constraint and control.

In 'excellent' organisations there is a willingness to try things out and an ability to handle ambiguity and paradox. Some chaos is permissible in return for quick action and regular experimentation. This research has drawn attention to some very important behind-the-scenes processes.

Griffiths Report on the NHS

Nurses have generally been disappointed with the results of the implementation of the Griffiths Report (1983; Buchan, 1987; Chudley, 1989; Robinson & Strong, 1989). However, the Report itself and its accompanying letter echoed several of the ideas set out above. For example, the authors emphasised that

responsibility should be pushed as far down the line as possible, i.e. to the point where action can be taken effectively.

They were concerned that devolution of responsibility was too slow, that it lacked necessary direction and dynamism and that change was difficult to achieve. They wanted management to be concerned with staff motivation and

to capitalise on the existing high levels of dedication and expertise among NHS staff of all disciplines, and to stimulate initiative, urgency and vitality.

They were anxious there should be a keen sense of how well 'customers' are being looked after.

FOUR REAL-LIFE EXAMPLES

These documents have given extra ammunition to forward-looking managers anxious to see innovation and to discover and respond to local people's particular requirements. There are many examples of this enabling management style in health visiting and four are provided here.

The first describes the experience of two health visitors involved in group work on management planning issues and the second is about a health visitor working with the elderly. She was encouraged to plan for and to implement new initiatives. The third example is about the enabling management approach of a neighbourhood nurse manager and the fourth describes the staff-developmental philosophy of management in the city of Oxford. Each example includes a health visitor cycle model showing elements of this participative management approach, which makes the staff feel valued and well motivated and enables them to be more effective.

EXAMPLE ONE: GROUP PROJECTS

A community unit in the north of England is encouraging staff involvement in management planning processes aimed at improving the service. A teamwork approach is being used. A management consultant was brought in to facilitate the early stages.

Representatives of midwives, health visitors, school nurses, clinical medical officers and administrative and clerical staff were invited to a meeting. Liz Winder and Sue Roberts (see Fig. 14.1) each represented the health visitors in their health centre. Everyone at the meeting was asked to suggest issues of concern to the staff.

An ingenious questionnaire, drawn up from this information, was designed to show the degree of concern on each of the thirty issues raised. Every member of the community staff was asked to complete and return it. Use of a computer made it possible to chart the level of concern in each professional group.

Having identified the four most worrying issues:

- staff safety whilst visiting
- increased feedback from all disciplines
- support for staff (care for professional carers)
- consultation before changes,

four working groups were set up to consider them. Staff most anxious about particular issues were naturally assigned to that group. Sue and Liz became members of the 'safety' and 'support' groups.

These two issues are important on account of their influence on work with clients. For example, Liz and Sue know just how much staff support groups can help health visitors gain a better insight into their everyday work and how 'sharing' problematic experiences with supportive colleagues can lead to greater understanding of particular clients who are facing major difficulties. These groups can also gently incorporate more formal peer-group review, thereby further influencing the quality of our work.

The problem of violence to staff is not taken seriously by many employers (Dingwall, 1984). By implementing 'bottom-up management', this health authority is using the expert knowledge and enthusiasm of its staff to plan and take practical action.

Once the objectives for the working groups were set, target dates were arranged. Sue and Liz are both reading widely on the issues they are tackling. Liz is hoping to arrange for a community psychiatric nurse to become involved with their group-work counselling. Feedback sessions with the staff, mainly the health visitors and midwives, have enabled good suggestions to be brought forward. The 'pros' and 'cons' of various possible solutions are being well debated and generally acceptable compromises considered. Some while ago there was a lunchtime peer-support group, but this did not give enough time. The health visitors are hopeful about getting a regular group during working hours.

Fig. 14.1 Health visitor cycle outlining Liz Winder's and Sue Roberts' involvement in a particular style of management.

Managers have been very supportive of the ideas already presented by the groups. Arrangements are being made for those proposals to be put into action. However, investigations, for example into personal alarm equipment and into police interest in staff safety, are getting slow responses. In order to get any action, it has been necessary to follow up initial inquiry letters with repeated phone calls. Having deadlines — certain intermediate dates and a final feedback session — provides a stimulus for action and achievement.

The final feedback and evaluation day is in a month's time. All four groups will be reporting back and everyone is looking forward to hearing what the others have achieved. This 'bottom-up' style of management, drawing out and using fieldworkers' ideas about chosen key

professional matters, is encouraging innovation and strong team participation.

This approach will be very valuable as the community unit increasingly makes use of community health profiles (the subject of another working party) and adopts more effective ways of providing health promotion services. For example, health visitors might wish to work on new ideas such as having a market stall to 'sell health', and/or to consider a minimum level of 'contact with families' rather than the current count of 'home visits'. The staff now has a framework for working together to present managers with well reasoned and thoroughly researched proposals, tailor-made for the locality. This will be particularly helpful now 'patch management' is being planned.

Even though, for both the health visitors, the

groupwork and the feedback sessions have had to be fitted into a busy workload, they are clearly enjoying the experience. They have one regret. This is that the district nurses, who will become a much closer part of the team in 'patch management', are not yet participating in these planning activities.

Teamwork skills are being built up and a forward-looking, proactive style of management is being developed. Clients will benefit and the staff are clearly appreciating and enjoying the group work.

EXAMPLE TWO: A SUPPORT TEAM FOR THE ELDERLY

Moving into a newly created post in a Support

Team for the Elderly is proving to be a very positive experience for Elisabeth Rogers. It is an attractive challenge after many years of the traditional child-centred, 'routine visiting' approach. In this new post, the management style, shown in Figure 14.2, encourages full use of professional skills. It provides opportunities to take initiatives and to implement up-to-date ideas.

The teamwork, in which district nurses and health visitors provide a health promotion and prevention service, is for the elderly in a Health Authority which covers two outer London Boroughs. Elisabeth is assigned to the theoretical care of about 30 000 people over the age of 60 in one of those Boroughs. She is part-time and has recently been joined by a part-time district nurse. They are now working out programmes together.

Fig. 14.2 Health visitor cycle showing some of the ways that the team manager is encouraging innovation by Elisabeth Rogers and the rest of the Support Team for the Elderly.

There was a great deal to learn on joining the team. There were many people to meet and much thinking to be done on how to approach such a broad remit. After a few weeks' induction, Elisabeth was given the freedom to find her way around, making contacts, picking up ideas and planning her first strategies. The team manager was very supportive. She trusted Elisabeth's professional expertise and judgement, leaving her free to do anything that was 'for the benefit of the elderly'. It was a good foundation for innovaton. Verbal progress reports were given. As trials and schemes have progressed, they have been written up. Each programme has helped, along with background reading, to increase understanding of the special needs of older people. The schemes have provided indicators for what should be tried next. Some of the activities are shown in Table 14.1.

Table 14.1 Prevention model showing some of Elisabeth Rogers' activities with the Support Group for the Elderly

Aim	Through	Examples
Prevent occurrence of problems	Health education	'Look After Yourself' tutor and 'Extend' courses for talks with Age Concern and other groups. 'Time to Act' film shows people how they can help themselves
Prevent development of problems	Monitoring/ search	Home visits in pre-war housing estate: discovers grass roots health and welfare needs and dificulties, e.g. form filling to claim eye test & dental fees. Adviser to GP and HV wishing to screen elderly on practice list
Prevent deterioration where problems already exist	Support	Follow up of casualty department home accident cases finds many people needing aids and services, bereavement counselling and care for carers . . .

The team members are based in one centre. They are perpetually learning from each other and sharing their discoveries. They give each other a great deal of valuable support and encouragement. Their team manager has changed but management style has remained the same.

An early idea when the team was set up, was

that a supportive service should be offered to all old people recently discharged from hospital who were not visited by a district nurse or health visitor. Wanting to concentrate on positive health promotion, one of Elisabeth's early activities was to follow up home accident cases of elderly people who attended the local Casualty Department, but who were not admitted. The hospital is adjacent to a large pre-war housing estate. It has many low income elderly residents.

When followed up, quite a few of the old people were found to need services, for example, chiropody, walking aids or meals on wheels. Advice aimed at helping them maintain their independence was also an important part of the work. Box 7.5 in the chapter on work with the elderly (p. 134), lists some of the factors included in the assessment.

The high levels of local use of the casualty service led to Elisabeth's visiting many of these homes. This 'random sampling' helped build up a picture of that area's grass roots needs and difficulties and gave direct knowledge of particular problems there. For example, it became clear that the complexities of form filling prevent many old people from claiming the costs of eye tests and dental care. This and other by-products of this work are already helping to decide further strategies.

The philosophy of the team has gradually altered. It is now felt that it would be better to concentrate much more on providing a service at an earlier stage, to promote the health of the well elderly and to initiate screening. Already a local general practitioner and health visitor have become interested in screening their elderly and Elisabeth has helped them research and plan this.

Health education accounts for about a third of Elisabeth's time. Funds were made available for her to go on 'Look After Yourself' and 'EXTEND' tutor courses. She goes into Age Concern and other existing groups. After attending these courses, many old people have gone on to take regular exercise, which they had not done before: activities such as swimming, walking and dancing.

The General Manager was speaking publicly about these courses and the concurrent screening. It was reported in the press. The Health Authority phones became jammed with enquiries. Many ideas for team projects arose out of this public interest.

However, the team members are aware that problems can arise where public expectations are raised and a service cannot be provided. At the moment, it is a question of attempting to make the best possible use of the available resources.

With this in mind, Elisabeth is planning to put on a health education course in the pre-war housing estate, which will help to respond to the particular needs there. Also, the public interest in screening, brought to light by the press report, led to the idea of taking these services to swimming sessions and to other suitable places where old people are meeting together. In the light of the enormous task of trying to provide a service for 30 000 old people, this may not seem much. However, having been encouraged to make their own investigations and to implement and monitor their own ideas, the team is clearly moving gradually towards its goal.

Neighbourhood nursing teams are being set up in the District and it is proposed that the Support Team be separated and posted out with these. However, it is also intended that these 'specialists' continue to meet very regularly to share ideas and to provide mutual support.

Elisabeth is convinced that the team members will increasingly act as an advisory resource for the generalist health visitors as they move forward and away from the current traditional 'routine' child-centred approach. Perhaps a similar enabling management style for neighbourhood nursing will help them to do this.

EXAMPLE THREE: A NEIGHBOURHOOD NURSE MANAGER

Two years ago Sue Machell became a neighbourhood nurse manager in Wandsworth. Neighbourhood health care teams, based on ideas from the Cumberlege Report (Department of Health and Social Security, 1986), were being introduced throughout the Community Unit. The management style had already been established as democratic and biased towards action, during the previous year's planning stage. For example, health visitors and other field-level staff had been included in the planning committees. They channelled in their colleagues' suggestions and reactions. These committees generated a minimum of reports and everything was concentrated on getting an early start.

When Sue arrived, the district nurses, health visitors and school nurses in her patch still had separate offices and separate nurse managers. Accommodation for the teams was not perfect, but it was decided to go ahead with the new scheme. The nurses moved into offices with their particular team. The move had its

difficulties. Sue likened forming a team to having a baby: you cannot be totally prepared for it, though it helps to have given the matter a good deal of thought.

Putting nurses together does not automatically make a team. Sue said staff can be quite upset about changes. The individual way people will *feel* about it cannot be foreseen. Some show distinct signs of bereavement, such as phases of anger which come and go. These people need a chance to talk the problem through, just like anyone else in a bereavement situation.

Health visitors in particular found it hard. They are not used to working in teams and are much more used to identifying with their own profession. Also, general practice (GP) attachment is encouraged locally and has been increasing. Some of these health visitors found they did not feel so much part of the team. It is a question of helping them confront and talk through these issues.

The main difficulties are now sorted out. The benefits of successful team building and common goals for neighbourhood health care have been evident for some time. Team members pool their ideas, share local knowledge and work together for their community, and morale is much improved. For example, one health visitor, working there in the normal, isolated way for the past 20 years, had little feedback from colleagues. Now in a team, she gets a great deal of appreciation of her wide experience and her specialist local knowledge.

The success also shows in even more fundamental ways. For example, prior to the new democratic and team approach, there were problems in attracting staff. The Unit was regularly one third short of health visitors, but now has the full number. For many years, the money not spent on staff was diverted for use by the acute unit. That money has now been returned to the Community Unit.

In this fieldworker-centred management approach, all team members are encouraged to develop their own ideas, to formulate objectives and to be involved in self and peer assessment. The Community Unit employs a staff development officer to help staff achieve this. The 'plodders' as well as the 'high fliers' are nurtured and appreciated. In the past, the latter have attracted all the attention and have then moved away seeking promotion. Sue explained that the backbone of the work in a District is provided by so-called 'ordinary' nurses and health visitors. They are now supported and educated proportionately more.

Everyone is encouraged to spend a half day in the library once a month. Most of the team members are receiving assertiveness training to help them to achieve the changes that they seek. Days off are given for relevant education. For example, one health visitor is studying family therapy, which is particularly relevant in her neighbourhood. She is having a day a week in term time for two years.

The aim is to concentrate on what can reasonably be achieved, to find out what staff are good at and to help them develop that. Sue gave examples of health visitors working with groups in which they had a special interest and said that group work has been increasing significantly.

This democratic and flexible management style helps the health visitors and other team members to plan their individual and joint objectives. Sue says it is a question of negotiation with the staff. For example, when there is a management objective to be tackled, first an explanation is given of what is intended. Then the team is asked what they want to do to achieve this.

When it is the other way round and team members come to Sue with a new idea, she will often say, 'That sounds an interesting idea, would you like to look into and develop it?' She then asks for a note of exactly what is wanted and for a list of the good and bad points about it. This way, well thought out ideas are presented by the staff, perhaps along with some preliminary criteria for team and self-assessment.

The adult learning model of quality assurance (Wilson, 1987) is used locally. It mirrors the

Fig. 14.3 Health visitor cycle showing some important factors in Sue Machell's work as a neighbourhood nurse manager in Wandsworth.

style of management. Sue feels strongly about clarity of objectives and says, 'If you have no plan and aim at nothing, you will certainly hit it. But, aim at something and you will get there.'

Managers also need support and education. Sue has gained much from other managers in the District and from the Health Visitors' Association's (HVA) Senior Managers' Network (see Useful Addresses). She goes on various courses and undertakes a great deal of management reading. She has a day off each week to study for a degree.

As shown in Figure 14.3, this management style has paid off. The team members have been able to provide a more thinking and responsive service, morale is high and staffing levels are at last correct. At the time of writing, Sue's neighbourhood nurse management post is being taken over by somebody else. She has been promoted to Locality Manager.

EXAMPLE FOUR: HEALTH VISITOR DEVELOPMENT

Three years ago, Jackie Carnell became Assistant Director of Nursing Services in Oxford City. Her remit includes the professional development of health visitors and school nurses for Oxfordshire and the management of community nursing services in Oxford City. The now well-known Oxfordshire strategy for health visiting was being formulated by field staff, clinical practice development workers and managers when she came into the post.

Jackie is a firm believer in the so-called 'bottom-up' management, but says it should be known as 'top-down'. This she explained, is because *service delivery* is the most important factor and therefore the staff actually delivering the service are the key people. They and the clients should be seen as at the top. The purpose of management is to nurture, empower and to support these field workers and, Jackie argues, the management hierarchy is inversely able to do this (see Fig. 14.4). The lower the level of management and closeness of contact with field staff, the greater is the ability to fulfill this nurturing role.

The most important management relationship is the one between health visitors and their immediate nurse managers. It is at this level that staff self-esteem is most effectively nurtured and that a sensitive assessment can be made of the resources the health visitors need in order to do their work properly. These include adequate:

- explanation of what is expected of them

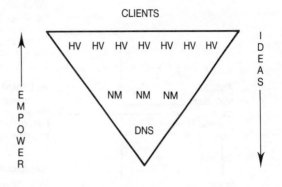

Fig. 14.4 A diagram depicting Jackie Carnell's idea of 'top-down' management, in which the health visitors (HV) as service providers are at the top. Nurse managers (NM) or senior nurses come below. This model inverts the standard picture of nursing hierarchy and puts the clients first. The innovation and ideas come from clients and field-level practice, and 'empowerment' through management.

- education
- work accommodation and equipment
- time
- professional support
- and systematic assessment of their individual needs for professional development.

In order to enable a closer and more productive management style in the city, the four nursing officers have developed into a team of six senior nurses who are responsible for fewer staff. One fifth of the time in this new post is spent in practising field-level health visiting. As shown in Figure 14.5, this side-by-side work between health visitor and senior nurse enables these new managers to experience the effects of change and get more immediate feedback on the feelings of staff.

It is too easy, Jackie observes, for management to be seen as a separate part of the service. She has been aware of situations where new ideas and innovations are bubbling up in the practice of community nursing, whilst management has stayed unmoved and unchanged. It is like a heavy sea crashing against great bureaucratic rocks, but swirling on and around, despite them.

Managers need to be a proactive part of change. That does not mean taking an autocratic or dogmatic approach, feeding information and instructions to staff. What is

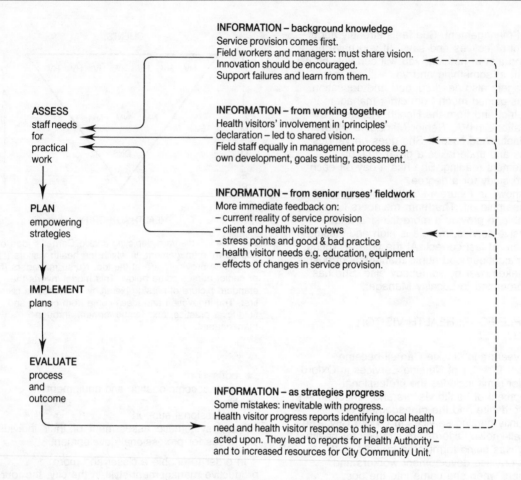

Fig. 14.5 Health visitor cycle showing some important aspects of Jackie Carnell's staff-development approach to management.

wanted is an interactive and empowering approach. The aim is that managers should act towards their health visitors in the same way that they hope health visitors are behaving towards their clients. This involves, for example:

- giving them confidence in their own ability
- working on their strengths
- starting where they are at
- encouraging self-reliance and
- having an open and honest relationship.

Honesty is important. For example, child-abusing parents are less able to improve if health visitors are not diplomatically honest about their concern. In the same way, less-than-adequate health visitors need an open and truthful relationship with management, in order to improve the quality of their work. Jackie

says the senior nurses are encouraged to practice openness over records and reports on their staff. This style of management does not come easily to everyone. The senior nurses too, need the support and the encouragement of *their* managers.

Valued and nurtured within this 'staff-developmental' ethos of management, individual health visitors are free to use their professional judgement. They can mould their service to fit in with the clients' perceptions and with the health needs found in their particular caseload. This freedom is possible because the boundaries of their responsibilities are clearly laid out.

The tasks expected of the health visitors are described from two main viewpoints. Firstly, there is an underlying 'shared vision' within the

Oxfordshire health visiting service. This has been clarified and written up as their basic philosophy. There is also a clearly stated job description for health visitors that really does reflect their work (Health Visitor Development Group, 1989, p. 29–33). These wider parameters of the work were drawn up and agreed as part of the Oxfordshire health visiting strategy, through working parties in which field-level health visitors were the main representatives. Secondly, working from annually compiled practice health profiles, each health visitor selects priorities and achievable goals, also recording and reporting what identified health needs are being left out of the programme. These narrower parameters are self set. They are measured against the Unit and District objectives which are also beginning to be more clearly stated.

The health visitors are given authority to practise in the way their caseload dictates and are encouraged to be creative and innovative. Jackie explained that change cannot go ahead without some mistakes occurring. She says that in good management this is accepted as a necessary part of progress. The alternative, professional stasis, is clearly to be avoided.

On account of all these factors, staff anxiety levels are being reduced. Health visitors are now truly able to work together with their clients, planning strategies of care. The health visitors are expanding their ways of working. For example, there has been an increase in group work and also a great deal of inter-professional teamwork, particularly regarding the Healthy Cities Project in Oxford.

The health visitors' work is now being acknowledged. The annual evaluation of their work enables regular detailed reports to be submitted to the Health Authority. The Unit General Manager has been able to present a good case. Extra resources have been assigned to the City, including two more health visitors, two more district nurses and clerical staff. Health visiting has achieved a much higher profile and the programme continues very positively.

Jackie likens both managers and health visitors to jugglers' spinning plates, each balanced and turning at the top of a pole. Like the plates, we all tend to wobble a bit. Each of us needs a little touch and some attention to keep us on course and working well. Jackie feels strongly that no one should work alone. Practice and management need to go forward together in a direction that has been agreed and set in action by team effort. This is the key to staff development — and success.

HELP AND HINDRANCE

In this section, we look at practical help available and at the difficulties for some managers. The subsequent sections look more specifically at ways health visitors and their managers can help each other achieve an enabling style of management. The format is outlined in Figure 14.6.

BACKGROUND KNOWLEDGE AND PERCEPTIONS

There can be little disagreement about the need to capitalise on the dedication and expertise amongst staff and to employ an enabling, participative style of management. It is obvious that staff should be provided with supportive attention, an exciting and creative working environment and all the other features of an excellent management style listed at the beginning of the chapter. The question is: how can this be achieved and what help and guidance is there?

Help

There is a great deal to learn in the small amount of time generally allotted to formal health visitor management training (Bowden, 1987). There is no research to show how health visiting management style is acquired. Perhaps it has mainly to do with a combination of personality and the general management ethos locally. Whichever way, enabling and participative management is more easily said than done!

Books can provide a very good medium for handing on relevant advice. Patricia Slack (1987) regretted the lack of literature by nurse managers describing practical aspects of their work. She felt

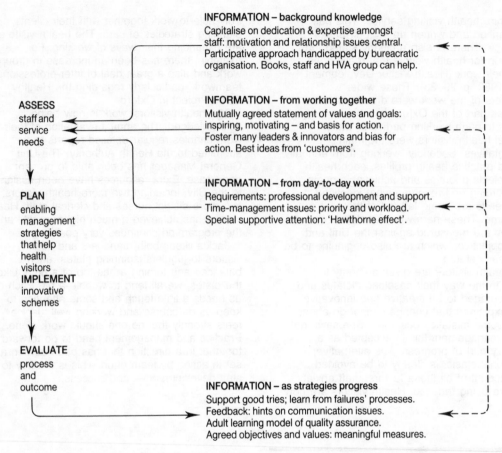

INFORMATION – background knowledge
Capitalise on dedication & expertise amongst staff: motivation and relationship issues central. Participative approach handicapped by bureacratic organisation. Books, staff and HVA group can help.

ASSESS
staff and service needs

INFORMATION – from working together
Mutually agreed statement of values and goals: inspiring, motivating – and basis for action. Foster many leaders & innovators and bias for action. Best ideas from 'customers'.

PLAN
enabling management strategies that help health visitors

INFORMATION – from day-to-day work
Requirements: professional development and support. Time-management issues: priority and workload. Special supportive attention: 'Hawthorne effect'.

IMPLEMENT
innovative schemes

EVALUATE
process and outcome

INFORMATION – as strategies progress
Support good tries; learn from failures' processes. Feedback: hints on communication issues. Adult learning model of quality assurance. Agreed objectives and values: meaningful measures.

Fig. 14.6 Health visitor cycle showing several important features of an enabling community management style.

each new manager has to start from scratch rather than being able to build on others' experience. Some recent books which may help are listed in Box 14.1.

There are three introductions to management style and employee relationships that are well worth recommending. Like the Peters and Waterman (1982) book referred to earlier in the chapter, they are American. They are easy and quick to read. One is written specifically for nurse managers and provides very practical advice and many examples (Pugh and Woodward-Smith, 1989). Another is amusing and provides a very clear description of how to motivate people (Blanchard & Johnson, 1983). The third takes a 'health' perspective (Blanchard & Tager, 1986). These books would be useful both to health visitors and their

managers. The problems need to be understood and the relevant skills practised on both sides.

Health visitors and other community staff can make a significant contribution towards an appropriate management style. Research into nurse managers' stress drew attention to the managers' tendency to lack of self confidence (Hingley et al, 1986). With this in mind and recalling her own management experience, Eileen Kay (1988) described how staff can help by providing their managers with positive feedback and constructive suggestions. Ms Kay said that it facilitates the managers' ability to come out from behind 'a safety screen of authority' and perform well.

Another source of help for managers is the Health Visitor Association Senior Management Network (see useful addresses). It provides the

Box 14.1 Some recent books on nurse management

Dauncey J. Twinn S & Carnell J 1990
Managing change in clinical practice
Health Visitors' Association, £1.95

Winn L, Quick A 1990
User friendly services. Guidelines for managers of community health services
King's Fund Centre, £9.75

Scammell B 1990
Communication skills
Macmillan Education, £6.99

Broome A 1990
Managing change
Macmillan Education, £6.99

Marson S, Johnston R, Hartlebury M & Scammell B 1990
Managing people
Macmillan Education. £6.99

Pugh J B & Woodward-Smith M A 1989
Nurse manager. A practical guide to better employee relations
W B Saunders Company, £7.50

Dodwell M & Lathlean J (eds) 1988
Management and professional development for nurses
Harper and Row, £9.95

Hyett K 1988
Nursing management handbook
Churchill Livingstone, £11.95

Marriner-Tomey A 1987
A guide to nursing management, 3rd edn
Blackwell Scientific, £18.50

---

opportunity for exchange of ideas and support. Practical experiences can be handed on — even though there is no time to write about it!

Hindrance

Managers working in a highly bureaucratic organisation may face extra difficulties. These can be associated, for example, with higher management, limited personal experience and/or the characteristics of the staff with whom they work.

Task-oriented directives from the upper echelons of management can provide significant hurdles. It is, of course, easiest for a manager to decide one-sidedly a course of action, then set tasks and monitor to see if these tasks are achieved. When this happens, the tasks tend to be based on the more readily measured criteria and crude statistics, for example, immunisations, screening tests and numbers of clients seen. These decisions can overrule action on sensitive but less visible criteria, such as personality and relationship matters. It is these latter factors that keep the organisation running well. More importantly, they are the key to a good health visiting service.

Sometimes health visitor managers have been promoted on a basis of seniority rather than aptitude (Health Visitors Association, 1985, p. 42). Those with no personal field-level experience of trying to innovate, may find particular difficulty in adjusting to the ambiguities associated with an environment of change.

Table 14.2 Comparison of some features of the 'bottom-up' (enabling and participatory) and the 'top-down' (controlling and bureaucratic) styles of management

	'Bottom-up' communicative/ participative management style	'Top-down' hierarchical/ bureaucratic management style
Main emphasis	Enablement and staff development	Control and command
Knowledge	Aware each health visitor is a specialist on own locality and develops own particular expertise	Assume know more than field-workers and must decide for them
Approach	Flexible: attempts response to stated local need. Encourages use of staff initiative and further education and development	Rigid: limited to knowledge at top management level. Task oriented. Resists new ideas 'not invented here'
Planning	Based on mutually agreed goals. Negotiated decisions: staff encouraged to demonstrate case for change of approach	Decisions made according to particular interest of dominant manager or advisor — or current fashion
Staff meetings	Forum for exchange of ideas	Formulated ideas 'handed down'
Staff motivation	Excellent: relevance of work obvious, and *feeling* of control & being valued	Poor: not convinced of importance of what asked to do

In a very bureacratic organisation, people who take risks and challenge the status quo are seen as a nuisance. This may lead to high staff turnover and leave behind a large proportion of staff well-schooled in meekly carrying out tasks proposed by people further up the hierarchy. Staff who have adjusted to this management style may have difficulty in adopting a new, more flexible approach. Table 14.2 shows some of the features of the two opposing styles of management.

Hindrances such as these make achieving an enabling and participative style of management more of a challenge. However, there are many positive steps that managers and staff can take to help each other attain it. We shall consider some in the following sections. First we shall look at the creation of a mutually agreed statement of goals and values. This will help top managers and others understand the purpose and parameters of the work. We shall also discuss some aspects of staff involvement in drawing up their own suggestions on more effective ways of working.

CREATIVE PLANNING

INFORMATION — FROM WORKING TOGETHER

Working parties provide one way of helping health visitors to be drawn into the planning processes. Volunteer health visitors delegated by the staff from their health centres work along with representatives of management on some particular issue. It has been a fairly common strategy. Groups without management can also get together formally or informally and be very effective. Vari Drennan (1988) has provided several examples.

Shared goals and values

The fifth Peters and Waterman (1982) basic feature in our introduction, noted the importance of being clear about the organisation's basic philosophy. Oxfordshire has provided a very good example of a group working to make explicit their shared vision of their work. The subsequent statement describing a set of fundamental principles formed the basis of their new strategy (Dauncey, 1987; 1988; 1989; 1990; Health Visitor Development Group, 1989; Deacon, 1989; Jackson, 1989a; Nashe, 1990). Their achievement has shown that paying specific attention to what the organisation stands for, has indeed helped to create an exciting environment in which to work.

A health visiting shared ideal and vision was found to be a major motivating force (West, 1989a). There are many advantages in having it written and made explicit in terms of philosophy and goals mutually agreed by staff and management. Liz Winn (1987) described how a grass roots attempt to change the way of working failed because the objectives did not match those of the local policy framework.

The Royal College of Nursing (1989) sees a written statement as the first requirement in the management of nursing. However, it is not always easy to achieve. Practical advice on working through the ideas may be obtained, for example, from Gawlinski and Graessle's (1988, pp. 35–46) workbook and from *The One Minute Manager*'s approach to goal setting (Blanchard & Johnson, 1983, pp. 27–34). Brief and readable advice on how to improve writing skills is provided by Health Care Education Associates (1986).

Fostering many leaders

Once a mutually agreed written statement of values and goals is achieved, it becomes less frightening for managers to allow greater freedom to innovate, within those parameters. Autonomy and entrepreneurship can be encouraged. Staff can develop their own special skills, helping to maximise the pool of expertise available within the limited community resources. Leadership qualities of relevant members of the general public can be harnessed.

Groups of community staff can work together pooling their local knowledge and ideas for action and they can draw up community and caseload profiles. These issues will be discussed in Chapter 15. As the best ideas come from the customers, the staff need to be free to 'network' in the community and to use their initiative in gaining and maintaining good contacts. These factors have already been mentioned in Chapter 12.

Creativity and early action on ideas depend on an organisational and a decision-making approach that does not impede or obstruct. The first, third and seventh of the basic features listed in our introduction (Peters and Waterman, 1982) clearly demonstrate this. However, group work and other aspects of 'working together' do not always fulfil these requirements.

Groupthink or teamwork?

Robert Waterman (1987) looked at the difference between teamwork and what he called 'groupthink'. Teamwork was defined as existing where there is healthy discussion open to new ideas. In groupthink, on the other hand, there is an expectation of agreement with the dominant view. Dissension is discouraged. There is a tendency to 'cover-up' and a fundamental assumption that participants will not 'create waves'. Groupthink has basically a suppressive nature. Waterman's analysis helps managers and staff to look critically and constructively at the processes taking place in their group and other planning work.

It is important that a fair hearing is given to all proposals and ideas, that there is the ability to negotiate and that a reasonable level of mutual agreement is reached. In any group there is likely to be a significant diversity of opinions and priorities. A certain amount of give and take is inevitable.

Assertiveness training

Many health visitors and managers are finding that assertiveness training increases their confidence and their ability to state their case. It helps them cope with the various conflicting pressures and the underlying ambivalences involved. Figure 14.7 provides a simple picture of the value of an assertive management style and the unfortunate outcomes of passive and aggressive approaches.

Some of the books describing assertiveness techniques and associated factors are listed in Box

MANAGEMENT STYLE

PASSIVE	ASSERTIVE	AGGRESSIVE
staff goals only	mutually agreed goals	organisational goals dominate
no respect from staff or organisation	cooperation and respect from staff	poor morale: high staff leaving rate

Fig. 14.7 A continuum showing the range of management style from passive to aggressive. It is based on Pugh and Woodward-Smith's (1989, pp. 3–12) description and outlines some of the effects on goals and staff morale.

14.2. Self-help schemes and advice are available both for individual and/or for group use (Lindenfield, 1986; Bond, 1987; 1988a; 1988b; 1988c; 1988d; 1988e; 1988f; 1988g; 1988h; 1988i; Pugh & Woodward-Smith, 1989).

It is well worth practising these skills. There are so many sensitive issues around. For example, staff need to be aware that their new ideas may be

Box 14.2 Some books discussing assertiveness and self-awareness issues.

Pugh J B & Woodward-Smith M A 1989
Nurse manager. A practical guide to better employee relations
W B Saunders Company, Philadelphia

Bond M 1986
Stress and self-awareness: a guide for nurses
Heinemann Nursing, London

Dickson A 1982
A woman in your own right: assertiveness and you
Quartet, London

Alberti R & Emmons M 1983
Your perfect right. A guide to assertive living
Impact Publishers, United States

Lindenfield G 1986
Assert yourself
Thorsens Publishing Group, Wellingborough

Tschudin V & Schober J 1989
Managing yourself
Macmillan Education, Basingstoke

Burnard P 1985
Learning human skills. A guide for nurses
Heinemann Nursing, London

lampooning some dearly-held philosophy and/or their manager's proud success of a few years back. It can be very difficult for these managers not to be defensive. They probably spent just as much time and effort on getting their scheme implemented as the current generation is spending now.

These and other skills involved in interpersonal competence are seen by Field and Larson (1989) as a key matter in the preparaton of staff for management. These researchers' in-depth study of one manager's work, demonstrated that such skills are central to every aspect of management.

The qualities of leadership were considered by Jane Salvage (1989). She listed the attributes of 'good' and 'bad' leaders and demonstrated that successful leaders do not necessarily have wide formal powers. It is more a question of being able to convince others of a vision of the future and to cope with the practicalities of achieving it. These skills are needed amongst staff and managers alike, so that they are able to plan and work together towards shared goals.

SUPPORT AND DEVELOPMENT

INFORMATION — FROM DAY-TO-DAY WORK

The equivalent of this section in earlier health visitor cycles, has been used to highlight information from health visitor observations and client opinion. In this particular case it looks at managers' observations and health visitors' views about their everyday functioning and the way they are feeling. This is very important information for managers planning support and development for health visitors.

A good quality service depends on the provision of professional requirements, such as relevant accommodation, equipment and support, a clear remit, education, adequate time, and a systematic and sympathetic assessment for individual professional development (West, 1989a; 1989b). Managers need clear and regular feedback on these issues.

Limited space allows us to consider only one of these requirements. Time management has been chosen to provide an example of how management and staff can work together towards a suitable work environment and help overcome everyday-work tensions and difficulties. Time management is a key issue regarding professional standards.

Time management

More than a quarter of the health visitors taking part in a research project (West & Savage, 1988a; 1988b; 1988c; 1988d; West et al, 1988) identified pressures of time as a major source of stress. This was caused by, for example, general work overload, including telephoning and clerical pressures. Other sources of stress were 'difficult' cases and visits, low morale and feelings of inadequacy and isolation, and managers who did not understand the work. Gough and Hingley (1988) found a similar pattern.

One way to help overcome work overload problems is for health visitors to take positive steps to demonstrate visually (see Figs. 14.8a and 14.8b) how their time is spent. Clarity about this issue is important for increased:

- management understanding
- health visitor morale and
- professional standards for both.

Time management is a basic key to good proactive health visiting and to being able to put the basic principles into practice. A visual presentation of workload obligations can be a powerful tool. It is something health visitors can provide for their managers to help them argue more lucidly for resources. It can also help to focus on the important differences between:

- priority and urgency
- caseload and workload.

The quality of a health visitor's work and the related implications for professional competence/incompetence may depend on being clear about these issues.

Priority and urgency

When health visitors have far too many demanding

	MONDAY	TUESDAY	WEDNESDAY	THURSDAY	FRIDAY
8.30	C L E R I C A L W O R K				
10.30 11.30 12.30	Staff meeting /visits	Child protection liaison meeting /visits		Primary H.C. team meeting. Talk in school.	etc etc etc
1 pm 2 pm 3 pm	Child health clinic		Child health clinic	Market stall	etc etc etc
4 pm	C L E R I C A L W O R K				

Fig. 14.8a An example of part of a timetable format to demonstrate a health visitor's workload. Overlays such as that in Figure 14.8b can be used to demonstrate the workload implications of extra caseloads or 'acting up' for managers.

	MONDAY	TUESDAY	WEDNESDAY	THURSDAY	FRIDAY
8.30	C L E R I C A L W O R K				
10.30 11.30 12.30	Staff meeting /visits	Child protection liaison meeting /visits	Primary H.C. team meeting /visits		etc etc etc
1 pm 2 pm 3 pm		Elderly assessment clinic		Child health clinic	etc etc etc
4 pm	C L E R I C A L W O R K				

Fig. 14.8b An example of part of a timetable overlay showing the reassigned workload of an absent colleague. It is placed on top of the health visitor's basic timetable to demonstrate time-allocation problems and the related implications for professional standards. Further caseloads or 'acting up' would need further overlays.

problems filling their day, there is no time left to step back and take a professional look at *priorities*. The *urgency* of innumerable pressing issues can crowd out the really important part of the work (Lakein, 1985; Cowley, 1989). Where the health visitors allow themselves to take on too many

responsibilities, their professional competence can become endangered.

Caseload and workload

The solution is to be quite clear about the difference between caseload and workload. Differing somewhat from the English National Board (1986) definition, *caseload* tends to be identified with reference to the filing cabinet and health visitor record cards (Piggott, 1988). This gives no indication of the actual work involved, especially with regard to the many time-consuming, behind-the-scenes activities such as:

- report writing
- lengthy handwritten records
- telephone calls seeking immediate aid
- teaching visiting students
- form filling and
- liaison work.

Fortunately, in-depth, qualitative research into health visiting practice, such as Luker and Chalmers' (1989) study of referral activities, is emerging. This research will help managers and others gain a better understanding of the complex processes underlying everyday health visiting tasks, and the time and skills needed for them.

Workload, then, looks at the actual tasks undertaken. A timetable presentation similar to the charts at school or college, is the best way to demonstrate it. This chart shows the major activities throughout the day, each week or each month, using colour or marking codes as shown in Figures 14.8a and 14.8b. This can then be compared with a pie chart like that in Figure 14.9. The pie is drawn to show the percentages of time that, in an ideal situation, would be allotted to important health visiting activities such as:

- planning
- recording
- professional reading
- research
- contact with manager
- peer group evaluation
- liaison
- networking
- group work
- clinic work
- visiting.

Charting in this way makes a good exercise. For example, health visitors who accept second caseloads or who 'act up' for managers in addition

For example :

visits
planning and research
contact with manager
peergroup evaluation
liaison
clinic work
et cetera, et cetera

Fig. 14.9 Pie chart format demonstrating how it can be used to show time allocation in an 'ideal' workload. As there is no absolute ideal, the sizes of the sections and the items included would vary somewhat between individual health visitors.

to their caseload, will soon be able to gauge to what extent they are, or are not, leaving themselves time to undertake good quality work. Some part of their work must be left unattended to (Brown, 1987).

Professional competence

The danger is that health visitors who mildly and unthinkingly accept more and more work, are hazarding their professional competence. They risk being disciplined for poor quality work, *and* without their overloaded work schedule being taken into account.

It is the individual responsibility of all health visitors, and of their managers once they know of the situation, to make sure work practice conforms with the United Kingdom Central Council (1984) code of conduct. Clauses 4, 10 and 11 are those of concern in this particular context. The standard against which to measure is basically that set in the health visitor qualifying examinations and in the period of supervised practice. Cath Jackson (1989b) describes the importance of writing to managers and requesting a meeting in cases where workloads could endanger standards of practice.

Where time-management difficulties are due to staff shortages, the question is why? In some cases the vacancies remain unfilled because the money for them has been transferred into the acute sector and away from preventive care. Another reason could be associated with the reputation of the community nursing services. June Andrews (1989) advises managers to market what they are doing in their authority and to make sure staff feel wanted.

Hawthorne effect

Staff need to be nurtured. Eileen Kay (Dopson, 1984) stressed the importance of informal, regular contact with staff. Opportunities for professional education and development and good management support are important factors in staff retention (Darbyshire, 1988; Nursing Times, 1988b; Shenton & Hamm, 1988; Willkin, 1988; Andrews, 1989; Barratt, 1989) as well as for standards of practice.

High levels of feedback, good knowledge of results and supportive senior nurses have distinctly positive effects on health visiting practice (West et al, 1988): the 'Hawthorne effect' of Peters and Waterman's (1982, p. 6) fourth basic factor. Like the researcher's influence in the experimental situation, high levels of interest and regular personal attention from management stimulate exceptional effort and achievements from staff.

It also facilitates two-way communications about professional needs for support and development, including workload issues.

A POSITIVE APPROACH

INFORMATION — AS STRATEGIES PROGRESS

Regular two-way communications and 'nurturing' become particularly important when health visitors and managers are trying to study what has been achieved and what can be learned from the processes underlying their work. The ability to be frank with each other and, at the same time, to be supportive and emphasise the positive, is a key factor. This section looks at some intercommunication issues in evaluation, firstly of health visiting and then of management style.

Feedback on innovations . . . .

Encouragement from the manager helps to keep motivation and morale levels high, for example through:

- 'one minute praising' (Blanchard & Johnson, 1983)
- supporting 'good tries'
- helping staff see
  — 'failure' as a positive learning experience and
  — some mistakes inevitable with progress.

Pugh and Woodward-Smith (1989, pp. 62–69) provide seven guiding principles to guide managers providing performance feedback. They suggest there should be:

- staff expectation of performance evaluation, both formal and informal
- well-timed, that is, early feedback
- sensitivity to individual circumstances
- feedback on specific issues, stated in measurable objective terms
- tactful communication — 'I-messages' (pp. 13–19) recommended
- honest and constructive feedback and
- checking that the *intended* message was received.

This analysis tends to ignore the active part which the nurse or health visitor takes in her own evaluation. However, the authors draw attention to many important issues. For example, the traps that managers with a nursing background may fall into, such as trying to be a 'super-nurse' (pp. 35–41) or tending to 'nurse' employees (pp. 73–79).

Many managers and senior nurses have responsibility for 30 or more staff (Health Visitor, 1987; West, 1989a). Some are overloaded with many administrative tasks and have difficulty in keeping in touch with their staff (West, 1989a; West & Savage, 1988c; 1988d).

Increasingly, staff development officers are being employed to help provide in-service support and education. Assessment of staff performance is a natural part of this. For some health visitors, this non-managerial post may provide a less threatening setting for evaluation than that with a manager or with someone employed specifically as a quality assurance officer.

Formal evaluation, discussed from different perspectives in Chapters 8 and 12, is becoming increasingly popular. Quality assurance and individual performance review techniques are proliferating (Dickson, 1987; Balogh & Beattie, 1988; Brown, 1988; Harvey, 1988a; 1988b; Kitson, 1988; Nursing Times, 1988a; Rowland, 1988). However, many of the schemes are found to be confusing and/or irrelevant.

Adult learning model

One particularly lucid and practical approach is Christopher Wilson's (1985; 1987) adult learning model (ALM) of quality assurance (QA). The scheme follows the basic tenets of enlightened adult education. It starts by discovering people's current perspectives on the issue and offers a participative, self-paced inquiry backed up by support and coaching. It provides a strategy for growth and not, as many of the alternatives appear to, the imposition of a new system.

Dr Wilson points out that everyone makes judgements about the quality of work in which they are involved. The first step then in ALM, is to find out how those informal judgements are currently being made. The next is to get people to document that and then to make regular reports. In the later stages, standards and criteria are developed, as tools and servants and not masters of the process. Seven 'dos and don'ts' are offered for guidance on standards and criteria (Wilson, 1985, p. 13; 1987, p. 75). The reports describe:

- the topic reviewed
- how it was measured
- what the findings were
- why the topic and the findings are important
- the consequent action taken.

Rubbish in = rubbish out

It is important that any QA communication is meaningful to the staff sending the information. If it is not, it cannot have meaning for the recipients, whatever boxes have been filled in or reams of statistics have been sent. Only information seen as important by and to the reporter should be included (Wilson, 1985, p. 20).

This is related to the fundamental need for clarity and agreement about basic objectives and values. Measures for one philosophy can be totally invalid for judging another. For example, criteria for assessing client-centred, self-help-based health-promotion work are quite different from those for the professional-centred, conform-to-my-expert-opinion approach. Also, no subject can ever be totally evaluated. Comprehensive assessment is neither feasible nor is it an economic proposition. The objective therefore is to study 'what it is most important to know' (Bruce-Quay et al, 1986).

.... and management strategies

These same factors are just as relevant in self-, peer- and staff-assessment of a manager's style and strategies. For example, managers need positive feedback from, and appreciation shown by, their staff. Managers need to be told what they are doing right (Kay, 1988)!

Staff will be making informal judgements of management style (Fig. 14.10) and Chris Wilson's (1985; 1987) adult learning model for assessment may provide ideas for keying into this wealth of observation. Also, Dr West's questionnaire, used in the research into the main sources of stress in health visiting, is available (West et al, 1988). This could provide very useful feedback from staff right across the District.

Differences in basic objectives and values are very important in assessments of management strategies. If for example, individual performance reviews concentrate mainly on administrative tasks, then this implies an expectation of a style in which instruction and control dominate. Where this prevails, health visitor managers need to talk through the issue with their managers.

A good review will encourage in-depth description of strategies and achievements in 'human resource management', including key issues of staff motivation and enablement such as:

- staff self-esteem

Fig. 14.10 Showing health visitors comparing management style.

- clarity about 'what we are here for'
- actively seeking staff view
- trust of staff expertise
- increasing that expertise
- enabling staff to follow particular interests
- supportive attention.

In essence, it is managers approaching staff as they hope the staff approach their clientèle.

This section has looked at some of the ways health visitors and their managers can work together to review management strategies that aim to encourage innovation.

The chapter has described aspects of the spirit underlying positive change and new ideas in health visiting. It has not revealed the recipe for an elixir that would solve all management problems! However, it has introduced ideas from industrial management and has directed readers towards useful literature. It has provided four examples of participative management schemes and has discussed, through the health visitor cycle format, some of the factors associated with an enabling management style.

USEFUL ADDRESS

Health Visitors' Association Senior
Managers Network
c/o Jane Naish
Professional Officer
Health Visitors' Association
50 Southwark Street
London SE1 1UN
Tel 071 378 7255

REFERENCES

Andrews J 1989 I need you. Nursing Times 85, 24: 26

Balogh R, Beattie A 1988 Performance review. Nursing Times 84, 18: 67–69

Barratt E 1989 A survey of why nurses remain in employment in one health authority. Nursing Times 85, 1: 52

Blanchard K, Johnson S 1983 The One Minute Manager. Fontana/Collins, London — Strongly recommended.

Blanchard M, Tager M J 1986 Working well. Managing for health and high performance. Wildwood House Ltd, Aldershot — Recommended.

Bond M 1987 Being assertive. Pack 18 of the Managing Care series. Distance Learning Centre, South Bank Polytechnic, London

Bond M 1988a Setting up assertiveness training groups. Nursing Times 84, 5: 57–60

Bond M 1988b Understanding assertiveness. Nursing Times 84, 9: 61–64

Bond M 1988c When and why assertive? Nursing Times 84, 10: 69–72

Bond M 1988d Assertive rights and body language. Nursing Times 84, 11: 67–70

Bond M 1988e Assertive discussion. Nursing Times 84, 12: 73–76

Bond M 1988f Making requests assertively. Nursing Times 84, 13: 77–80

Bond M 1988g Saying no assertively. Nursing Times 84, 14: 63–66

Bond M 1988h Giving compliments and criticism. Nursing Times 84, 15: 75–78

Bond M 1988i Responding to feedback. Nursing Times 84, 16: 75–78

Bowden H I 1987 Manpower planning and health visiting survey. Health Visitor 60, 12: 403–406

Brown K 1987 Stand together. Nursing Times 83, 42: 70

Brown P 1988 First fix your goalposts. Health Service Journal 98, 5103: 618–619

Bruce-Quay M, Burton M, Heafford G 1986 Self-help guide to evaluation. North Manchester Health Promotion, Manchester — Recommended.

Buchan J 1987 Reporting on Griffiths. Nursing Times 83, 29: 34–35

Chudley P 1989 Confusion in common. Nursing Times 85, 15: 18

Cowley S 1989 The tyranny of crisis intervention. Senior Nurse 10, 3: 11–13

Darbyshire P 1988 Thinly disguised contempt. Nursing Times 84, 20: 42–44

Dauncey J 1987 (letter) Health visiting in Oxfordshire. Health Visitor 60, 6: 181*

Dauncey J 1988 A positive response. Nursing Times 84, 42: 75–77*

Dauncey J 1989 (letter) Oxfordshire's health visiting strategy. Health Visitor 62, 12: 388*

Dauncey J 1990 (letter) A plea for the future of health visiting. Health Visitor 63, 3: 104*

Dauncey J, Twinn S, Carnell J 1990 Managing change in clinical practice. Health Visitors' Association, London — Recommended: articles also associated with this scheme are labelled with an asterisk, i.e.*

Deacon G 1989 (letter) Metamorphosis of a health visitor. Health Visitor 62, 5: 165*

Department of Health and Social Security 1986 Neighbourhood nursing — a focus for health care. Report of the Community Nursing Review. HMSO, London

Dickson N 1987 Do you measure up? Nursing Times 83, 44: 25–28

Dingwall R 1984 Who is to blame, anyway? Nursing Times 80, 15: 42–43

Dopson L 1984 The nurse's tale. Health visitor and nursing officer. Nursing Times 80, 19: 36–37

Drennan V (ed) 1988 Health visitors and groups — politics and practice. Heinemann Nursing, Oxford

English National Board 1986 Guidelines for fieldwork placements. English National Board, London, Appendix 1

Field P A, Larsen J 1989 Management behaviour of one community health nurse supervisor. Journal of Advanced Nursing 14: 234–239 — Essential reading.

Gawlinski L, Graessle L 1988 Planning together. The art of effective teamwork. Bedford Square Press, London

Gough P, Hingley P 1988 Combating the pressure. Nursing Times 84, 2: 43–45

Griffiths Report 1983 NHS Management Inquiry. Letter to Secretary of State, Department of Health and Social Security, London

Harvey G 1988a The right tools for the job. Nursing Times 84, 26: 47–49

Harvey G 1988b More tools for the job. Nursing Times 84, 28: 33–34

Health Care Education Associates 1986 Professional writing skills for health care managers. A practical guide. Williams & Wilkins, London (ISBN 0-8016-2123-2) — Strongly recommended.

Health Visitor 1987 Stress and the workloads of health visitors in Sheffield. Health Visitor 60, 6: 201 — Recommended.

Health Visitor Development Group 1989 A change for the better. Oxfordshire's strategy for health visiting, 2nd Edn. Oxfordshire Health Authority, Oxford c/o Jane Dauncey, East Oxford Health Centre, Cowley Road, Oxford OX4 1XD — Recommended reading, alongside the articles labelled with an asterisk, i.e.*

Health Visitors' Association 1985 Health visiting and school nursing: the future. Health Visitors' Association, London, p 42

Hingley P, Cooper C 1, Harris P 1986 Stress in nurse managers. King's Fund, London

Jackson C 1989a Wherefore to Oxfordshire? Health Visitor 62, 5: 159–160*

Jackson C 1989b The last straw . . . excessive workloads. Health Visitor 62, 10: 317

Kay E 1988 Finding the manager behind the mask. Nursing Times 84, 23: 40–41 — Essential reading.

Kitson A 1988 Raising the standards. Nursing Times 84, 25: 28–32

Lakein A 1985 How to get control of your time and life. Gower, Aldershot — Recommended.

Lindenfield G 1986 Assert yourself. Thorsens Publishing Group, Wellingborough — Quick and easy to read.

Luker K A, Chalmers K I 1989 The referral process in health visiting. International Journal of Nursing Studies 26, 2: 173–185 — Strongly recommended.

Nashe S 1990 (letter) Oxford responds. Health Visitor 63, 3: 104*

Nursing Times 1988a Economic, efficient and effective. Nursing Times 84, 18: 66

Nursing Times 1988b Editorial. Nursing Times 84, 44: 3

Orr J 1989 The blueprint already exists. Health Visitor 62, 8: 238 — Recommended.

Peters T J, Waterman R H 1982 In search of excellence. Lessons from America's best-run companies. Harper and Row, New York — Basic reading.

Piggott M 1988 Making the numbers add up. Nursing Times 84, 1: 36–37

Pugh J B, Woodward-Smith M A 1989 Nurse manager. A practical guide to better employee relations. W B Saunders Co, Philadelphia — Essential reading.

Robinson J, Strong P 1989 Griffiths and the NHS. Health Visitor 61, 9: 283

Rowland V 1988 Getting results from IPR. Health Service Review 98, 5106: 710

Royal College of Nursing 1989 Standards of care for management in nursing. Scutari Projects Ltd, Harrow

Salvage J 1989 Take me to your leader. Nursing Times 85, 25: 34–35 — Recommended.

Shenton H, Hamm C 1988 How to retain nurses. The Professional Nurse, June: 360

Slack P 1987 Winds of change. Nursing Times 83, 9: 40–41

United Kingdom Central Council 1984 Code of professional conduct for the nurse, midwife and health visitor, 2nd edn. United Kingdom Central Council for Nursing, Midwifery and Health Visiting, London

Waterman R 1987 The renewal factor. Bantam Books, New York, p 312 (1989 for paperback ed)

West M A 1989a Prescriptions for health visiting. Health Visitor 62, 12: 378–381 — Essential reading.

West M A 1989b Innovation in health visiting. Health Visitor 62, 2: 46–48 — Essential reading.

West M A, Jones A, Savage Y 1988 Stress in health visiting: a quantitative assessment. Health Visiting 61, 9: 269–271 — Essential reading.

West M A, Savage Y 1988a Visitations of distress. Nursing Times 84, 31: 43–44 — Essential reading.

West M A, Savage Y 1988b Stress in health visiting: qualitative accounts. Health Visiting 61, 10: 305–308 — Essential reading.

West M A, Savage Y 1988c Satisfactions of health visiting. Health Visiting 61, 11: 336–338 — Essential reading.

West M A, Savage Y 1988d Coping with stress in health visiting. Health Visiting 61, 12: 366–368 — Essential reading.

Willkin P 1988 Someone to watch over me. Nursing Times 84, 33: 33–34

Wilson C R M 1985 Quality assurance: getting started. Ontario Hospital Association, Toronto — Recommended booklet, but not as good as the same author's book below.

Wilson C R M 1987 Hospital-wide quality assurance. Models for implementation and development. W B Saunders, Toronto — Essential reading.

Winn L 1987 Learning through mistakes. Senior Nurse 7, 6: 13–14

Articles pertaining to the Oxfordshire strategy are labelled with an asterisk, i.e.

Chapter 15 uses a community perspective family health needs model in each of the examples. Community and caseload health profiling, the foundation for well-planned, cooperative health promotional work, is followed by a brief look at teamwork initiatives. Finally, we return to the family health needs format to present a range of health promotion issues.

15

The Cumberlege approach

MAKING PROGRESS

The Cumberlege inquiry team was able to report and to build on the good practices in community nursing that they found at the time of their investigation (Brown & Gordon, 1987). They carefully documented useful ideas and practical schemes. This has helped to speed up experimentation and wider implementation of initiatives in well-planned community nurse services. This chapter concentrates on two of the aspects of health visiting which the Cumberlege Report (DHSS, 1986) helped to influence. These are community and caseload profiling and teamwork in community nursing.

There are many variations on these themes. Elements of them ran through the previous three chapters. The first half of this chapter provides four particular examples. The first is of a health visitor single-handedly implementing these principles of analysis and teamwork. The second shows how a group of health visitors organised caseload and community profiles. The next example, a pilot scheme built on already successful teamwork, progressed well but was not easily replicated. The last shows how neighbourhood teamwork with appropriate management and educational support, transformed an inner-city working environment and significantly improved health promotion services.

The model

Each of these examples includes at least one

community perspective family health needs model, following a format similar to that found earlier in Chapters 12 and 13 (Box 12.1, Boxes 13.1a & 13.1b, Boxes 13.2a & 13.2b). In this model, health needs or problems in the caseload, patch or community are classified, sometimes rather arbitrarily, under the health heading of 'environmental', 'physical', 'mental/emotional' or 'social aspects'. Where appropriate, a second model lists health visitor responses to some of the health needs or problems that were found.

When analysing our work using these frameworks, the exact category under which issues are listed is not of prime importance. There are many interrelated and interlinking factors within any single issue. The value of the classification activity lies in the questioning it raises and in the consequent stimulation of further thought.

Following the real-life examples, the second half of the chapter provides some general guidance on profiling and considers teamwork initiatives. It finishes with a brief look at some important health promotion issues. These are classified under the family health needs headings and include unemployment and low income, coronary heart disease, stress management and AIDS.

FOUR REAL-LIFE EXAMPLES

EXAMPLE ONE: CATERING FOR LOCAL NEED

This example shows how the Cumberlege ideas can be implemented with great effect by an individual health visitor.

Having been given a geographically assigned inner-city caseload, Sandy Blakeborough started to plan a health profile and to investigate current use of available services. Her aim was to discover where need was greatest, to provide appropriate health-promotional services and to monitor the results (Fig. 15.1).

It is an interesting 'patch'. At one end is an older area of back-to-back houses (Area III), mostly populated by well-established Caucasian families with a high level of unemployment. These residents have a high attendance rate at their nearby health centre. At the other end, a mile from the health centre, is an area containing city-centre pubs and high-rise flats

with a mainly Afro-Caribbean and Caucasian mix, many single-parent families and a high proportion of older people. This is Area I, from which there is a low level of clinic attendance. In between is Area II, a rather higher income area.

Office of Census and Population mortality statistics for the caseload showed a well-above-average early death rate. A caseload count of families with children showed 55% to be single parent and nearly a quarter of the population is over 60.

Being concerned about levels of nutrition,

Table 15.1 Prevention model outlining Sandy's drop-in centre and group work with clients, school governors and health and welfare workers

Aim	Through	Examples
Prevent occurrence of problems	Health education	Targeting area where people not attending existing formal facilities Providing environment which encourages learning about rights, entitlements and health knowledge.
	Increased awareness	Using statistics to inform decision-makers and influence allocation of resources towards areas of need
Prevent development of problems	Monitoring/ search	Gleaning statistics and mapping, to discover whereabouts of main clusters of problems Changing own work practice to provide more appropriate facilities
	Early care	Explaining to fellow school governors the facilities and services required by children with special needs
Prevent deterioration where problems already exist	Support	Providing supportive listening and peer-support structure Morale-boosting occupations for group, e.g. video work for young, and 'work bees' for older clients 'At risk' families pop in to maintain contact or to request visit Liaison with other workers in area to ensure best possible help available

Sandy created a questionnaire that would enable the community dietitian and health visitors to assess the level of nutrition in each of her three sub-areas. She hoped it would also help evaluate health visitor achievement in this field.

As it might be assumed that low uptake of health services reflects a negative attitude towards health, two questions were included in the format which were intended to demonstrate this. The questionnaires were filled in at the health assessment mornings. The best nutritional score was in Area III, the one close to the health centre. The worst was in Area I, but negative attitudes towards health were not found. We shall return to this.

There are many people working in the area in one way or another. Sandy made contact with representatives from:

- Adult Education
- Health Education Department
- neighbourhood social work team
- community centre management committees
- probation services
- police services
- health visitor assistant for the elderly
- school nurses
- community midwifery service
- local schoolteachers
- social services voluntary coordinator
- community programme workers
- various other voluntary services.

INFORMATION – background knowledge
Of 'Cumberlege' approach: survey levels of health and use of facilities currently provided; close liaison with other local workers; take services to the public and strong client involvement.

INFORMATION – from liaison & OPCS records
With many local statutory and voluntary workers: becoming monthly lunchtime meeting. Local social, morbidity & mortality statistics.

INFORMATION – visits, clinic and group work
HV observation: nutrition questionnaire; clinic attendance and groups monitored.
Client view: drop-in centre attenders hungry for knowledge; respond to informal setting and client-led discussions.

INFORMATION – when projects under way
Sandy's home visits did most to stimulate initial interest and group attendance.
Drop-in centre attendance established and growing, and spawned new groups.
Increased use of health visitor as resource.
Client-led health promotion successful: keep requesting more topics; improved nutrition.
Sandy appointed as school governor, later at school for children with special needs.

ASSESS area

PLAN drop-centre

IMPLEMENT ideas

EVALUATE project

Fig. 15.1 Health visitor cycle showing Sandy Blakeborough's approach to planning and monitoring health promotion requirements in her inner city geographic patch.

This linking together was so successful that now all these people gather for a regular monthly lunchtime meeting. Sandy heard all about what services already existed and what was planned, and everyone else learned about her aims (Table 15.1).

Having got to know the people living and working in the 'patch', and having demonstrated the area with the lowest levels of health, parenting skills, family support, nutritional levels and also poorest health facilities (Box 15.1a), Sandy set about trying to provide suitable health promotional opportunities.

A mother and toddler group was set up in a room in a city-centre pub, for lonely young mothers living over city-centre premises.

Box 15.1a Family health needs model showing examples of what Sandy found in area I. (Box 15.1b provides examples of what she did about it.)

Environment	Physical health	Mental/emotional health	Social aspects of health
What found in area I			
Mobile population, housed in LA high-rise flats. Many single-parent families and 23% of population over 60 years	Standard Mortality Ratio comparisons for several causes of death: above average death rate for that city and for England and Wales	Poor parenting skills common: high potential for child abuse	Many people have poor or no family support
Nearest health clinic one mile away	Scores on level of nutrition from first questionnaire: lowest of the three areas within caseload	Low self-esteem	Isolation for young mothers
Area has under-utilised community centre		Apparently negative, but actually positive attitude towards health	Isolation for carers of very elderly
Ignorance of rights and benefits		Lack of knowledge about human body functioning: hence difficulty in understanding normal, formal health service	Lack of life skills
			Low use of health service provision

Box 15.1b Examples of what Sandy provided in area 1 through drop-in centre and group work

Environment	Physical health	Mental/emotional health	Social aspects of health
What provided in area I			
Drop-in centre for all age groups at community centre. Congenial setting — no white coats, no insensitive clinic officials, no formality. It spawned other groups for: single parents; carers of the very elderly; mothers and toddlers	'Family Health Mornings': personal goals related to smoking, diet, weight etc, after health profile assessment	Child health and development requested as health topics	Expression of fears, e.g. about isolation: provides release of tension and realisation that others also have these same problems
	Clients' choice of health-education topics: relevant; trigger videos useful	Turnover of membership within discussion session leads to frequent recapping: natural reinforcement of ideas under debate, hence easier learning	Empathy and trust built up in group, leading to network of support for individuals with personal crises
As requested: information on rights and benefits	Improved scores for nutritional level in second questionnaire	Mothers able to video themselves interacting with their children: improved self-esteem	Carers' 'work bees' provide social contact
		Carers' group 'work-bees' on own unfinished favourite handicrafts boost morale and facilitate health promotion.	

A drop-in centre was established in the under-utilised community centre. Here, a weekly all-age 'Family Health Morning' provided health profile assessments from which personal goals were chosen, for example, on smoking, diet or weight. Participants were then invited to join informal groups to discuss these issues.

This style of health promotion, outlined in Box 15.1b, helped improve knowledge, for example, of rights and benefits, child health and development, to boost self-esteem and to improve nutritional levels — as measured by a second questionnaire.

The group discussions led Sandy to have a much better idea of the motivations and needs of her clientele in Area I. It seems the previous lack of uptake of health services was not only related to the distance from the health centre. Low self-esteem, poor life skills and lack of understanding about human body functioning made the normal, formal health education service inappropriate.

It is interesting to note that although community programme workers helped create a handbill advertising the Family Health Morning, and delivered a copy to every household, it was Sandy's personal contact with clients and then word of mouth, which was the most successful way of bringing people to the service.

The groups that grew out of the drop-in

Fig. 15.2 Health visitor cycle outlining Sandy's work as school governor with particular remit for children with special needs.

sessions (see Box 15.1b) had a great deal of help and support. For example:
- Adult Education, the cost of the hall
- community health workers provided a crèche
- Health Education, displays and video equipment
- Pre-school Play Association covered insurance.

Being asked to become a school governor, before long with a remit for children with special needs, was clear evidence of appreciation of the quality of Sandy's work. Again, she took a broad approach to the task (Fig. 15.2), working closely with the:

- educational welfare officer
- special needs teacher
- educational psychologist
- school nurse and
- community social worker.

This was both on individual cases and on drawing up local health and welfare statistics on children with special needs in order to influence the allocation of resources. This group now has a regular termly meeting.

A report for management is being followed up by an article for the *Health Visitor* (Blakeborough, 1990). Sandy has the satisfaction of knowing that by changing local health visitor practice, she has become more accessible and useful to her clients. Through these informal services, she has helped people to become confident, to learn about what they wish to at their own particular level and at their own pace. These people have become able to do something early, preventing the development (and maybe the occurrence) of problems (Table 15.1) in their health and welfare.

This outline and the accompanying models concentrate on what has been happening in Area I. Needless to say much good health-promotional work has also been achieved in the other areas of this caseload!

EXAMPLE TWO: CREATING COMMUNITY AND PRACTICE PROFILES

Southampton and South West Hampshire Health Authority is implementing 'A Charter for Change' in its health visiting services. A key part of this is to be the development of community and caseload profiling by the health visitors. The managers aim to give:

- help — from a coordinator/facilitator
- time — to complete the profiles and analyse findings

- freedom — to negotiate changed patterns of work and
- education — to enable these initiatives.
The possibility of clerical support and support workers is being investigated.

The programme has already started. The idea grew out of meetings between health visitor management and Margaret Buttigieg, a lecturer in health visiting from the local university. They were discussing formulation of the way forward for Southampton health visiting. Workshops were set up for all health visitors. A group of

Table 15.2 Prevention model outlining a few of Chris Pidduck's plans for future work. Her community and practice profiles highlighted the relevance of spending a greater proportion of her time on activities for the elderly

Aim	Through	Examples
Prevent occurrence of problems	Health education	At a screening clinic for the middle-aged run by practice nurse
	Increasing awareness	Lobbying: using profile statistics to demonstrate need for day care; continuing teamwork with other HVs to pressure Social Services Dept for provision of services[†]
		Lobbying re chiropody services.[*]
Prevent development of problems	Monitoring/ search	Further information to clarify which old people needing attention; who already receiving what services from whom, e.g. district nurse, social worker, voluntary agency, family carer
	Early care	Chiropody waiting list 12 months: aim to help improve this — see above[*]
Prevent deterioration where difficulties already exist	Support	Day clubs for elderly, long waiting list: aim to improve this — see above,[†]
		Carers' groups: liaison with worker from Age Concern aimed at helping to set up local groups

interested health visitors (Box 15.2) then began to meet with Margaret at the university. They wanted to draw up some guidance for health visitors setting out to create community and practice profiles. They decided on the key factors (Box 15.3) and listed them on forms to be filled in. Chris Pidduck was a member of this 'think tank' and was also one of the first to undertake the task. She described it as having been fascinating.

The exercise (Fig. 15.3) was very hard work, but it had brought everything into focus more

clearly. For example, the statistics have given a more concrete base from which to make decisions and to demonstrate need, both in lobbying (see Table 15.2) and to managers. The figures have confirmed Chris' feelings about the health status of the community.

There are more benefits. Chris says that the local contacts that she made were particularly worthwhile. These have helped her get more of an idea of what local people are wanting. For example, a neighbourhood group compiling a directory of local information provided a very good source. These contacts mean that more activists in the community have learned about health visiting. Many will be very useful in future work. Chris already feels more closely involved with and welcomed into the nearby community.

The community profiles were undertaken by nine health visitors, covering between them the whole of the District. They were given two weeks for this project which was to include their own practice profile. Health visiting cover was provided for their caseload.

Background help was available from a special projects manager (SPM) who had built up a very useful file of statistics. It was not comprehensive, but she was able to meet the health visitors regularly and to gather more in response to their requests.

Box 15.2 Health visitors taking part in The Southampton and South West Hampshire District Health Authority Profile Pilot, May, 1989

Kathy Dowland	Totton, Hampshire
Di Fletcher	Lymington, Hampshire
Gill Gallagher	Romsey, Hampshire
Sue Gee	Southampton
Hilda Lemon	Southampton
Jenny Mills	Totton, Hampshire
Meg Mulady	Southampton
Chris Pidduck	Southampton
Stephanie Ramsey	Southampton
Barbara Smith	Southampton

Box 15.3 Family health needs model showing examples of the factors affecting health included in Chris Pidduck's community profile

Environment	Physical health	Mental/emotional health	Social aspects of health
Maps showing facilities e.g. shopping, schooling, health clinics, Housing Dept, Environmental Health Dept & other LA depts	Population size and age distribution	Suicide rate	Group activities
	Birth and infant death rates	Psychiatric services	Halls
		Libraries	Churches
Dept of Social Security	Death rates e.g. 0—1	Educational establishments	Information systems e.g. local newspaper, notice boards
Types of housing	2—4 5—15	Health promotion initiatives and programmes	
Transport patterns:	16—64 65—74	Clinics: e.g. sleep, child behaviour, speech therapy	Recreational facilities
• bus, train	75+		Mobility of families
• frequency & cost	Incidence & prevalence of various diseases	Voluntary services: e.g. Relate	Cultural patterns
Socio-economic mix		Alcohol related crime figures	Carers' self-help groups (none)
Occupational patterns	Health services: e.g. chiropody clinics, immunisation rates, audiometry		
Main employers			
Unemployment			
Homelessness	Clinics: e.g. family planning, well woman, child health		

INFORMATION – background knowledge
Profiling clarifies picture and helps HV to show managers where work emphases should be.
Need: help in planning and in finding statistics; time; clerical support; cover for caseload; to learn as you go along; freedom to work in new ways.

INFORMATION – from liaison
HVs' teamwork: support & coordination.
HV tutor: 'think tank'. SPM: statistics.
Various: e.g. LA depts, voluntary groups, church.
Within practice: PHC teamwork.

ASSESS
relevant
factors

INFORMATION – from community
Observations: of community (validated by statistics) and of families with under 5s (noted in records).
Consumer views: families' re local facilities e.g. lack of playgroups; community forum (vol. group) compiling directory of local information.

PLAN
community
& practice
profiles

IMPLEMENT
plan

EVALUATE
process
outcome

INFORMATION – from profiles
Brings local situation into clearer focus.
Shows need for more information re elderly.
Provides written evidence:
to back up HV's proposed changes of practice;
to lobby for improved local services.
New GP computer will add information.

Fig. 15.3 Health visitor cycle showing some of the important factors that helped Chris Pidduck create community and caseload profiles and that enable relevant changes in practice.

The neat forms devised earlier provided excellent guidance. However, they were inadequate for actually recording the information. Each profile needed significantly different spacing for its particular relevant data. This emphasised just how different is each community.

The nine health visitors were able to work as a team. They supported each other and organised their searches so that they were not all bothering each institution for the same information. Some time was wasted over arrangements to visit the various agencies. Consequently, guidance for future health visitors will suggest that these appointments are organised well in advance.

The local authority (LA) Housing Department was visited by one health visitor and another contacted the Environmental Health Offices. This Department supplied information about important factors such as the number and whereabouts of housing in multiple occupancy (HMOs) and houses in disrepair. HMOs are now spreading into Chris' area.

The information from the Community Development Department, which deals with leisure and amenities, was very practical. Improvements in parks and in children's play area equipment and safety were noted, as were adventure parks and areas for informal recreation. The Department was able to identify

Box 15.4 Lists of some of the characteristics recommended for inclusion in the practice profile. Note: Chris points out that in non-zoned GP practices, the profile boundaries need to be clearly stated. They need to encompass the main clusters of people on the practice list

A brief statement of:
- members of PHCT
- type of environment
- social mix of population

Information available: e.g.
- age: sex register
- computer
- access to GP notes

Accommodation:
- facilities
- HV equipment

Practice population statistics 0–1; 2–4; 5–15; 16–64; 65–74; 75+

Vulnerable: e.g.
- single parents
- elderly living alone
- handicapped — physical, mental
- ethnic minority
- bereaved

HV caseload statistics:
- classified as above
- transfers in/out
- movement within area
- vulnerable families
- vulnerable elderly

Current HV work: e.g.
- clinics
- health education sessions
- group work
- committees

Practice statistics: e.g.
- births — FT, prem, LBW
- infant mortality rate
- termination of pregnancy
- stillbirth
- SIDS

Mortality statistics: male, female 0–1; 2–4; 5–15; 16–64; 65–74; 75+

Morbidity statistics: e.g.
- coronary heart disease
- ischaemic heart disease
- cerebrovascular accident
- hypertensive disease
- Ca lung, breast, cervix
- motor accident
- suicide
- AIDS

Children at risk: e.g.
- on child abuse register
- case conference children
- case discussed children
- at risk, not on register
- number children in care

Referrals to: e.g.
- Social Services
- speech therapy
- hearing clinic
- vision screening
- clinical medical officer
- child guidance
- sleep clinic

Comments as appropriate:
- at end of each section above

Finally, notes on: e.g.
- what achieved in previous year
- priorities for coming year.

the buildings available for community use, in many cases, when they were used/not used and even which groups took which room! Chris now has a much clearer picture of local group activities. She also knows where people can look for accommodation, for example, for future groupwork.

It seems the practice GPs have shown particular interest in the profiles. They will soon be having to create their own, on account of the recent White Paper (Department of Health,

1989) and are installing a computer for practice information. Chris' file of neat maps drawn up to show, for example, health education and social facilities, the statistical tables with comments, and the timetables and local directories provides a valuable resource.

Members of the primary health care (PHC) team were available to help provide information for the practice profile (see Box 15.4). Chris says it took three or four days to go through the caseload health visitor records. In this exercise, she was able to demonstrate, for example, the percentages of the 450 children under five registered with the practice who had a:

- single parent
- mother aged 19 or younger
- step parent
- homeless family
- childminder

and the percentages who:

- moved within the last year
- attended casualty
- breast fed at six weeks
- breast fed at six months
- were immunised.

The practice profile showed 840 people aged 65–74 and 588 aged over 75. The community profile showed:
- 29% lived alone
- 17 private rest homes in the area
- 2 Part III homes
- chiropody waiting list 12 months
- long waiting list for day clubs
- no carers group in that half of the city
- high percentage of casualty attendances after falls at home.

Table 15.2 shows some of Chris' plans for future work for the elderly.

Some information suggested for the profile was not available, for example, morbidity rates in the practice for coronary and ischaemic heart disease, various accidents and cancers (see Box 15.4). The practice has just acquired a computer which will make much more information available. However, Chris is aware that the social statistics which she now has and her information about the environment give much better guidance to levels of health of the community. She knows that trying to compare between the morbidity and mortality statistics of small patches is not generally very valuable anyway. The pilot project health visitors (Box 15.2) are currently critically rethinking their practice profile format and new ideas are emerging.

Clerical assistance was able to be given for typing up the profiles only because the SPM's typist did it in her own time. However, the pilot trial has ironed out most of the difficulties and demonstrated the positive value of profiling. Chris hopes to implement some new initiatives early in 1990, by which time she will have gathered further information. Along with the others involved in the pilot project, she will provide background support for other health visitors building profiles and rethinking their caseload patterns. They are fortunate that there has been so much preparatory work.

EXAMPLE THREE: A SUCCESSFUL PILOT, BUT. . . .

The managers of a largely urban Community Unit, impressed by the ideas in the Cumberlege Report (Department of Health and Social Security, 1986), decided to introduce a neighbourhood approach into the community nursing services. They began with a pilot scheme. A nurse manager described how the area chosen has an easily defined neighbourhood as it is surrounded by the green belt and the boundaries coincide with that of an electoral ward. She said it has a very active community. The nurses there were already community oriented and well motivated and it was felt they would enjoy the challenge.

The pilot has been a great success. When it started, there was already good primary health care teamwork. There was also a great deal of cooperation between the two health visitors, the two district nurses, the school nurses and the various other nurses. However, the new scheme's regular and more frequent meetings forced a much closer working relationship, particularly between the health visitors (HVs), the district nurses (DNs) and the health centre manager (HCM). The latter specialises in the neighbourhood team's administrative and clerical work, of which there is a great deal.

Originally they were supposed to have a team leader, but they found they work much better together under a democratic scheme. Each member has equal status and equal say. They have frequent lunch-time meetings to 'thrash out' issues on which they need to agree. They have drawn up for themselves basic, achievable objectives.

One aim was to improve communications. The HVs, DNs and HCM started making contact with as many voluntary and statutory organisations as they could think of. There are now inter-disciplinary meetings every two months, averaging about 40 at each gathering. The same democratic your-idea-is-as-good-as-mine approach is used. The original people who came suggested more people who should, and the

Box 15.5 Family health needs model showing a few of the issues discussed within the pilot scheme multi-disciplinary meetings thereby stimulating greater cooperation and understanding between group members

Environment	Physical health	Mental/emotional health	Social aspects of health
Housing problems and homelessness	Mobility of the elderly	AIDS/HIV preventive strategies	Drug Unit Work
Social work dilemmas	Strokes	Community psychiatric care	Lack of accommodation for playgroups
Social Security difficulties	Exercising for fitness	Bereavement counselling	Problems of carers
Unemployment	Accidents in the home	Psycho-geriatrics	Luncheon clubs and other groups for the elderly
	Meals on wheels		

success has snowballed. The meetings have provided the opportunity to learn about other people's work and to cross-fertilise ideas and to exchange information (see Box 15.5).

Many new schemes and joint activities have emerged as a result. For example, services for the elderly have now improved in many ways. Prior to the pilot scheme, the team had acquired demographic information from the local authority statistics department. Putting this information together with their work experience and with the views of the multi-disciplinary group and from a clinic questionnaire, it was decided that the elderly should be assigned highest priority. This guided the group's cooperative efforts in their first year.

During the second year, it was decided that a joint-effort 'Health Day' should be arranged. A stall or demonstration was provided for every aspect of preventive health care that the group could muster. It took six months' preparation and these efforts were rewarded on the day by a public attendance of about 800 and a great deal of interest in the health promotional messages, This cooperative activity turned the multi-disciplinary group into much more of a team. It is a good omen for preventive health care in that neighbourhood.

Early in the trial, the pilot area had demonstrated optimism and progress. It was decided to implement the neighbourhood nurse scheme in other parts of the District. Specific HVs and DNs were assigned to go out to 'make community links' in particular 'neighbourhoods' which were, in fact, electoral wards. They found this work conflicted with their other workload obligations, such as compulsory visiting

schedules and clinic work. Some district nurses experienced difficulty in trying to make this sort of community contact, as it was not a normal feature of their work.

The nurse manager described how, in the meantime, she set up regular inter-professional meetings with as many of the voluntary and statutory organisations as was possible. She had worked for years in this part of the District and knew many of the personalities interested in or involved with health promotional or supportive work. She brought them together and initially chaired the meetings. Many good and new initiatives have spun off from this coming together.

However, the health visitors and district nurses assigned to making links, came to meetings with their nurse manager with few ideas and little progress. They were confused and not a little disheartened when they compared themselves with the success of the pilot area and with their manager's achievements.

The full implementation of the scheme was not going well. The nurse manager tried to analyse what had been happening. Firstly they had chosen to start with the easiest neighbourhood, which had already been achieving a great deal. All the others were bound to be more difficult. Some possible reasons for this were that staff were:
1. working in different type of area with
   - less clearly defined neighbourhoods
   - greater levels of deprivation
   - less clearly visible social networks
   - apparently fewer local activists;
2. less experienced in community interaction and therefore need

Fig. 15.4 Health visitor cycle outlining implementation of a pilot 'neighbourhood' scheme, followed by District-wide implementation.

- staff development education and support directly related to new practice requirements
- encouragement to take time to implement the new initiative
- a clear management statement about ending 'you-*must*-visit' policies
- to work as a team for mutual support and to use all nurse skills
- to volunteer rather than be directed/assigned.

The nurse manager felt, in retrospect, that it would probably have been better if she had not been so active herself and if she had enabled her staff to 'discover' the community workers of whom she knew, She was optimistic about finding a solution to the current difficulty. She said there was much to learn from what had happened (see Fig. 15.4) and a great deal to

discuss, both with her staff and at managers' meetings. If this story were published, she added, other people might also learn something from it.

EXAMPLE FOUR: A NEIGHBOURHOOD TEAM

Some Wandsworth health visitors described how they work within one of the new neighbourhood health care teams (NHCT). This scheme has brought radical changes to the provision of Wandsworth community health care. Staff education and support are given high priority and there is management encouragement to take well considered risks in efforts to provide client-centred care. The smaller units of the neighbourhood scheme enable much closer communication between the professionals working there and greater sensitivity to client wishes.

The NHCT nurses have been brought together, either by moving office, or through administrative rearrangement. For example, the district nurses, now based in the clinic, used to work from a central base. Community midwives are still attached to the hospital, but are assigned to a particular neighbourhood. Community psychiatric nurses, medical officers and physiotherapists, speech therapists and dentists are also assigned to teams. The neighbourhood and locality boundaries were broadly aligned with those of the Local Authority social work teams, enabling an extremely close working relationship. There is regular contact with other statutory and with voluntary organisations working within the neighbourhood. The GPs are becoming increasingly involved.

The health visitors in this NHCT include a part-timer, Joy, and three full timers, Adele Rutledge, Ann Sullivan and Liz Wombwell. Ann has been working in this area for nearly seven years. Her first job was based at this clinic with a geographic patch caseload. For the past five years she has been GP-attached, with a caseload spread right across the neighbourhood. Ann described how the atmosphere in the clinic has changed. For many years there was an enormous shortage and a heavy turnover of health visitors. Now it has a stable, enthusiastic and proactive team with an infectiously high morale.

This clinic was included in the pilot scheme for the Wandsworth neighbourhood teams. At that time there were only two part-time health visitors based at this clinic. Other health visitors from different areas were sent in to cover the clinics, new birth visits and emergencies. It was far from satisfactory. Then Liz and Adele came to work at the clinic. That was two years ago, soon after neighbourhood teams were set up throughout the Community Unit. They were both newly qualified and found it difficult at first because they met local resistance and hostility. The clients' feeling was that, like the previous health visitors, they would not remain more than six months: it was not the sort of place that people stayed if they could help it. But they *have* stayed. Furthermore, Liz, Adele and Joy are able to put into practice the sort of client-centred, needs-based health visiting they learned about in college and, like all the rest of the NHCT staff, they are clearly enjoying the work.

The Community Unit employs a professional development officer for support, education and quality assurance. Because she is outside management and is approachable, staff feel able to discuss issues freely. She holds support sessions monthly for newly qualified staff, which are strictly confidential. Adele and Liz attended. Now, during their second year, these sessions have dropped to three-monthly.

Education is given high priority. There are some mandatory topics. Other subjects are available for those who feel it is relevant to their work. Everyone in this team has taken assertion training.

Communications are remarkable. This applies within the team and with clients, other agencies and management. The health visitors said that with all these people, they feel there is no longer a 'them and us' situation. Almost symbolic of this is the team's neighbourhood nurse manager. She has a habit of leaving her office door open. She sees her role as that of a facilitator and is clearly approachable.

The community midwife said that clients remark on the smooth running of the services and on the way that everyone from the various services knows the others' names and mode of work. The midwife added that it is now easier to work together on antenatal care. Also, communications are much improved, for example, over contact with social workers or regarding continued care when midwifery problems persist after the tenth day.

The health visitors are encouraged to make contact with other health and welfare organisations. There is now a regular meeting of representatives of most statutory and voluntary agencies active within the area Liz attends. She also works with a multi-disciplinary group planning HIV and AIDS education for the neighbourhood workers and local volunteers, such as crèche staff, community workers, clergy, housing department workers and local activist young mothers. The health authority HIV education advisor is playing a key role in this.

The Save the Children Fund has set up activities in the very poorest of the estates in the neighbourhood. This is Adele's patch and she is working very closely alongside them. In order to fully benefit from Adele's influential position within the estate, and to provide continuity, she has arranged with Ann to work with Ann's clients who live there.

A Community Unit steering group is looking at new initiatives in health visiting. Ann attends and brings back the ideas discussed so that the team

INFORMATION – background knowledge
Client comes first.
Communication a key factor. More effective
in small unit: enables closer contact.
Education and support for staff increases
their ability to provide good quality work.

INFORMATION – from liaison
Social work teams: similar neighbourhoods.
Nearby statutory & voluntary organisations:
frequent and informative gatherings.
Health visitors on Community Unit steering &
work groups: 'bottom-up' decision-making.

ASSESS
client
needs

PLAN
teamwork
strategies

INFORMATION – from community
High levels of social deprivation and low
levels of health: many crises.
Clientele were insulted by '6 month health
visitors': women's and other groups now
request health promotion.

IMPLEMENT
plan

EVALUATE
process
and
outcome

INFORMATION – as teamwork progresses
Clients feel valued. They help evaluate the
work and appreciate smooth running teamwork
and response to their wishes.
Health visitors feel valued, free and able to
provide relevant service, Körner statistics excepted.
HV: 'There is so much to be achieved .....'

Fig. 15.5 Health visitor cycle showing some of the important issues associated with the Wandsworth neighbourhood
health care teamwork planning.

health visitors can then feed in their views. In a
similar way, she attends a quality assurance
working party which is drawing together the
other health visitors' perceptions on 'aims and
objectives' and on measuring quality.

The Wandsworth style of management,
already described in Chapter 14's Example
Three, is geared to develop and to make full
use of staff expertise. It encourages modification
of traditional practice and then experimentation
in teamwork service provision.

A great deal of teamwork and liaison is going
on, but only a few examples can be mentioned
here. Figure 15.5 shows several important
issues in this Wandsworth teamwork planning.
Box 15.6a shows examples of the
neighbourhood characteristics and Box 15.6b
lists some of the NHCT responses, with Table
15.3 highlighting some of the team members'
preventive strategies. Together these give a brief
introduction to the progress that is being made
in this neighbourhood health care team.

Box 15.6a Family health needs model showing examples of local neighbourhood factors evident from the Neighbourhood Nurse Manager's community profile and from the health visitors' caseload profile, observations and knowledge. Note: See Jarman (1983; 1984; 1989) for information about the scoring system mentioned under mental/emotional health

Environment	Physical health	Mental emotional health	Social aspects of health
Exceedingly large number of substandard dwellings Very high level of unemployment Very long waiting list for housing Those housed (transfers in) are mainly from bed and breakfast accommodation and have innumerable problems	1. High infant mortality rates 2. Elderly living in deprived circumstances: little help or support 3. GP has age/sex register	Poor Jarman score shows multiple problems and high stress levels Many mothers clearly depressed and anxious	1. A quarter of the children on LA's Child Protection Register from this tiny neighbourhood 2. Residents' and many other organisations already exist in neighbourhood 3. National and local figures on AIDS: increasing

Box 15.6b Family health needs model showing some of the Wandsworth strategies of care in response to the examples of the neighbourhood factors shown in Box 15.6a

Environment	Physical health	Mental/emotional health	Social aspects of health
Staff caseloads kept low Try to provide walk-in service: preferred by clients Work very closely with voluntary and statutory agencies Pilot scheme: visit newcomers and inform about local services	1. Close teamwork: HV/midwife antenatally and with 'handover' Applying for family planning clinic (enabling pre-conceptual care too) in very poor estate Group work, especially within this poor estate 2. After unsuccessful multi-profession health education sessions, jumble sale promotion planned: DN & HV 3. Well Person Clinics and opportunistic work by HV and district and practice nurses	Teamwork with outreach group: Community Mental Health Unit based at clinic. Work with groups and referrals Mother and toddler group work Most health visiting action in this neighbourhood has large mental health element — support and listening	1. Health promotion work within Save the Children Fund Group on neediest estate and concentrated work on that estate Good knowledge of 'procedures' and close work with social workers and child minding advisors 2. Health promotion within existing groups 3. Team staff and statutory and voluntary services cooperative learning about AIDS: will prevent staff fear (and prejudice) and improve service

Table 15.3 Prevention model showing some of the strategies of this Wandsworth neighbourhood health care team

Aim	Through	Examples
Prevent occurrence of problems	Health education	Group work with existing groups on requested topics; A/N & P/N too
		Jumble sale popular with elderly: plan health promotion stall there
	Increasing awareness	Plan to use local statistics to make case for new family planning clinic
		Wrote to MP & local council re lack of play space; to MP re families' inability, now, to acquire safety equipment, e.g. fireguard, safety gate
Prevent development of problems	Monitoring/ search	Adult health assessments and introductory visits to newcomers on practice list: pilot scheme
	Early care	Close teamwork for early referral to appropriate health/ welfare service
Prevent deterioration where problems already exist	Support	Planning AIDS education for team with other local workers for *future* care, decreasing fear and increasing knowledge and cooperation, hence power to help
		Multi-disciplinary liaison meetings: work together to find best help for clients in crisis

KNOW YOUR PATCH

This section looks at community and caseload profiling and at some of the underlying issues. Brief descriptions of profiling are backed up by many references, chosen to provide health visitors with broader guidance. We start with recent history of the subject.

The Cumberlege Report's (DHSS, 1986) basic suggestion that nurses should work together in neighbourhoods, drew attention to the need for population profiles to be drawn up. They were needed for planning community health care and would be based on health and social data, and take public perceptions into account. Many profiles are now being undertaken.

AN 'EPIDEMIOLOGICAL' APPROACH

Earlier in the 1980s, wide variations in local need had led Baroness MacFarlane (1982; Nursing Times, 1981) to suggest that health visitors should become the epidemiologists of the primary health care team. She also questioned the value of 'attachment' to GPs and suggested that health visitors might identify local health trends and health needs and find ways of improving them, perhaps on a 'patch' basis. There has been no shortage of ideas and guidance on epidemiological concepts and practices (Richards, 1980; McCarthy, 1982; World Health Organisation, 1982; Farmer & Miller, 1983; Waters & Cliff, 1983).

Caution

However, Jane Robinson (1983) proposed caution over the idea of health visitors becoming epidemiological missionaries and going out and seeking new health needs based on these sorts of studies. Firstly, her research had made her very aware of the heartfelt needs amongst families at an individual level and she defended the traditional generalist approach in health visiting. Professor Robinson was also concerned about the 'spurious scientific respectability' implicitly endowed upon such small scale epidemiological studies, which would in fact be far too small to be able to produce statistically reliable conclusions.

Broader idea

The meaning of 'an epidemiological approach' was taken by Muir Gray (1983) to mean something rather broader. He saw it as a population-based approach as opposed to the more common approach in medicine, which is concerned only with those individuals who happen to have made contact with the services. He said health visitors' interest in the wider population is a distinct attribute. Dr Gray emphasised that the challenge in health care is to attend to problems where there is currently nothing being done. He agreed about the importance of personal attention to individual families. However, he pointed out that health visitors' ability to focus attention on community wide factors make them aware of those people with a need for preventive care, but who tend to make contact with the health services too late.

A community health profile is an important tool in this work. The seeking out and documenting of relevant statistics and local people's views helps to identify the more vulnerable groups and their main health needs. It also helps to discover which health promotion strategies are acceptable to them. Many well established health visitors carry in their heads an excellent knowledge of their area and caseload clientele. Even so, studying the statistics and/or more actively and systematically seeking clients' opinions, can lead to a new perspective. It can reveal factors of which the health visitor has been unaware (Wilson, 1986).

There are other advantages to drawing up health profiles. For example, an easy-to-understand outline of a caseload and the neighbourhood, with simple statements about the priorities chosen and why, helps to provide continuity. Staff taking over the caseload, for whatever reason, have this direct link through to the health visitor's great fund of knowledge. Also, it is helpful to nurse managers, pressed to justify the expenditure of resources on preventive health services. Profiles can give them written evidence of our actual work, incorporating understandable explanations and descriptions of the processes involved, possible alternatives and what is intended. This is what the many, many reams of Körner statistics, limited to counting the numbers of contacts and hazily defined activities, can never do. There are implications also for the evaluation of health visitor work practices (Hunt, 1982c).

SETTING ABOUT PROFILING

The idea of trying to draw up a health profile can seem very daunting. Describing something as nebulous and at the same time as complex as 'a local community' certainly presents a challenge. However, it becomes much less frightening when would-be profilers come to terms with the fact that it can and should only be a limited picture. If the presentation is too complex and tries to involve too much data, it becomes very confusing and informs no one.

It is a question of making choices. Anyone involved in creating a health profile, has to make value judgements about which issues and statistics might best describe the health of their particular area. On account of this, there needs to be clarity about the purpose of including the chosen indicators. Decisions on the relevance or otherwise of any data will mostly be guided by the extent to which that information helps towards planning health promotion strategies and/or highlighting unmet health needs.

It is also necessary to accept that statistics and the issues chosen can only act as indicators. There is no magic 'total truth' that can be described. Any statistical or other gathered data is to some extent limited in the information that it can provide. Common inadequacies for purposes of analysis are, for example:

- out-of-date statistics
- small sample
- classification difficulties
- weighting system questionable
- under-estimation for reasons such as
  — only those *currently* receiving care counted
  — low level of notification or
  — inclusion relies on self-reporting.

In view of the inevitability of choices having to be made and of some defects in the data, it is wise to be critical of prescribed formulae for 'how to do health profiles'. The inherent value judgements of the authors will be contained in their format. It is worth remembering that it was designed for their area and for *their* service objectives. A locally *imposed* format may warrant being considered in a similarly critical way.

The conclusion is that there is no perfect scheme. It is a question of doing the best possible, given the limitations. The great advantage of health visitor health profiles, unlike the one undertaken during the HV course, is that they are not a once-and-for-all project. The annual updates of the profiles give plenty of opportunity for additions, amendments and any new surveys or observations that come to health visitors' attention, or form part of their work, during the year.

Inevitably, the quality of District-wide community and caseload profiles will depend on the priority they are given by local management. As Sheila Twinn and others (1990) make quite clear, there need to be, for example:

- health visitor involvement in planning (see Chapter 14)
- specific and caseload-free *time* set aside for the project
- educational and statistical backup
- clerical help and,
- support of someone such as a professional development officer.

Health visitors who have undertaken a profile during their training have an advantage, although Maura Hunt (1982a) pointed out that the old style neighbourhood studies tended to be rather too idealistic.

Community profiles

Outline guidance on community profiling is available from the Cumberlege Report (DHSS, 1986, Part Two, p. 3) and from McClymont and others (1986). Jean Orr (1985a; 1985b) looked at the subject in depth. She discussed many issues and put forward ideas that would help give health visitors courage to use their imagination and initiative. The 'Oxfordshire strategy' is a practical scheme which has been written up (Health Visitor Development Group, 1988; Twinn et al, 1990). It has been very influential and their pamphlets offer basic and valuable guidance on health profiling.

Very practical advice has been made available by Sue Blennerhassett (forthcoming publication/ 1991). In a review of community health surveys in which the client viewpoint is central, she describes researchers' experiences and some of the ways they overcame difficulties. Many key issues are discussed and the review is well referenced. The

National Community Health Resource library (see Useful Addresses) holds a very wide range of published health profiles and surveys. Box 15.7 gives examples, many of which can also be studied through the library of the Health Visitors' Association (see Useful Addresses).

Box 15.7 Examples of published health surveys and profiles, showing contact addresses and telephone numbers, and costs

Anti-Poverty Strategy Team 1987 Fair shares? The Southwark poverty profile. Public Protection Department, London Borough of Southwark, 19 Grange Road, London SE1 3BE Tel 071 231 7331 ext 2181 £5.00

Ashton J 1984 Health in Mersey. A review. A report produced for the first Mersey Health Promotion Conference, 4th April, 1984. Department of Public Health, University of Liverpool, PO BOX 147, Liverpool L69 3BX Tel 051 794 2000 ext 5575 £5.00

Barnes J, Bickler G 1987 Southwark's health. A report on the health of the Borough of Southwark. Public Protection Department of the London Borough of Southwark/Department of Community Medicine of King's College School of Medicine and Dentistry. Available from Public Protection Department, London Borough of Southwark, 19 Grange Road, London SE1 3BE Tel 071 237 4551 ext 2181 Free

Denning S 1986 Barriers to health. A survey of the health care needs of Bengali people in King's Cross. King's Cross Centre Campaign, 62 Marchment Street, London WC1 1AB Tel 071 278 5069 £3.00

Griffiths R K, Kyle D R, Cooper R F, Kemm J R and many others 1987 Picture of health? A report. Department of Public Health Medicine, Central Birmingham Health Authority, District Offices, Vincent Drive, Edgebaston, Birmingham B15 2TZ Tel 021 472 2294 ext 3750 £6.95; photocopies £4.50

Ginnety P 1985 Moyard. A health profile. Report of the health needs of the area. Findings of the Moyard health survey. Health Promotion and Education Unit, 12–22 Linenhall Street, Belfast BT2 8BS Tel 0232 321313 ext 2015 Free

Ginnety P, Kelly K, Black M 1985 Moyard. A health profile. Final Report. Health Promotion and Education Unit, 12–22 Linenhall Street, Belfast BT2 8BS Tel 0232 321313 ext 2015 Free

Hayes M G 1989 Health inequalities in Liverpool. Liverpool City Planning Department, Wilberforce House, 25 The Strand, Liverpool L2 7QA Tel 051 225 5671 ext 5624 £3.00

Johnson I S, Coyne A-M, Milner P C, Coupland A I, Watts M, Reid G T, Heesterman R A, Harrison J, Thomas G, Todd J N 1985 A profile of health care and disease in Sheffield. Department of Community Medicine/Information Section of Sheffield Health Authority, Westbrook House, Shantervale Road, Sheffield S11 8EU Tel 0742 670333 ext 6188 £2.00

Leeds City Council 1986 Health in Leeds. The Health

Unit, Leeds City Council, 3rd Floor, Dudley House, 133 Albion Street, Leeds, LS2 8PS Tel 0532 462340 Free

Sainsbury P 1990 Croxteth health action area: developing a small area database. Department of Public Health, University of Liverpool, PO BOX 147, Liverpool L69 3BX Tel 051 794 2000 ext 5575 £5.00

Tower Hamlets Health Inquiry Team 1987 Tower Hamlets Inquiry Health Report. Community Health Council, 23 New Road, London E1 Tel 071 247 7858 Free

Townsend P, Simpson D, Tibbs N 1984 Inequalities of health in the City of Bristol. A preliminary review of statistical evidence. Department of Social Administration School of Applied Social Studies, University of Bristol, 40 Berkeley Square, Bristol BS8 1HY Tel 0272 303030 £3.00

Time spent in preparation is well worthwhile. For example, reading widely helps to avoid possible traps already discovered by others. Also, liaison with workers in other local agencies who may already have prepared a health profile helps to avoid unnecessary duplication. Many local authorities (LA) planning departments have published health profiles (Leeds City Council, 1986; Anti-Poverty Strategy Team, 1987; Barnes & Bickler, 1987; Nursing Times, 1987; Anti-Poverty Strategy Working Group, 1989; Hayes, 1989). Some are taking part in the Healthy Cities Project (Ashton et al, 1986; Delamothe, 1988; Grice & Fryer, 1988; Moore, 1988).

There are great advantages to be gained from teamwork with other agencies interested in profiling. For example, it adds to perspectives and expertise and provides a good basis for cooperative health promotion strategies which result from the studies. Where possible, the public view should be represented. The Pimlico Patch Committee (Dunford & Hughes, 1988), the Moyard experience (Ginnety et al, 1985) and Zana Rae Higgs (1985) provide ideas and examples of what can be achieved when local people are drawn into profile planning.

Teamwork may help with another basic task: the decision about the boundaries of the community/neighbourhood. Finding convenient and appropriate borders can present problems. For example, health authority and local authority boundaries, and therefore their statistics, do not always coincide. Decisions are likely to be influenced by factors such as the way the 'neighbourhood' is perceived and the availability of appropriate small area, post-coded or ward-based statistics and other surveys and information. It will also depend on whether the 'community' to be reviewed is a convenient sub-division of the District Health Authority, an electoral ward, 'a patch' or an area that serves to provide a background setting for a GP list.

There is no lack of statistics and data. It is a question of seeking out the most indicative. The Office of Population Census Statistics and *Social Trends* are good starting points. Perhaps the best single measure of workload and health need is Professor Jarman's (1983; 1984; 1989) underprivileged area scoring system. The values for electoral wards in England and Wales are available on request (Jarman, 1989, p. 108).

When the profile is being written up, it is necessary to state the source of the statistics or survey and to interpret the findings for the reader, for example:

- what the statistics are
- why they were chosen and
- the meaning of these particular figures.

Commonly, the aim is to concentrate attention on the weakest groups in the community/neighbourhood/area/electoral ward. An outline is therefore provided of, for example:

- population — structure
        — changes
- unemployment
- single parent families
- pensioners living alone
- ethnic background/origin.

Indicators are needed for the sort of issues listed earlier in this chapter in Example Two's Box 15.3 and in Figure 1 of Christina Edwards' (1990) description of locality management in West Suffolk.

Caseload profiles

Early in the '80s, Maura Hunt (1982a; 1982b; 1982c) drew attention to the value of caseload profiling and outlined how to set about constructing one (Hunt 1982b). Heather Wilson (1986) described how her colleagues helped her gather information from her health visitor records for a caseload profile and how she devised a questionnaire. She used very simple survey techniques and found it increased her awareness of people's lack of knowledge about personal health and the services available. A working party of health visitors and fieldwork teachers in Pontefract drew up caseload profiles using health visitor records, clinic records and age/sex registers. Their work was used to demonstrate the client groups most needing health visitor input (Houghton, 1987). More and more health visitors are undertaking these profiles.

Gradually, systems are being developed that help to key into some of the great wealth of information that exists. For example, Carr-Hill and others (1987) describe how data held by family practitioner committees could be used together with other information available, to help form detailed profiles of practice populations.

Computers are likely to be increasingly involved in helping to map community health (Thomas, 1990). Health visitors could help to influence which particular criteria are monitored. For example, they may feel, like John Catford (1983), that the time has come for greater use of positive health indicators, such as the percentage of population who are *not* smoking or who *are* taking exercise.

Quick access to health visitor record card information is important. This is made much easier where it is clearly placed on the face sheet. For example, where annual counting is intended of factors such as immunisation status, breastfeeding duration or whether or not the parents are employed, records can be prepared appropriately.

Just as in the community profile, there is no absolute formula for a caseload profile. Some of the basic features would be likely to be the number of:

- families
- children
  - total; age structure
  - on 'at risk' register
  - on 'of concern' list
  - handicapped
- single parent families

- pensioners
  - in the caseload
  - total: age structure
  - on GP list/in patch or area
- homeless families
  - adults
  - children
  - unregistered with GP
- unemployed.

Other basic factors might include indicators of:

- social class
- type of employment
- housing type
  - council/private rented or owner occupied
  - with parents or homeless
- environment
  - transport
  - facilities
- ethnic background or origin

and mortality statistics, compared with health district/LA and national figures, such as those for:

- coronary heart disease
- cancers
- chronic respiratory disease
- accidents
- strokes
- suicides
- AIDS and
- infant mortality rates
- perinatal mortality rates.

The basic statistics and descriptive data may advantageously be augmented by in-depth surveys of particular subgroups or samples, and/or of specific investigation of client attitudes and knowledge. Planning for client-centred strategies cannot take place without good indicators of consumer opinion. It is interesting to note that the Cumberlege inquiry team found that where nurses had researched what was wanted, excellent work was indeed achieved.

In writing up the caseload profile, unusual features such as a very mobile population, a very high percentage of elderly people living alone or of homeless families, would naturally need to be highlighted. Issues raised by the results of client opinion and other caseload surveys can be discussed. In Example Two, the caseload profile in

Box 15.4 (see page 305) included a brief outline of the primary health care team and facilities, the health visitor's current work patterns and her referrals. The description ended with what had been achieved by the health visitor the previous year and her priorities for the coming year. In the 'Oxfordshire Strategy', a statement is made each year of identified health needs which health visitors are unable to attend to (Dauncey, 1988). Where relevant, a note could also be included comparing health visitor establishment figures with the number actually employed, alongside an indication of closed or double caseloads and how long that situation has existed. This would help give a clearer picture of what *could* be achieved.

This description of community and caseload profiling has not tried to propose an ideal model. The aim has been to provide an introduction, to offer reassurances and also cautions, and to indicate where some further information and guidance can be found. The profiles can then be tailored to particular local circumstances.

WORKING TOGETHER

The chapter now takes a brief look at the emergence of neighbourhood health care schemes, at team building and provides examples of teamwork. It concludes with a selection of practical health promotion issues in which teamwork may be involved.

Neighbourhood health care emerges

In the year following publication of the Cumberlege Report (1986), around half the English health authorities were organising decentralisation of their community services (Daley, 1987). Early in 1988, the King's Fund was able to report that 74 health authorities had implemented, or were planning, neighbourhood nursing (Nursing Times, 1988a).

Pilot schemes were being set up and accounts of several of the strategies appeared in the journals. Examples are Sally Malin's (1987) description of patch work on the Isle of Dogs, Kathy Elliott's (1988) of the Haggerston estate project and various

reports on the progress of decentralisation in Islington (Daley & Shepherd, 1987; Malin & Shepherd, 1988; Brown P, 1989).

Dr Deborah Hennessy (1987) wrote an informative, succinct account of the Wandsworth strategy. This article also provides good background reading for our Wandsworth examples, Example Four earlier in this chapter and Example Three of the previous chapter. The West Suffolk locality-based nursing service was given a NT/3M award for management. Their scheme included high profile local contact, 'Cooperation for Change' days to draw workers together and a commitment to provide appropriate professional backup for field staff (Smith, 1989; Edwards, 1990).

These examples provide evidence of the need to spend time, effort and other resources on the *processes* involved in, for example, profiling and planning health care strategies and in teamwork. Jean Orr (1989) pointed out that in many places, implementation of Cumberlege has been concentrating on *structural* changes only. That is, they have merely moved health visitors and district nurses into the same office!

As was evident in the previous chapter, it is attention to the underlying processes which is the key to successful change. New ways of working need well-planned preparation and management backup. Health visitors require, for example, appropriate:

- in-post education and training
- equipment and accommodation
- professional support
- open and honest assessment of achievements
- opportunities for staff development.

TEAMWORK

One of the needs is for time and opportunity for teambuilding. Everyone agrees that working together brings many advantages. For example, it brings:

- improved communication
- mutual support
- exchange of ideas and information
- increased confidence
- peer-group motivation and
- access to peer-group evaluation.

However, working closely with people from other professional backgrounds and training, with distinctly different goals and attitudes, can be confusing. This is true even within the same profession. In Example Three of Chapter 14, Sue Machell remarked that putting nurses together does not automatically make a team. She also noted bereavement reactions to change and the need to help health visitors talk through their difficulties. Weighill and others (1986) wrote about their multidisciplinary cooperative efforts during a series of weight-loss groups. They described the teamwork problems they encountered and how frankness and willingness to debate the differences enabled them to provide a good service and to develop professionally.

In some circumstances, particularly when the changes are imposed, teambuilding programmes or exercises may help. It may be worth trying out either some activities carefully planned by Gawlinski and Graessle (1988) or parts of the Maddux (1988) programme. For health visitors who prefer to read about the practicalities and the processes involved in working together, there are, for example, descriptions of health visitor teamwork in a shared workload (Rowe, 1989) and ideas from members of a multi-disciplinary community forum (Community Forum, 1990).

Teamwork examples

June Clark (1986) predicted that it would be the nurses themselves who determined whether or not the ideas of the Cumberlege Report (1986) would be implemented. She was right. With or without the formal changes, teamwork is increasing. However, only a few health visitors involved in teamwork have found the time to write about it. Some have recounted how they worked with other health visitors, for example, to establish health market stalls (Brierley et al, 1988; Jackson, 1990) or a women's health education discussion group (Dobson, 1987). Others have described how they teamed up to make sure that child health clinics are available when and where people would like them (Betts & Betts, 1990; Tully 1990; Husain, 1990).

Health visitors have also described their team-work with other workers in the community. For example, some set up stalls at a local trade fair (Astrop, 1987) or a health fair (Begg, 1989). Others ran a stall and various health promotion sessions at a market (Coppenhall, 1990). There have been accounts of cooperative work over a family health unit (Cubbin, 1987), a family centre (Koris, 1987) and drop-in centres (May, 1989), as well as teamwork for lone-parent groups (Brown G, 1989) and for parents of children with sleeping problems (Balfour, 1988). One health visitor has described how she stepped beyond the confines of the GP practice population and worked with local volunteers to set up a village care scheme (Enticknap, 1987). The 'Cumberlege approach' is becoming well established.

SOME HEALTH PROMOTION ISSUES

Teamwork and community and caseload profiling are encouraging and guiding the use of new initiatives in health promotion, which are particularly responsive to clients' perspectives and needs. Relevant issues embrace the entire range of environmental, physical, mental/emotional and social aspects of health. A few important examples follow.

Environmental aspects of health: an example

Unemployment and low income

The profile unemployment statistics might reveal surprises, although family visiting gives most health visitors a fairly clear idea of the degree of that problem in their area. Unemployment and/or a marginal income affect the nature of families' circumstances and immediate environment and hence their future health. Many people do not take up their full entitlements. One health visiting aim is to increase awareness of what these are and how to claim them.

Advice on how to help the families has been offered by Shirley Goodwin (1988), particularly with reference to contacts with social fund officers.

The *Health Visitor* frequently provides clearly explained benefits updates (Ravetz, 1988; Henwood, 1989a; 1989b; 1989c; Health Visitor, 1990a; Lakhani, 1990), which clients may find useful. Many of these articles also note the Child Poverty Action Group's (CPAG) telephone advice line. The CPAG guides to benefits (Chapman et al, 1989; Kennedy et al, 1989) are found invaluable by many health visitors and are small enough to be kept accessible in a briefcase.

Groupwork may provide a good environment for exploring the difficulties encountered. For example, application forms such as those for payment for NHS services or for claiming community care grants, are very complicated. The guidance notes provided can be very confusing. Meeting other people in similar circumstances who also find these forms difficult, can be reassuring. Group efforts at filling in a spare set of forms might produce some hilarity and light relief. However, a visit to the group from someone from a local advice centre or welfare rights unit would bring enlightenment.

There is a great deal of potential in groupwork. For example, health visitors might suggest use of the *Unemployment and health* resource pack (Black & Laughlin, 1987). This publication starts with an introduction to the way unemployment affects health and goes on to provide ideas for a range of actions that a group can take. The resources section was devised specifically for the use of people in the Glasgow area. However, the section provides guidance on the sort of information that groups could usefully gather for their own area. The pack offers a very practical and positive approach to promoting health.

Physical health: two examples

Pet-associated health problems

When people are asked what health issue causes them greatest concern, they may, like those answering a questionnaire in Chapter 12's Example Three, give a particularly high rating to medical hazards from dogs, or other pet-associated health problems (Lissauer & Pollock, 1984; Bewley, 1985; Elliot et al, 1985). Health visitors are currently attempting to influence policies both nationally and locally on dog-related health issues (Health Visitor, 1990b).

Coronary heart disease

From a statistical point of view, the greatest health problem is coronary heart disease. It is the major killer of our time and is an enormous burden on NHS resources. The National Audit Office (1989) has written a report which is scathing about the lack of proper planning for prevention programmes. The authors regretted the lack both of coordination between government departments and of guidance to health authorities on the development of programmes. In stark contrast, many other countries have achieved significant reductions in premature deaths from the disease (Nutbeam, 1987).

There is a coordinated prevention programme in Wales (Parish, 1987) in which health visitors are taking part (Edwards, 1987). In most of the United Kingdom there is reliance on local liaison with health education officers and on health visitors' own initiatives, such as those at the fairs and market places mentioned in the teamwork section above. The Nursing Times 'MOT for Humans' day provided a similar scheme. It concentrated particularly on issues such as:

- height and weight
- blood pressure
- alcohol
- exercise
- nutrition
- smoking and
- stress.

Pamela Holmes (1987) described the project and provided a guide for others organising their own day. Health visitors may also find helpful Tudor-Hart and Stilwell's (1988) workbook and Goodliffe's (1987) guide.

In one forward-looking GP practice, two health visitors were employed specifically to provide a screening and education service for practice patients, aimed at preventing coronary heart disease (Fitzpatrick & Ridley, 1988). Vari Reynolds and Helen Hay (1988) undertook a survey and discovered a great deal of support for a health education and screening service for men, both amongst health visitors and from potential clients. These authors offer advice for health visitors planning to set up a scheme.

There are still many gaps in our knowledge and there is inevitably some guesswork about exactly what factors lead to coronary heart disease. In simplifying information for consumer understanding, care has to be taken that it is not made over simple. For example, dietary advice is seen as being essential (Cameron, 1989; Scott, 1989), but it is in fact a complex issue. Historically, advice on nutrition has been gradually changed and refined over the years as further evidence has become available. The part played by fat in the diet is not now a clear-cut issue (Holmes, 1988; 1989). Health visitors need to keep themselves as up to date as they can with the latest range of views.

Approach is also important. For example, we can take lessons from commercial advertisers and learn to accentuate the positive and to keep 'thou shalt not' out of health education issues (Gray, 1984). Also, connotations of 'victim blaming' are to be avoided (Sadler, 1989).

Mental/emotional health: an example

Stress management

Anxiety is an important influence on levels of health. Mark Payne (1989) sees stress as the most underrated factor causing heart attacks. Both he and Christine Bundy (1988) have explained very simply, how psychological factors can lead to heart disease. The Consumer Association has provided practical advice on stress and appropriate helping agencies (Rudinger, 1988).

The stress factor has not been underestimated at the Steyning health centre. Their 'human MOT' scheme offers three stress management classes at monthly intervals to people whose 'MOT' anxiety-levels assessment shows they might benefit (Martin & Duncan-Grant, 1989). An eight session group stress-management programme, its planning, dynamics and evaluation, were outlined by Christine Howden and Anita Levison (1987).

The tranquilliser support group in which Sarah

Forester (1988) was a joint group leader, did not have management support and had to be run 'on the quiet'. Marion Tyler and Sue Barnes (1986; 1989) had the reverse experience. The value of their courses was clearly recognised. Subsequently other health visitors in their area have been trained and have now set up similar support groups.

Some health visitors will be lucky enough to be/have been a member of a work-based stress-management group (Goldblatt, 1988). These groups are particularly important in the light of the clear need for strategies to cope with our occupational stress (Goodwin, 1987; Gough & Hingley, 1988; Rowe, 1988; West et al, 1989). This kind of experience could help with later co-leadership work. The group may, for example, have tried out tapes (Burnard, 1988; Wood, 1989), taken part in distance learning (Holland, 1986; 1987) or assertiveness training (see Chapter 14), or used stress-check schedules for monitoring the effect of programmes (Bailey, 1985).

Social aspects of health: an example

AIDS/HIV

The chapter finishes with a very brief look at HIV/AIDS. This is somewhat provocatively included under 'social aspects of health' because social behaviour is so great a factor in its spread (Wells, 1989). It is also because stigmatisation and non-acceptance so significantly affect how HIV/AIDS sufferers and the people who look after them are treated (England, 1990; Pownall, 1990). Health promotion which overcomes the myths, prejudices and complacency is sorely needed.

It is not easy to predict exactly how many AIDS cases the future will bring (Kmietowicz, 1990; Nursing Times, 1990). However, the government's chief medical officer feels AIDS could make the worst fatal epidemic in history (Dickson, 1989). Now is the time for getting together with others, taking stock and implementing relevant initiatives (Smits, 1987; Carlisle, 1989; Pye et al, 1989; Thompson, 1989).

In order to have enough practical knowledge, it is necessary to keep up to date. There is a wide range of relevant literature available (e.g.: Pratt,

1986; Gordon & Mitchell, 1988; McMullen, 1988; Miller & Bor, 1988; Richardson, 1989), but new research and ideas are emerging all the time. Good sources of up-to-date information are the most recent

- booklets from the Terence Higgins Trust (see Useful Addresses)
- copies of *Aids Newsletter*, a three-weekly magazine
- Department of Health leaflets and figures

which may be available from your local

- medical library and/or
- Health Education/Promotion Department.

Putting on lectures (Neale, 1987) and attending conferences can help (Burke, 1987; Jones, 1987a; 1987b; Thompson, 1987). There are now several relevant videos available for purchase or on five days' free loan from CFL Vision (see Useful Addresses; Nursing Times, 1988b; 1989).

We have now looked very briefly at health profiling, at teamwork and at some health promotion issues. Many references have been given so that readers can study these issues more deeply. Real-life examples concentrated on teamwork and health profiling, this chapter's themes from the 'Cumberlege approach'.

USEFUL ADDRESSES

CFL Vision
PO Box 35
Weatherby,
Yorkshire LS23 7EX
Tel 0937 541010

Health Visitors' Association library
50 Southwark Street
London SE1 1UN
Tel 071 378 7255
Ring for appointment to visit

National Community Health Resource
library
57 Chalton Street
London NW1 1HU
Tel 071 383 3841
Ring for appointment to visit

Terence Higgins Trust
52–54 Grays Inn Road
London WCIX 8JU
Tel 071 831 0330
Helpline tel 071 242 1010
3 p.m.–10 p.m. daily

REFERENCES

Anti-Poverty Strategy Team 1987 Fair shares? The Southwark poverty profile. Public Protection Department, London Borough of Southwark, London

Anti-Poverty Strategy Working Group 1989 Developing an anti-poverty strategy. Southampton City Council, Southampton

Ashton J, Grey P, Barnard K 1986 Healthy cities — WHO's new public health initiative. Health Promotion 1, 3: 319–324

Astrop P 1987 All the fun of the fair. Health Visitor 60, 6: 189

Bailey R D 1985 Coping with stress in caring. Blackwell Scientific Publications, Oxford — Recommended, Appendices 1–5 can be used to help monitor progress before and after stress-control programmes.

Balfour A 1988 A group for parents who have children with sleeping problems. Health Visitor 61, 10: 316–318

Barnes J, Bickler G 1987 Southwark's health. A report on the health of the Borough of Southwark. Public

Protection Department of the London Borough of Southwark, London

Begg E 1989 Planning a health fair. Nursing Times Community Outlook 85, 41: 19–22

Betts G, Betts J 1990 Establishing a child health clinic in a deprived area. Health Visitor 63, 4: 122–124

Bewley B R 1985 Medical hazards from dogs. British Medical Journal 291: 760–761

Black D, Laughlin S (eds) 1987 Unemployment and health: resources, information, action, discussion, 2nd edn. Greater Glasgow Health Board Health Education Department, Glasgow — Recommended. Available from Belvedere House, 1362 London Road, Glasgow G31 4QY Tel: 041 556 2201

Blakeborough S 1990 Health mornings in the inner city. Health Visitor 63, 10: 344–345

Blennerhassett S (forthcoming publication/1991) A review of community health surveys. National Community Health

Resource/Health Education Authority, London

Brierley H, Goddard P, Wildbore A 1988 Yes, we have no bananas, but plenty of health care today. Health Visitor 61, 12: 369–370

Brown G 1989 A lone parent group in Yorkshire. Health Visitor 62, 6: 187–188

Brown P 1989 Challenges for community nursing in a decentralised community service. Senior Nurse 10, 3: 9–10

Brown P, Gordon P (eds) 1987 Cumberlege in action. A directory of good practice that influenced the community nursing review team. KFC 87/62 King's Fund Centre, London

Bundy C 1988 Making sense of stress and coronary heart disease. Nursing Times 84, 44: 35–37

Burke E 1987 AIDS and community care. Health Visitor 60, 8: 271

Burnard P 1988 Stress and relaxation in health visiting. Health Visitor 61, 9: 272

Cameron J 1989 Wholesome Britain. Nursing Times 85, 7: 20

Carlisle D 1989 Working on the edge. Nursing Times 85, 45: 27–29

Carr-Hill R, Kirby P, Fordham R, Houghton K 1987 Locality health planning: contibuting a data base. Discussion paper 34. Centre for Health Economics, University of York, Heslington

Catford J 1983 Positive health indicators — towards a new information base for health promotion. Community Medicine 5, 2: 125–132 — Recommended.

Chapman V, Lakhani D, Read J, Wood P 1989 National welfare benefits handbook 1989–90, 19th edn. Child Poverty Action Group — Very useful, clearly written and well presented. Available from CPAG (Pubs), 4th Floor, 1–5 Bath Street, London EC1V 9PY

Clark J 1986 A lesson in politics. Senior Nurse 5, 3: 6–7

Community Forum (ed) 1990 Working together. Innovations in group work for primary health care. Parkside Health Authority, London — Recommended.

Coppenhall K 1990 Raising health visitors' profiles. Health Visitor 63, 1: 26–27

Cubbin J 1987 Sharing the burden. Nursing Times Community Outlook 83, 32: 11–14

Daley G 1987 Decentralisation: a new way of organising community health services. Hospital and Health Services Review 83, 2: 72–74

Daley G, Shepherd G 1987 'Going local' gathers speed. Health Service Journal 97, 5060: 850–851

Dauncey J 1988 A positive response. Nursing Times 84, 42: 75–77

Delamothe T 1988 First United Kingdom Health Cities conference, Liverpool. British Medical Journal 296: 1117–1120

Department of Health 1989 Working for patients. HMSO, London

DHSS 1986 Neighbourhood nursing — a focus for health care. Report of the Community Nursing Review. (Chairman, Julia Cumberlege) HMSO, London

Dickson N 1989 A monstrous deception. Nursing Times 85, 51: 22–23

Dobson E A 1987 Good health for women. Health Visitor 60, 11: 363

Dunford H, Hughes J 1988 Pimlico Patch Committee. An experiment in locality planning. Primary Health Care Group, King's Fund, London — Recommended.

Edwards C 1990 Neighbourhood networks. Nursing Times 86, 5: 36–38 — Recommended.

Edwards J 1987 Passports to health. Nursing Times 83, 15: 27–28

Elliot D L, Tolle S W, Goldberg L, Miller J B 1985 Pet-associated illness. New England Journal of Medicine 313, 16: 985–995

Elliott K 1988 Health and the inner city. Health Service Journal 98, 5088: 212–213

England V 1990 (letter) Insensitive treament. Nursing Times 86; 19: 13

Enticknap B 1987 Village volunteers. Nursing Times Community Outlook 83,38: 19–22

Farmer R D T, Miller D L 1983 Lecture notes of epidemiology and community medicine. Blackwell Scientific Publications, Oxford

Fitzpatrick S, Ridley M 1988 Heart disease: a contemporary issue. Health Visitor 61, 4: 110–111

Forester S 1988 A tranquiliser support group. In: Drennan V (ed) Health visitors and groups: politics and practice. Heinemann Nursing, Oxford — Describes behind-the-scenes factors.

Gawlinski G, Graessle L 1988 Planning together, The art of effective teamwork. Bedford Square Press, London — Recommended.

Ginnety P, Kelly K, Black M 1985 Moyard. A health profile. Final Report. Health Promotion and Education Unit, Belfast, pp 11–17 — Recommended.

Goldblatt P 1988 Connections and adaptations. Health visitor 61, 9: 273–274 — Recommended: Group for newly qualified health visitors.

Goodliffe C 1987 How to avoid heart disease. Blandford Press, London

Goodwin S 1987 Stress in health visiting. In: Hockey L Recent advances in nursing: 15. Community nursing. Churchill Livingstone, Edinburgh

Goodwin S 1988 Clients must come first. Health Service Journal 98, 5094: 364

Gordon P, Mitchell L 1988 Safer sex: a new look at sexual pleasure. Faber, London

Gough P, Hingley P 1988 Combating the pressure. Nursing Times 84, 2: 43–45

Gray F 1984 Accentuate the positive. Health and Social Service Journal XCIV, 4890: 380

Gray J A M 1983 Role dilemma of health visiting (letter). Health Visitor 56: 83–84

Grice D, Fryer P 1988 Giving good counsel on health. Health Service Journal 98, 5098: 480–481

Hayes M G 1989 Health inequalities in Liverpool. Liverpool City Planning Department, Liverpool City Council, Liverpool

Health Visitor 1990a New benefits rates: from 9 April 1990. Health Visitor 63, 4: 133

Health Visitor 1990b Curbs sought. Health Visitor 63, 6: 182

Health Visitor Development Group 1988 Oxfordshire's strategy for health visiting: a change for the better. Oxfordshire Health Authority, Oxford — Helpful.

Hennessy D 1987 Developing a strategy for neighbourhood health care. Primary Health Care April: 13 — Recommended.

Henwood J 1989a The health visitors' guide to new benefits' rates 1989–90. Health Visitor 62, 4: 127

Henwood J 1989b Claiming community care grants. Health Visitor 62, 6: 190

Henwood J 1989c Benefits for children and young people in education. Health Visitor 62, 7: 225

Higgs Z R 1985 The community assessment project. In: Higgs Z R, Gustafson D D (eds) Community as client: assessment and diagnosis. F A Davis Company, Philadephia

Holland S (ed) 1986 Stress in nursing: reader. Distance Learning Centre, South Bank Polytechnic, London

Holland S 1987 Stress in nursing: workbook. Distance Learning Centre, South Bank Polytechnic, London

Holmes P 1987 MOT for humans. Nursing Times 83, 10: 35–38

Holmes S 1988 Does a high fat diet cause health disease? Nursing Times 84, 13: 34–35

Holmes S 1989 The hazards of health eating. Nursing Times 85, 26: 49–51

Houghton D 1987 Development of caseload and community profiles. Health Visitor 60, 9: 298 — Recommended.

Howden C, Levison A 1987 Coping with stress — sharing and learning. Senior Nurse 7, 2: 6–8

Hunt M 1982a A critique of the neighbourhood study in health visitor training. Health Visitor 55, 10: 521–525 — Essential reading.

Hunt M 1982b Caseload profiles — an alternative to the neighbourhood study. Health Visitor 55, 11: 606–607 — Essential reading.

Hunt M 1982c Caseload profiles: their implications for evaluating health visiting practice. Health Visitor 55, 12: 662–665 — Recommended.

Husain M 1990 Parents' attitudes to a child clinic. Health Visitor 63, 3: 84

Jackson C 1989 Still killing after all these years. Health Visitor 62, 8: 254

Jackson C 1990 To market, to market. Health Visitor 63, 3: 95–96

Jarman B 1983 Identification of underprivileged areas. British Medical Journal 286: 1705–1709 — Recommended.

Jarman B 1984 Underprivileged areas: validation and distribution of scores. British Medical Journal 289: 1587–1592 — Recommended.

Jarman B 1989 General practice. In: While A (ed) Health in the inner city. Heinemann Medical Books, Oxford — Recommended.

Jones J 1987a AIDS and the community nurse. Health Visitor 60, 8: 270

Jones J 1987b AIDS in childhood and adolescence. Health Visitor 60, 8: 270

Kennedy C, McMullen J, Rowland M 1989 Rights guide to non-means-tested social security benefits, 12th edn. Child Poverty Action Group — Very useful, clearly written and well presented. Available from CPAG (Pubs), 4th Floor, 1–5 Bath Street, London EC1V 9PY

Kmietowicz Z 1990 Pattern of AIDS set to change. General Practioner 16th February: 12

Koris J 1987 Health visitor involvement in a family centre. Health Visitor 60, 2: 43–44

Lakhani B 1990 A hole in the budget. Health Visitor 63, 5: 170

Leeds City Council 1986 Health in Leeds. The Health Unit, Leeds City Council, Leeds

Lissauer T, Pollock I 1984 Animal bites in infants and young children. Modern Medicine 29, 5: 22–24

MacFarlane of Llandaff 1982 Responsibility for future development of health visiting. Health Visitor 55: 273–277

McCarthy M 1982 Epidemiology and policies for health planning. King Edward's Hospital Fund for London, London

McClymont M, Thomas S, Denham M J 1986 Health visiting and the elderly. Churchill Livingstone, Edinburgh, Appendix 5 — Recommended.

McMullen R 1988 Living with HIV in self and others. GMP Publishers Ltd, London

Maddux R B 1988 Team building. An exercise in leadership, 2nd edn. Kogan Page, London

Malin S 1987 Bridging a healthcare gap. Health Service Journal 97, 5038: 218

Malin S, Shepherd G 1988 Hats off to going local. Health Service Journal 98, 5108: 762–763

Martin M, Duncan-Grant A 1989 The Steyning way. Nursing Times 85, 21: 36–38

May K 1989 A new venture in health care. Health Visitor 62, 7: 211–213

Miller R, Bor R 1988 AIDS: a guide to clinical counselling. Science Press, London

Moore W 1988 Healthy cities: are they on the horizon? Health Service Journal 98, 5095: 382–383

National Audit Office 1989 National Health Service: coronary heart disease. HMSO, London

Neale S 1987 Babies with AIDS. Health Visitor 60, 8: 271

Nursing Times 1981 Baroness looks for new role for the HV. Nursing Times 77: 1867

Nursing Times 1987 Edinburgh's poor fall through NHS net. Nursing Times 83, 31: 10

Nursing Times 1988a No time to lose on patch nursing. Nursing Times 84, 10: 10

Nursing Times 1988b Plain clothes district nurses to visit AIDS patients. Nursing Times 84, 35: 8

Nursing Times 1989 Two AIDS teaching videos launched. Nursing Times 85, 16: 9

Nursing Times 1990 Pattern of AIDS increase. Nursing Times 86, 9: 10

Nutbeam D 1987 Controlling a killer. Nursing Times 83, 15: 24–26

Orr J 1985a The community dimension. In: Luker K, Orr J (eds) Health visiting. Blackwell Scientific Publications, Oxford — Good background reading.

Orr J 1985b Health visiting and the community. In: Luker K, Orr J (eds) Health visiting. Blackwell Scientific Publications, Oxford — Recommended.

Orr J 1989 The blueprint already exists. Health Visitor 62, 8: 238 – Recommended.

Parish R 1987 Wales paves the way to heart health. Nursing Times 83, 16: 34–36

Payne M 1989 How to take care of your heart. Your survival and lifestyle handbook. Northcote House, Plymouth — A well-written book which outlines the basic issues: useful for clients.

Pownall M 1990 Testing question. Nursing Times 86, 19: 18

Pratt R J 1986 AIDS: a strategy for nursing care. Edward Arnold, Sevenoaks

Pye M, Kapila M, Buckley G, Cunningham D 1989 Responding to the AIDS challenge: comparative study of local AIDS programmes in the United Kingdom. Longman, Harlow

Ravetz A 1988 Income support. Health Visitor 61, 4: 117

Reynolds V, Hay H 1988 Primary prevention of coronary heart disease. Health Visitor 61, 4: 108–109

Richards I G D 1980 The epidemiology of disease in

childhood. In: Mitchell R G (ed) Child health in the community, 2nd edn. Churchill Livingstone, Edinburgh

Richardson D 1989 Women and the AIDS crisis. Pandora Press, London

Robinson J 1983 The role dilemma of health visiting. Health Visitor 56: 22–24

Rowe J 1988 Health visitors talking. In: Drennan V (ed) Health visitors and groups: politics and practice. Heinemann Nursing, Oxford — Recommended: health visitor mutual support group.

Rowe J 1989 New Ideas notebook. Hillingdon Primary and Community Health Care Services, Hillingdon Health Authority, London

Rudinger E (ed) 1988 Understanding stress. How to recognise the causes and effects of stress and what steps to take to come to terms with them. Consumers' Association/Hodder and Stoughton, London — Recommended: useful for clients.

Sadler C 1989 Fat chance. Nursing Times 85, 25: 18

Scott A 1989 Diet combats coronaries. Nursing Times 85, 22: 29–30

Smith S 1989 Community patchwork. Nursing Times 85, 3: 29–31

Smits A 1988 Community outreach. Nursing Times 84, 46: 71

Thomas E 1990 Mapping community health. Nursing Times Community Outlook 86, 8: 6–8

Thompson A 1989 Crisis on the streets. Nursing Times Community Outlook 85, 2: 8–9

Thompson L 1987 AIDS, ethics and medicine. Health Visitor 60, 8: 271

Tudor-Hart J, Stilwell B 1988 Prevention of coronary heart diseases and stroke: a workbook for primary care teams. Faber, London

Tully C 1990 Saving a clinic. Health Visitor 63, 3: 87–88

Twinn S, Dauncey J, Carnell J 1990 The process of health profiling. Health Visitors' Association, London — Essential reading.

Tyler M, Barnes S 1986 The group approach to living with stress. Health Visitor 59, 1'4–16 — Recommended: Describes course and measurement of progress.

Tyler M, Barnes S 1989 The group approach to living with stress: four years on. Health Visitor 62, 10: 309–311 Recommended: Outlines course, reading list and independent assessment.

Waters W E, Cliff K S 1983 Community medicine: a textbook for nurses and health visitors. Croom Helm, London

Weighill V E, Tilley S, Keenan G C 1986 Weight groups: reflections on working together in primary care. Health Visitor 59, 4: 106–108

Wells R 1989 AIDS: is the danger exaggerated? The case against. Nursing Times 85, 42: 53

West M, Jones A, Savage Y 1988 Stress in health visiting: a quantitative assessment. Health Visitor 61, 9: 269–271

Wilson H 1986 Caseload profile. Health Visitor 59, 2: 40 — Recommended.

Wood C 1989 Relax with a tape. Nursing Times 85, 23: 52–54

World Health Organisation 1982 The place of epidemiology in local health work: the experience of a group of developing countries. World Health Organisation, Geneva

In this last chapter, we look at some of the administrative changes that have affected health visiting in recent years, some of the challenges that face the profession and the need now for greater political awareness. Some of the current underlying debates are mentioned. Finally, our three basic models are considered in the light of a health visitor's work in a community-based initiative.

16

Health visiting — which way now?

INFLUENCES AND CHALLENGES

Administrative changes over recent years have meant that, despite high levels of agreement that prevention is better than cure, health visiting, alongside other community services, has had to fight for funds in competition with more prestigious and powerful medical lobbies. Naturally, there are fears that expenditure on community health services would not be adequate to enable proper care if the demands for limitless resources for high technology medicine prevail (DHSS, 1986, p. (i)).

The purpose and the nature of health visiting is not always easily understood by people oriented to acute care. However, an increasing number of health visitors are writing and explaining about their work and about the results of new initiatives they have been undertaking. There are plenty of debates within the profession. We will take a brief look at some of the issues such as those in the specialist-versus-generalist and the groupwork-versus-home-visiting arguments. The book concludes with the three frameworks used in the earlier chapters, showing their three perspectives of an award-winning community-based project.

RECENT ISSUES

The reorganisation of the health service in 1974 brought health visitors from the relative obscurity of the Medical Officers of Health Local Authority departments into mainstream nursing and funding through the NHS. They moved from a unit that clearly sympathised with and fully supported their preventive role, into the much larger arena of the Health Authorities, which were, until then, almost totally concerned with acute clinical care.

The debate and 'identity'

There was an obvious need to be able to explain the health visitor's role in clear terms. In 1974, tutors were expressing concern about the definitions associated with the theoretical aspects of the course that described the practice of health visiting (Council for the Education and Training of Health Visitors, 1977). A wide ranging debate was set up by the Council for the Education and Training of Health Visitors (CETHV) (1977, 1980, 1982) in which many health visitors participated.

The self-questioning and the discussions of the CETHV's 'Investigation' coincided with a new phase in which more health visitors were prepared to write about their work and to try to find ways of evaluating it. Clear evidence of this trend can be seen in the significant improvement over recent years of the quality and content of the *Health Visitor* journal.

In the changing times of the mid-seventies, this rigorous professional self-examination naturally engendered some feelings of professional insecurity. On the other hand, it did mean that these practitioners were not just unthinkingly continuing traditional patterns of practice. They were aiming to take a critical look at what they were hoping to achieve and at the significance of various aspects of the work and to find ways of explaining it.

Not all health visitors have been thinking and acting so systematically. The Community Nursing Review Team for England (Cumberlege Committee) felt community nurses in general were too limited by their traditional roles and 'in a rut' (DHSS, 1986, pp. 2–3; 11). They suggested that health visitors, district nurses and school nurses should work together in groups providing neighbourhood nursing services. It was proposed, for example, that the nurses should undertake work based on more systematically identified health needs with improved nurse management closer to the consumer, that there should be more

involvement by the consumer and good team-work by primary health care team members.

The team felt that better organised and locally planned collaborative ventures could be significantly more responsive to the needs of each particular neighbourhood and to the individuals within it. The proposals provide an exciting challenge and some very useful pointers for the next phase in the history of our work. The role and skills of the health visitor were certainly appreciated by the team, a matter taken up later in this chapter (p. 329). The approach is well under way and many examples of this well-planned and collaborative work have been cited in the last few chapters.

For the most part, the move into the larger arena has made the work of the health visitor more widely and better understood. Their particular nursing role has been accepted. Evidence of this can be seen, for example, in their being specifically named alongside nurses and midwives in the Act of Parliament that unified the various aspects of the nursing profession (DHSS, 1979).

Competing for resources

The fight for funds presents a different problem. Factors such as structural changes, the apparent need to demonstrate dramatic success and the influence of the acute care model of health, mean health visitors need to make particular efforts to explain locally about the purpose and value of their work.

Peter Townsend (1982) explained the evident contradiction between the government's declared intentions to strengthen community health services and the reality, instead, of ever increasing resources in the field of acute care. He described important factors underlying this. One is that recent structural changes have led to a weakening of the already subordinate position of community health and community care. For example, the appointment of more consultants and the centralisation of management structures have meant that the political voice for acute sickness hospitals has been strengthened.

The dominance of the idea of health in which the body is seen as a machine for which a medical engineering approach is appropriate is another factor. Some managers tend to think in terms of this medical model 'health — illness' rather than the more complex social model of 'health — future health', which takes into account more the important non-medical factors such as the social and environmental influences on families. It is far more difficult for these people to speak for and explain about preventive health work such as health visiting. This has obvious implications for the allocation of funds for the service.

The Griffiths style of management has drawn another matter into the equation. The general managers' three to five year appointment puts pressure on managers, as well as government, to demonstrate their 'success'. This factor also favours the dramatic, readily quantifiable aspects of health care. It can be observed in the chosen patterns of expenditure and in governmental statements about, for example, more consultants' posts, reductions in hospital waiting lists and the number of hospitals being built.

There is a further problem. Wide-ranging identification of morbidity rates in various areas of the District, the logical approach to proper preventive health care, is unlikely to be encouraged by some of the new managers for whom visible 'success' is important. Instead of being seen as a sensible base from which to make health care decisions, it can be perceived as a potential Pandora's box, liable to throw into public focus and debate evidence of many preventable problems which require attention. To deal with these would need a re-allocation of funds which would have to be weaned away from the more powerful medical lobbies, a disincentive in itself. Also, there is no Dr Kildare type of dramatic appeal, the basis of good 'success' headlines, in work with people such as under-privileged young couples, the elderly, the handicapped and the unemployed.

It can be seen then that the system is loaded against prevention and community care at the moment. However, there are many people who wish to enhance the work. The managers likely to be most sympathetic to the public health needs are the new general managers for the community units. To a certain extent, they have become the successors to the Medical Officers of Health. They

are unlikely to be trained in public health matters, but will probably learn fast. There is an urgent need to help them understand about the purpose and value of preventive health care and it is up to health visitors to explain. It is worth remembering that these managers, too, will need ways of demonstrating 'success'. Let us hope they are made aware of criteria for measurement, such as home accident and breastfeeding rates, which are significantly more meaningful than, for example, the number of home visits undertaken by health visitors, and also the importance of a descriptive approach to evaluation and the clients' view of success. There were issues discussed towards and the end of Chapters 12 and 14.

Now they are out in the larger arena, health visitors must become more politically aware. However, as Sheila Jack (Health Visitor, 1984) pointed out, attributes such as competitiveness and power necessary for politics can be quite opposite to the qualities required in the practice of health visiting and other forms of nursing. However, Miss Jack's own example shows what can be achieved (Dopson, 1986).

MAKING THE MOST OF IT

Given the current economic climate and the increased activities in favour of acute care, it does not look as if there will be a significant and widespread increase in preventive health nursing in the short term. We have yet to find out if staffing levels will keep up with, for example, the rising birth rate and pressures to provide preventive health care in preparation for the increasing numbers of very old elderly people. However, there have been plenty of examples in recent years of health visitors using their initiative and organising their time in the best way they can for the particular community they serve.

Freedom to initiate

The question arises as to whether health visitors are normally free to use their professional knowledge and understanding in order to undertake the sort of work *they* see as most important for their locality. Some Health Authorities do restrict their health visitors to certain types of activities, by excluding tasks such as health education in schools or work with the elderly. Others restrict their ability to be innovative by insisting, for example, on a certain number of home visits to be completed each week.

All too often, though, it seems that myths arise about Health Authority policies for health visiting. Judith Fitton (1983, 1984a, 1984b) surveyed the views of the community nursing leaders of 45 Northern England Health Authorities about preventive care of the elderly. The results of her work led her to feel that health visitor practice was constrained by 'phantom policies'. She speculated that there are both health visitors and nurse managers who see themselves governed by the sort of policy they would find convenient, that is a policy reflecting traditional priorities and/or their personal views. In reality it seems that 60% of the Authority policies in the study were 'laissez-faire'. In these Health Authorities, the nursing leaders felt that the health visitors themselves should decide their priorities and whom to visit. The health visitors were in fact at liberty to do what they thought best.

It has been pointed out by Sue Grierson (1983) that health visitors should not feel controlled by management and that they should be free to plan their work on the basis of their up-to-date practical experience and their detailed knowledge of their particular locality. She also suggested that health visitors should make sure that enough time is made available for discussions with their managers on what can be done to improve the service.

The same principles apply to health visitors drawn into working even more closely with GPs on account of the new GP contract (Enticknap, 1987; Orr, 1988; Health Visitor, 1989a; 1989b; 1990a; 1990b; Cameron, 1990; Nursing Times, 1990; Spray, 1990), into newly set up Trusts (Potrykus, 1990) or into working as 'team leaders' (Johnston, 1989; Laurent 1989; Health Visitor, 1990c; 1990d; Robinson, 1990). These health visitors need to be sure that both their contract and their working environment enable them to seek and to respond to the clients' perspectives and to

provide acceptable and accessible services, including groupwork and community-based initiatives.

In this time of rapid change, there is a great deal of anxiety about what will happen to the service. It is all too easy to become nostalgic for our local authority days with employers who understood our work, and especially for the regular contact, support and encouragement to innovate provided by the Superintendents of Health Visitors. Their health visiting background enabled an empathetic hearing. Issues associated with a participative, listening style of management were discussed in Chapter 14. So much depends on this type of positive communication.

It is also important to understand managers' true position and intention. For example, the personal opinions of managers may, at first glance, mistakenly be taken to represent Authority policy. A health visitor was reported as telling a meeting how she had planned to present her views at a local public enquiry. On being advised by management against taking this 'political action', she enquired further and found out that, in reality, she was perfectly free to make her own decision about the matter (Health Visitor, 1981). It was worth discovering what was meant by the advice. However, any repercussions there might have been affecting her later relationship with the manager through not taking the advice, were not reported.

Professional decisions and modern management

Issues of control and the extent to which health visitors are individually able to decide their approach, their priorities and their methods of practice, become more important as health visitors and other nurses come under the wing of the newly appointed general managers. As part of their explanations about their work, health visitors need to describe to these managers how important it is to be able to respond, for example, to street level nuances of which they become aware in the course of their work and, as described at various points in this book, to the particular needs of the families in their locality.

However, it seems likely that the ability to respond to the local situation will remain. Firstly, it would be logical for these new-style managers to delegate the task of preventive health care to community nursing management. Secondly, a good manager will not knowingly quell initiative and stifle potentially useful innovation. Such a disaster is only likely if the manager is ill-informed or misinformed. It is up to the health visitors and other community nurses to ensure that the new managers are able to learn about the nature and purpose of their work. The brief given to the community nursing management can then incorporate that understanding.

This section has considered some implications of moving health visiting from the public health centred departments of the Local Authorities into the National Health Service. These include aspects of resource allocation and health visitors' ability to use their initiative and implement new, useful ideas.

IDEAS AND DEBATES

There have been many debates and discussion about what form initiatives should take and how best to use the scarce resource of health visiting. There is no shortage of people in medical and paramedical work who can see how health visiting could help in their particular speciality, for example, over alcoholism, drugs, ischaemic heart disease, pre-conceptual care, preventive health care for the middle aged and the problems of adolescence. There have been many interesting ideas put forward and many worthwhile projects undertaken. A variety of examples has been provided in the previous few chapters. There are many possible options and this has inevitably led to discussions and debates within the profession. For example, there is the debate as to whether health visitors should continue to maintain a generalist approach or should increasingly take on a more specialised remit, and discussions about the relative value of groupwork and home visiting.

There can be no single solution or any one formula for all time. The best course will be if health visitors continue to debate and undertake new initiatives and also put great efforts into explaining what they are doing and why. This way, objectives, achievements and any underlying problems will be better understood, responsiveness to local requirement will receive appropriate attention and a thinking profession will be making a progressive contribution to health care.

Specially assigned or generalist?

There has been discussion within the profession on the extent to which specialisation or generalism should be encouraged (Barratt, 1985). Each has merits and there seems plenty of room in health visiting for both. Some fear a two-tier profession (Davidson, 1979), but this seems to be based on a misunderstanding of the term 'specialist'. What is actually meant is 'specifically employed' or 'specially assigned' to certain duties, for example, for the elderly, the handicapped (see Box 9.3), for diabetics (Nursing Times, 1983; Jackson, 1981) in the Child Development Project (1984) or, as we have seen in the last few chapters, for group work (Drennan, 1984; 1985; 1988a) and community health development. In the Cumberlege Report (DHSS, 1986) it was suggested that these specialist health visitors should be brought into neighbourhood nursing services, in order to work closely with district nurses, school nurses and health visitors.

On training, the Cumberlege Report suggested a broad-based health visitor type of course for all these community nurses, in which students would opt for a specialist module. This would, for example, be in maternal and child health, health education, nurse practitioner work or the elderly. It was a relief to find that the authors stated emphatically that they were in no way proposing the introduction of a generic nurse and that they were particularly 'seeking to preserve the type of skills possessed by the health visitor' (p. 44). An all-purpose public health nurse would find it impossible to be well enough educated across the necessary range of preventive *and* acute care. Added to that, acute care would inevitably be rated as higher priority and preventive health care work would be sure to suffer (While, 1986). It was the potential for working together in order to share knowledge and approaches for the benefit of the clientele, that lay behind the Report's proposals.

There are advantages in specialisation. Specially employed health visitors are less likely to be side-tracked by crisis work or other health visitors' clinic sessions, and are therefore free to devote themselves to their particular client group. This can be especially useful in areas of deprivation, but only if theirs is an additional post.

These health visitors are not 'special'. Their range of basic skills is just the same. However, their narrower remit makes it easier for them to acquire a better depth of knowledge for the group they look after. As was suggested in Chapter 9 (Table 9.4), other health visitors may find them useful to turn to if they are also caring for the same sort of client group.

The disadvantage of the narrow remit and homing in on one care group is that it militates against an awareness of and an involvement with the wider community beyond that particular group. Here the traditional broader remit of the generalist health visitor is invaluable. Having a theoretical remit which has concern for the community as a whole enables, encourages and improves the potential in health visiting. There are several key factors. For example:

1. Acceptability

The universality of the service increases its acceptability and minimises the possibility of stigma. Specialist health visiting has a higher level of acceptability, even if it is concerned with a low status group, on account of the general image of health visiting.

2. Creativity

The wider remit and freedom to choose from a variety of ways to provide preventive health care, both for traditional and for new client groups, enables use of initiative in, for example, setting up pilot schemes to discover better ways of working.

3. Access

Being able to take the service to any group of people without their having to come forward and request it, encourages a search for acceptable and effective ways of taking preventive health care to vulnerable families or groups who are currently under-utilising the services or are unaware, for example, of the health problems of affluence.

Both specialists and generalists make timely use of skills and knowledge aimed at increasing people's independence in their health care. Both are versatile enough to be able to support individual and group work, whichever seems most appropriate. It seems very likely that the evolution of health visiting will see them both living in a symbiotic relationship for many years yet.

Home visiting versus group work

A large part of most health visitors' client-contact time is spent in one-to-one work in the privacy of people's homes. This basic approach has long been supplemented by clinic work and some fairly formal work with groups. Now, community-based health initiatives and a clearly participative style of group work are becoming increasingly popular.

The success of this modern group work has occasionally led to the assumption that it could provide the solution to all our health promotional problems. This arises, perhaps, out of an understandable over-reaction against recent trends. For example, some Districts' strict pre-set child surveillance programmes have fully taken over time which used to be spent on work with groups. Others have encouraged *increasing* home visiting *statistics* to become a prime objective. It is hardly surprising that as the spotlight comes back on to the group-work approach, it is receiving such an accolade! However, home visiting and group work each have their merits and advantages and each provide important and basic contributions to our work.

Home visits

Some of the more obvious benefits of home visits are that discussions are tailored to suit the individual family. The health visitor is able to give complete attention to that family, the issues which they choose to raise and to their perspectives of them. There are many examples in this book of how individual care can help to prevent the occurrence, development and deterioration of health problems. The Child Development Project (1984, O'Doherty, 1987) outlined in earlier chapters, is an excellent example of the value of personalised anticipatory guidance on health promotion. Walter Barker (1988; 1990a; 1990b) argues lucidly that providing positive support strategies in the home is also the best way to focus child abuse prevention strategies. Time is much better spent concentrating on, for example, building up vulnerable parents' self-esteem and parenting skills than on the distinctly questionable 'screening' strategies.

People with a low self-image and whose confidence levels are not yet good enough to cope with group dynamics need Child Development Project-style, one-to-one work in the home. Walter Barker described the pattern in group meetings with the parents in his earlier work with some 200 Brixton parents. Those who were least able to cope gradually dropped out of the groups. It seems that these parents were unable to face what they saw as the competition from the more successful group members (Barker et al, 1987).

The Children Act, 1989, brings with it an extra dimension on the need for home visiting. Jane Naish (1990) pointed out the implications of the Act's emphasis on 'parental responsibility', the requirement for parents to seek help over difficulties and the requirement for professionals to work 'in partnership with parents'. Health visitors will have an even greater need than now to share with the parents their professional view of the parents' childcare provisions. The sharing of negative opinion is a matter we touched on in Chapters 11 and 14. In Chapter 8 we discussed the value of open and, even better, parent-held records systems, which clearly facilitate an exchange of confidences of this nature.

If delicate issues are to be broached, there is much to be said for this happening on the parents' own home ground where they have greater control and an increased sense of dignity than they can have on the professional's territory at the surgery or clinic. Also universal visiting on a mutually agreed 'as needed' basis, such as that in the Oxford scheme (see Chapter 14), prevents people from being labelled and feeling especially singled out.

Early discovery of health-related problems can depend on being able to follow up families at home. For example, this may be necessary because a family included in District-wide services, such as hearing or child developmental tests, has been invited to a clinic screening session but has been unable or unwilling to attend. It might be because there was an indication of a problem too sensitive to be discussed at a clinic. Much of a health visitor's supportive care is reliant on privacy, at least initially, so that people can feel free to speak frankly. Home is usually the best place for this.

Often the health visitor is the only 'official' to be visiting in homes where there are great difficulties. Visiting individual families enables health visitors to become aware of trends amongst the families seen, for example, the emergence of health-related difficulties amongst the young unemployed or single parent families. Our earlier chapter on homelessness provides a good example of the key role of the health visitor in these sorts of circumstances.

Home visiting gives access to the realities and trends in difficulties that people are facing. This information can be incorporated with the health and welfare statistics and other data of the local health profile and can help lead to the planning and implementation of appropriate health visiting strategies. These are very likely to include various forms of, perhaps, community-based, group work. It is another case of a symbiotic relationship between two countervailing aspects of our work, this time between individual and groupwork approaches.

Group work

There are innumerable advantages to group work. Some of them include its confidence-building aspects, its strength to act, its maximisation of mutual help and the diversity of ways group work can be used to help achieve our objectives.

The best source of information about health

visiting aspects of group work is Vari Drennan's (1988b) book. It provides a wide variety of health visitors' practical group work experiences, including work with particular client groups and issues, group work aiming to influence policy and also groups aiming to improve health visiting practice. All this is backed up by clearly written explanations of recent changes in our professional practice and by useful ideas to guide health visitors newly venturing into group work.

Group work encompasses a very wide range of activities from discussion groups through to practical workshops. It can include particular matters such as women's health, stress management and 'Look After Your Heart' courses. The work may be aimed at the support and welfare of, and health promotion for, particular client groups such as carers, elderly people, homeless families or mothers and toddlers. Examples of groups planning to improve services and to influence health policies have been provided in the later chapters of this book. There is a great diversity of possible group work both with and for clients.

Learning in a group-work situation can be morale and confidence-boosting. For example, people can benefit from finding that others in the group 'do not know' either, or, perhaps, that they have faced similar experiences or feelings. In telling each other of their ups and downs of life, and of the way they see things, group members discover themselves to be 'normal', where they may previously have thought themselves to be lacking in some way. Even the provision of crèche facilities can help increase morale. It enables mothers to concentrate on themselves in time set aside especially for their own concerns, thereby helping to boost their image of their self-worth.

Related to this issue of confidence levels is the fact that in group work, just as in home visiting, an 'expert' can make people feel inadequate. There is inevitably some professional distance between a professional leader and the other group members. The aim is to shed or at least to minimise the inequalities. This is not easy to achieve and a good health visitor support system is needed. A multi-disciplinary approach to group work can also help with this issue. For example, a social worker and/or community psychiatric nurse might share leadership of a group along with a health visitor. Between them, these professionals are able to help each other interpret interaction within the group and so to improve group-work techniques.

The main purpose of multi-disciplinary group work is, of course, to provide an appropriate range of professional perspectives and skills for the various aspects of the difficulties faced by the group members. This breadth of service could not normally be available in home visiting. Group work is also a good way of helping people gain access to specialist information which they need. For example, a group of homeless parents might invite a lawyer who specialises in family rights or an environmental health officer from the Houses in Multiple Occupancy Department.

Groups can maximise on mutual help. Those whose members have a common problem have a great deal to gain by joining together. They can offer each other mutual help and support and this is especially valuable if a social stigma is attached to their particular situation. From collective decision-making, group members can gain the strength to *do* something about their difficulties, whereas an individual might feel very reticent. The group might contact people with influence and/or arrange to meet, for example, local authority officers from the department which would be able to provide greatest help. This kind of action needs assertiveness skills. These are now becoming more commonly encouraged and taught, especially in women's groups. A further dimension of the full use of mutual help is that independent self-help groups can develop from those originally 'midwifed' by the health visitor.

These then are a few of the special advantages of work with groups. However, in setting up new groups or in referring people to established ones, it is necessary to find people who can benefit from them. It will be recalled that the health visitor in Chapter 15's Example One, found that all the help she had with a circular put through people's doors, notifying them of the new health promotion service, had no effect. It was her contacts through home visiting which brought people to her new groups. The health visiting habit of universal home visiting makes it easier to discover people's particular problems and needs and to help those people who need it to set up an appropriate group or to become a member of an established one.

Many different schemes and programmes are being tried out, involving not only generalists, specialists, home visiting and group work, but also many other aspects of our work which, happily, also engender discussion. The rapid changes affecting the structure of the National Health Service are reverberating in the community health services. For example, the proposed emergence of Trusts and the changes in the GP Contract are making urgent the raising of issues such as those of accountability and the skills levels of people employed in our field of work.

The key factor will be whether changes in practice and choices of modes of work occur because they are believed in and pressed for on the evidence from field-level staff, or whether they are imposed 'from above' as part of a programme of cuts in budget allocation.

Health visitors looking for reassurance in these hectic times will gain much comfort and many good ideas from Tom Peters' (1989) *Thriving on chaos*. He emphasises the need for 'flexibility' and expands on some themes from his earlier book (Peters & Waterman, 1982), which was outlined in Chapter 14. Vari Drennan's (1990) work with the Islington community nurse services shows, coincidentally, how Peters' ideas, for example on what and how to measure, *do work* in our field too.

In this final chapter, we have looked at some of the administrative changes that have been occurring over the last few decades. The aim has been to provide a backcloth against which to discuss some of our current debates, difficulties and opportunities. We moved temporarily away from the underlying theme of the book, the three models. Now we take a last glance at them, in the context both of a modern initiative and their use in unison.

THE THREE MODELS

In conclusion

This final example of health visiting practice is of a health visitor's published and award-winning work in a community project. It rounds up the book by demonstrating in a nutshell how each of the three basic models presents a vehicle for highlighting a particular perspective of our work. However, there are limitations on the models' applicability. As we have said earlier, they are useful only as conceptual aids. The models are totally unsuitable for use as 'checklisting' tools either in practical work or in record-writing.

The book initially concentrated on the models from the point of view of face-to-face work with individual families. In the last few chapters, we have seen how the models can also be used to outline, and to help to marshal thought about, the broader aspects of our work. This concluding example shows the way a health visitor stepped outside her daily work routine and took a wider perspective, greatly to the benefit of her clients. We have already met this health visitor earlier in the book (see Ch. 9, p. 174 and Ch. 12, pp. 226–227). Sue Phillips (1986) started work in a south London housing estate as a newly qualified health visitor. Box 16.1 outlines some of the features affecting family health that struck her so forcefully. This is the 'what-problems' and 'what-particular-health-needs-there-are' model. Child safety and developmental progress, potential child abuse and maternal mental health were some of the particular concerns.

Miss Phillips started a project aimed at enabling a family centre to be set up. The model in Table 16.1 draws out the three aspects of preventive health care inherent in this work. It gives the 'why-it-needs-to-be-done' and 'how-it-might-be-achieved' perspective. Concerns here are for features such as a safe play area and child care facilities, meeting places and support for parents and for stimulation for the children.

The third model, seen in Figure 16.1, highlights the sources and sort of information that led to the project being undertaken and outlines a view of

Box 16.1 Family health needs model for Sue Phillips' community activity

Environmental factors	Physical and mental health	Social aspects of health
Poor and inadequate housing: high rise flats with frequent problems of access as lifts out of order	High incidence of depression amongst young parents	A great deal of isolation, especially amongst single parent families
Housing estate on the edge of two local authorities and allotted low priority by both	Marked level of developmental delay, especially delayed speech	No centre for community activities
No safe play area	Above average level of suspected and actual child abuse	No holiday play schemes
Miles from nearest local authority nursery (waiting list = 200)		No mother and toddler group
Child health clinic very small: no room for group work		

Table 16.1 Prevention model for Sue Phillips' community activity

Aspect of prevention	Through
Prevent occurrence of problems	Self-help support groups for young parents, especially single parents Safe play area
Prevent development of problems	Care of parental mental health and facilities for safe play to improve levels of developmental attainment, especially in speech Regular day care facilities
Prevent deterioration of established problems	Self-help support groups for depressed and lonely parents, especially single parents Day care facilities

'how it is planned and monitored'. The model draws attention to, for example, what was learned

in training, the clients' viewpoint and the results of the project.

Not for everyday tabulation

Demonstrating Sue Phillips' work in this form is not to suggest that she either did, or should have, listed these thoughts and observations. The models proposed in this book are merely ways of thinking about and approaching the work and are tabulated in this book in order to help explain them and for teaching purposes.

It is probable that it would be counter-productive to use these models in everyday health visiting in the form of complex charts or as multifactorial checklists for written records or planning schemes. Providing broad classifications, such as 'environmental factors', 'physical health', 'mental health' and 'social aspects of health' is no better than providing a blank piece of paper, and merely makes the presentation of the records unnecessarily complicated. If turned into lists of specific items, they would necessarily be limited, both conceptually and by the space available on the page. Sadly, checklists can channel concern and interest on to the listed items only and encourage an over-simplistic approach to the work.

Reality is extremely complex. Health visitor training and subsequent practical experience and study gradually build up a breadth of understanding and a wide-ranging knowledge of factors affecting health and welfare. The models provide a variety of ways of looking at the work. Whilst they remain simply a conceptual tool, they are likely to provide the means for creative thinking. This is by being able to be used in many individual ways to highlight and draw attention to important basic issues within the complexities of health visiting.

These models have been used throughout this book to classify and clarify various aspects of the work. Each has a particular perspective, and looking at them all within one example shows even more clearly the special contribution each can make.

This chapter has taken a look at recent influences and at some current challenges, debates and initiatives within the profession. It has rounded up

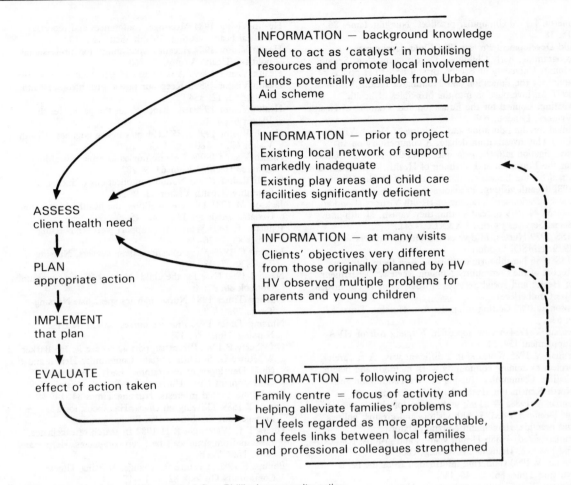

INFORMATION — background knowledge
Need to act as 'catalyst' in mobilising resources and promote local involvement
Funds potentially available from Urban Aid scheme

INFORMATION — prior to project
Existing local network of support markedly inadequate
Existing play areas and child care facilities significantly deficient

ASSESS
client health need

INFORMATION — at many visits
Clients' objectives very different from those originally planned by HV
HV observed multiple problems for parents and young children

PLAN
appropriate action

IMPLEMENT
that plan

EVALUATE
effect of action taken

INFORMATION — following project
Family centre = focus of activity and helping alleviate families' problems
HV feels regarded as more approachable, and feels links between local families and professional colleagues strengthened

Fig. 16.1 Health visitor cycle model of Sue Phillips' community action.

a basic message of the book by showing how the health visitor cycle, the prevention and the family health needs models provide a very useful way of describing a wide range of health visiting concerns.

It has not been possible to include all the arguments and possibilities in preventive health care in this book. However, the basic purposes and objectives of our work have been covered, and many references have been included so that these topics and debates can be studied further. There is so much to be learned about the perspectives and the health needs of the infinite variety of people that we meet in the practice of health visiting.

REFERENCES

Barker W 1988 Breaking the cycle. Nursing Times Community Outlook 84, August: 4–5
Barker W 1990a Practical and ethical doubts about screening for child abuse. Health Visitor 63, 1: 14–17
Barker W 1990b The aetiology of child sexual abuse. Nursing Times Community Outlook 86, April: 25–26

Barker W, Rowe G, Sutcliffe D (eds) 1987 Community health and the Child Development Programme. Early Childhood Unit, University of Bristol, Bristol, pp 66–67
Barratt L 1985 Generic versus specialist — the way ahead? Health Visitor 58: 155

Cameron J 1990 Unpopular practices. Nursing Times 86, 15: 18

Child Development Project 1984 Child development programme. Early Childhood Development Unit, Senate House, University of Bristol, Bristol BS8 1TH pp 25–27

Council for the Education and Training of Health Visitors 1977 An investigation into the principles of health visiting. Council for the Education and Training of Health Visitors, London, p 7

Council for the Education and Training of Health Visitors 1980 The investigation debate. A commentary on an investigation into the principles of health visiting. Council for the Education and Training of Health Visitors, London

Council for the Education and Training of Health Visitors 1982 Health visiting. Principles in practice. Council for the Education and Training of Health Visitors, London

Davidson N 1979 Spread so thin they vanish. Health and Social Services Journal LXXXIX: 1241

DHSS 1979 Nurses, Midwives and Health Visitors Act, 1979. HMSO, London

DHSS 1986 Neighbourhood nursing — a focus for care. Report of the Community Nursing Review. Department of Health and Social Services HMSO, London (Chairman, Mrs Cumberlege)

Dopson L 1986 Getting in on the Act. Nursing Times 82, 9: 64

Drennan V 1984 A new approach. Nursing Mirror HVA Supplement 159, 14: x–xi

Drennan V 1985 Working in a different way. A research project examining community work methods and health visiting. Community Nursing Service Paddington and North Kensington Health Authority, London

Drennan V 1988a Working with groups of elderly people. In: Drennan V (ed) Health visitors and groups: politics and practice. Heinemann Nursing, Oxford

Drennan V (ed) 1988b Health visitors and groups: politics and practice. Heinemann Nursing, Oxford

Drennan V 1990 Gathering information from the field. Nursing Times 86, 39: 46–48

Enticknap B 1987 Village volunteers. Nursing Times Community Outlook 83, 38: 19–20

Fitton J M 1983 Policy constraints on HV practice (letter) Health Visitor 56: 229

Fitton J M 1984a Health visiting the elderly: nurse managers' views. One. Nursing Times Occasional Paper No 10 80, 16: 59–61

Fitton J M 1984b Health visiting the elderly: nurse managers' views. Two. Nursing Times Occasional Paper No 11 80, 17: 67–69

Grierson S 1983 Caring for the carers (letter). Health Visitor 56: 44

Health Visitor 1981 Meetings, conferences and reports. Radical health visiting. Health Visitor 54: 406

Health Visitor 1984 Accept responsibility for 'professional politics'. Health Visitor 57: 360

Health Visitor 1989a A GP boss? Health Visitor 62, 4: 105

Health Visitor 1989b Keep our public health role. Health Visitor 62, 12: 364

Health Visitor 1990a A chance to set the pace. Health Visitor 63, 4: 107

Health Visitor 1990b UKCC issues new guidelines. Health Visitor 63, 6: 180

Health Visitor 1990c Generic nurses to replace health visitors? Health Visitor 63, 9: 287

Health Visitor 1990d National implications of increased flexibility. Health Visitor 63, 9: 287

Jackson M 1981 Diabetes mellitus: the health visitor's role Geriatric Medicine 11, 6: 42–45

Johnston C 1989 Who is the support worker? Nursing Times 85, 7: 26–28

Laurent C 1989 More questions than answers. Nursing Times 85, 7: 28–29

Naish J 1990 Care for the child. Nursing Times Community Outlook 86, 37: 46

Nursing Times 1983 Nurse diabetes specialist. Nursing Times 79, 37: 23

Nursing Times 1990 Practice nurses sacked by GPs. Nursing Times 86, 17: 5

O'Doherty P 1987 Parent support as we see it. In: Barker W, Rowe G, Sutcliffe D (eds) Community Health and the Child Development Programme. Early Childhood Development Unit, University of Bristol, Bristol

Orr J 1988 Vested interests. Nursing Times 84, 14: 34

Peters T 1989 Thriving on chaos. Handbook for a management revolution. Pan Books, London

Peters T J, Waterman R H 1982 In search of excellence. Lessons from America's best run companies. Harper and Row, New York

Phillips S 1986 A centre for change. Nursing Times Community Outlook 82, 7: 15–17

Potrykus C 1990 Trusts threaten jobs and services. Health Visitor 63, 9: 286–287

Robinson P B 1990 (letter) Health visitor 'major changes'. Nursing Standard 4, 41: 41–42

Spray J 1990 (letter) Greening health visiting. Health Visitor 653, 4: 137

Townsend P 1982 The policy implications of a positive approach to health. Health Visitor 55: 97–101

While A 1986 The value of health visitors, Health Visitor 59: 171–173

Author Index

Subject Index

Note: heavy type indicates subject looked at in greater depth